Sleep - Physiology, Functions, Dreaming and Disorders

nova
Medicine & Health
New York

Sleep - Physiology, Functions, Dreaming and Disorders

Human Health is a Matter of Timing: The Impact of Circadian Medicine on Disease and Health
Sumeyya Deniz Aybek, Gonca Gulbay, PhD
and Mucahit Secme, PhD (Editors)
2024. ISBN: 979-8-89113-467-6 (Hardcover)
2024. ISBN: 979-8-89113-559-8 (eBook)

Advances in Sleep Apnea: Detection, Diagnosis and Treatment
Francesco Lorusso, MD and Salvatore Gallina (Editors)
2021. ISBN: 978-1-53619-758-7 (Hardcover)
2021. ISBN: 978-1-53619-797-6 (eBook)

Sleep, Cognition and Emotion: From Molecules to Social Ecology
Ignacio Ramírez Salado, PhD, Ana Paula Rivera García, PhD
and Manuel Alejandro Cruz Aguilar, PhD (Editors)
2020. ISBN: 978-1-53617-561-5 (Hardcover)
2020. ISBN: 978-1-53617-562-2 (eBook)

Parasomnia Dreaming: Exploring Other Forms of Sleep Consciousness
James Frederic Pagel (Editor)
2020. ISBN: 978-1-53617-815-9 (Hardcover)
2020. ISBN: 978-1-53617-818-0 (eBook)

Children and Sleep: Management, Health Effects and Gender Differences
Olivie Gadbois (Editor)
2020. ISBN: 978-1-53618-074-9 (Softcover)
2020. ISBN: 978-1-53618-075-6 (eBook)

More information about this series can be found at
https://novapublishers.com/product-category/series/sleep-physiology-functions-dreaming-and-disorders/

Sumeyya Deniz Aybek
Gonca Gulbay
and Mucahit Secme

Human Health is a Matter of Timing

The Impact of Circadian Medicine on Disease and Health

nova
Medicine & Health
New York

Library of Congress Cataloging-in-Publication Data

ISBN: 979-8-89113-467-6

Published by Nova Science Publishers, Inc. † New York

To our precious families who shed light on us
in the rhythm of life

Contents

Preface

Life on Earth is adapted to our planet's 24-h rotation and orbital revolution around the sun. The circadian clock is organisms' natural timing devices, establishes a link between organism and its external environment to drive rhythms in feeding, activity and rest, body temperature, and hormones, from the level of cell to organism and from bacteria to mammals. The biological clock has emerged as a potent regulator of human physiology, which orchestrates cellular trafficking to achieve whole-body metabolic synchronization and thus, a temporary mismatch between this internal biological clock and our external environment could increase the risk for various diseases such as from cardiovascular diseases, diabetes, obesity, infertility, neurological disorders, and cancer. This book is comprised of twenty chapters written by experienced and passionate academics and professionals and will be a valuable source of information for scientists and clinicians. Collectively, this book has provided a comprehensive account of our current knowledge about emerging insights into the circadian rhythm in physiology and diseases, which will shed light on clinical and basic research and provide the development of new clinical strategies for therapeutic intervention.

Chapter 1

Introduction to the Circadian Clock

Mustafa Can Güler*, MD, PhD

Department of Physiology, Faculty of Medicine, Atatürk University, Erzurum, Turkiye

Abstract

All life forms have a systematic life cycle and are in a relationship with their environments to maintain life. Our spatial position is affected by the location and movements of our planet in the universe, which alter our biological activities. We may not sense changes in the earth's rote, but a parameter indicates the current situation, time perception. The existence or absence of light specifies the day and night concepts. The light-dark cycle is essential for the body to adjust and adapt. We continue our daily lives through the perception of the awake-sleep cycle. We designate a routine, a certain time for eating, working, resting, sleeping, and similar activities. Briefly, our all life is the summary of the 24-hour time zone. The circadian rhythm represents a 24-hour period. The circadian clock is the main regulator of the circadian rhythms of the body. The suprachiasmatic nucleus is the master clock of the circadian clock mechanism. It is associated with light, and it reacts due to its existence. The suprachiasmatic nucleus regulates several circadian rhythms, such as hormonal regulation, body temperature, and the sleep-wake cycle. Besides, there are other local clocks accompanying the suprachiasmatic nucleus. There are circadian clock genes that play vital roles in the expression of proteins as a part of the circadian rhythm and related physiological functions. A malfunction, a lesion, or a similar pathologic situation of the circadian clock influences the human body negatively. For example, impairment of the circadian sleep-wake cycle is one of the most common conditions in suprachiasmatic nucleus lesions. The

---

* Corresponding Author's Email: mcanguler@yahoo.com.

In: Human Health is a Matter of Timing
Editors: Sumeyya Deniz Aybek, Gonca Gulbay and Mucahit Secme
ISBN: 979-8-89113-467-6

circadian clock is a complicated mechanism, and it is strongly associated with both internal and external stimuli. Circadian rhythms mediate the lives of all organisms and are still a current issue to be explored. In this brief introduction, a general perspective of the circadian clock and its organization will be presented.

Keywords: circadian clock, circadian rhythm, master clock, suprachiasmatic nucleus

Introduction

Every living creature is subject to ongoing changes surrounding them depending on the position of the Earth in our universe. The "time" definition may be the key to understanding the reactions of organisms during exposure to fluctuant situations. Light and dark are the building stones of our perception of the sense of time. We adjust days, weeks, and even years with these terms. We work, sleep, relax, eat, and do numerous routines due to the existence or absence of light. As a result, the dark-light cycle evolves biological systems that can organize the activity, resting, and energy consumption. This evolution ends up with a circadian system. The circadian system regulates almost all essential physiological activities (Matveyenko, 2018). Circadian rhythmicity adjusts physiological mechanisms due to environmental conditions. Circadian rhythm describes fluctuant body activities within the 24-hours (24-h). Most of the body functions are carried out in this way. Circadian rhythms are responsible for our vital actions. The physiological mechanisms controlling circadian rhythms are complicated and constitute a 24-h molecular clock system. The circadian clock is the internal molecular mechanism controlling the physiological and behavioral responses to stimuli. There are clock genes associated with protein production for adequate cell function during a 24-h cycle (Greenwell et al., 2019). Thus, the circadian clock reacts through cellular mechanisms in a molecular pattern. The malfunction of the circadian clock causes serious health problems; therefore, it is essential to understand the main topics of the circadian clock.

The Historical Process of Circadian Clock

The day and night definitions have been noticed since the earliest humans. For example, the early Sumerians used time for agriculture. In Egypt, temples were constructed according to the direction of sunrise. Similar samples can be observed in ancient nations, examining time and considering its properties for viability and the maintainability of life. *Hippocrates* mentioned several situations, such as fevers that are related to a 24-h cycle. The true significance of the circadian clock was not realized until the eighteenth century. The circadian term is a Latin-based word composed of *circa* (nearly) and *dies* (day) words (Halberg, 1963).

A French astronomer observed the leaf movements of a plant during the light and dark in the 18th century, initiating the research on biological rhythms (de Mairan, 1729). He examined *Mimosa* and noticed that its leaves moved in a 24-h cycle independent of the existence or absence of light, indicating an endogenous biological clock. After this observation, several studies were carried out supporting that the circadian rhythms of plants are less affected by external stimuli than the endogenous clock.

Many scientists have focused on the main properties of the circadian clock. Bunning demonstrated that not only environmental stimuli regulate the circadian rhythms, but also genetic code influences the circadian clock (Chandrashekaran, 2006). There is a field of chronobiology interested in studying circadian rhythms, emphasizing the importance of the circadian clock. Pittendrigh and Aschoff contributed greatly to the chronobiology. They pioneered circadian rhythm research. Pittendrigh explained that a single light signal could restart or disrupt circadian rhythms (Pittendrigh, 1981). In addition, he studied the effects of light on the circadian clock periods. Aschoff demonstrated that external stimuli could organize internal clocks (Aschoff, 1960). In 2017, Jeffrey C. Hall, Michael Rosbash, and Michael W. Young were awarded the Nobel Prize in Physiology or Medicine for their contributions to circadian rhythm molecular mechanisms (Burki, 2017).

Organization of the Circadian Clock

The suprachiasmatic nucleus (SCN) is the major component of the circadian clock, "a master clock" that acts as an oscillator. It is located bilaterally within the anterior hypothalamus. The SCN includes about 20.000 neurons. CSN neurons serve as clock cells, representing spontaneous electrical activity as oscillatory and repetitive nearly every 24-h (Fox & Rompolski, 2018). The 24-h cycle is strongly related to dark-light duration due to the earth's rotation. Temperature also affects the circadian rhythm. As mentioned above, environmental changes alter (entrain) the SCN-related circadian rhythms and endogenous mechanisms. Various physiological processes, such as body metabolism, hormone secretion, and sleep, are regulated by the circadian clock through the SCN. Axon projections from the SCN to the hypothalamus play a vital role in these physiological processes. Melanopsin is a light-sensitive photopigment within intrinsically photosensitive retinal ganglion cells. The retinohypothalamic tract carries the signals from these cells. Retinohypothalamic fibers transport the information (light or darkness) to the SCN. The transmission of signals between SCN neurons is mediated by several neurotransmitters and hormones, including gamma-aminobutyric acid (GABA), vasoactive intestinal polypeptide (VIP), and arginine vasopressin (AVP) (Albrecht, 2012). SCN lesions result in many health conditions such as impaired circadian sleep-wake cycles. In addition, traveling in different time zones may lead to jet lag, a condition characterized by altered circadian rhythms, which may also affect the circadian sleep-wake cycle.

The pineal gland is related to the CSN and contributes to several circadian rhythms. It secretes the melatonin hormone. Melatonin synthesis is directly related to the dark-light cycle. Darkness stimulates, and light inhibits, melatonin secretion. During the day, SCN represses melatonin production through GABA (Kalsbeek et al., 2000), while glutamate induces the melatonin synthesis at night (Perreau-Lenz et al., 2004). Therefore, it participates in the sleep-wake cycle. Thereby, melatonin may be a messenger of reporting to the body about whether it is day or night to regulate its functions (melatonergic pathway). SCN is also a part of the regulation of the body temperature, feeding behaviour, and numerous hormonal processes (Hall & Hall, 2020).

The hypothalamic-pituitary axis (HPA) is a crucial mechanism for maintaining vitality and is an example of the endocrine rhythms of the circadian clock. SCN is involved in the working mechanism of HPA. It adjusts the activation of corticotropin-releasing hormone (CRH) neurons. CRH controls the production of glucocorticoids through the secretion of adrenocorticotrophic-releasing hormone (ACTH). ACTH is released as pulsatile. With this, the SCN directs the circadian oscillation of ACTH and glucocorticoid secretion as well (Balsalobre et al., 2000). Glucocorticoids are essential hormones for life and represent a wide range of physiological effects in the human body. Although 24-h dark-light cycle influences the SCN activity on body temperature, the sleep-wake cycle is ineffective. Human body temperatures are usually minimum between 3 and 6 a.m. and highest between 3 and 6 p.m. (Walter & Emile , 2016).

SCN neurons are connected to several regions of the brain comprising local (or peripheral) circadian clocks. Local clocks organize circadian gene expression for physiological rhythm regulation. They exist in almost all body tissues. Although SCN regulates them, they can control their circadian rhythms for a couple of days in the absence of SCN signals. There are circadian clock genes in SCN and other tissues performing the circadian oscillating activity. Brain and muscle aryl hydrocarbon receptor nuclear translocator-like protein 1 (BMAL1) and circadian locomotor output cycles kaput (CLOCK) proteins are transcriptional activators. They connect and activate the transcription of "cryptochrome genes" *(CRY1 and CRY2)* and "clock genes" *(PER1, PER2, and PER3)* (Hall & Hall, 2020).

Conclusion

The circadian clock is a vital feature for organisms maintaining a 24-h period mediated by molecular negative feedback mechanisms. The circadian clock adjusts the body and is related to internal and external stimuli. The day-light cycle is the leading environmental factor, and other stimulants, such as food intake and temperature, influence the circadian clock. The SCN and some other local clocks compose the circadian clock. Circadian clock genes contribute to these mechanisms maintaining oscillation for 24-h rhythmicity. For healthy cooperation with the environment and to maintain physiological processes, it is essential to provide the continuousness of the circadian clock.

References

Albrecht, U. (2012). Timing to perfection: the biology of central and peripheral circadian clocks. *Neuron*, *74*(2), 246-260. https://doi.org/10.1016/j.neuron.2012.04.006.

Aschoff, J. (1960). Exogenous and endogenous components in circadian rhythms. *Cold Spring Harb Symp Quant Biol*, *25*, 11-28. https://doi.org/10.1101/sqb.1960.025.01.004.

Balsalobre, A., Brown, S. A., Marcacci, L., Tronche, F., Kellendonk, C., Reichardt, H. M., Schütz, G., & Schibler, U. (2000). Resetting of Circadian Time in Peripheral Tissues by Glucocorticoid Signaling. *Science*, *289*(5488), 2344-2347. https://doi.org/10.1126/science.289.5488.2344.

Burki, T. (2017). Nobel Prize awarded for discoveries in circadian rhythm. *The Lancet*, *390*(10104), e25. https://doi.org/https://doi.org/10.1016/S0140-6736(17)32661-2.
Chandrashekaran, M. K. (2006). Erwin Bünning (1906-1990): a centennial homage. *J Biosci*, *31*(1), 5-12. https://doi.org/10.1007/bf02705230.
de Mairan, J.-J. (1729). Observation botanique. *Hist. de l'Acad. Royal Sciences*, 35-35. http://www.bibnum.education.fr/sciencesdelavie/biologie/observation-botanique
Fox, S., & Rompolski, K. (2018). *Human Physiology* (15th ed.). McGraw-Hill US Higher Ed ISE. http://ebookcentral.proquest.com/lib/abertay/detail.action?docID=6212551.
Greenwell, B. J., Trott, A. J., Beytebiere, J. R., Pao, S., Bosley, A., Beach, E., Finegan, P., Hernandez, C., & Menet, J. S. (2019). Rhythmic Food Intake Drives Rhythmic Gene Expression More Potently than the Hepatic Circadian Clock in Mice. *Cell Rep*, *27*(3), 649-657.e645. https://doi.org/10.1016/j.celrep.2019.03.064.
Halberg, F. (1963). Circadian (about twenty-four-hour) rhythms in experimental medicine. *Proc R Soc Med*, *56*(4), 253-257.
Hall, J. E., & Hall, M. E. (2020). Guyton and Hall Textbook of Medical Physiology E-Book. https://books.google.co.id/books?id=H1rrDwAAQBAJ.
Kalsbeek, A., Garidou, M. L., Palm, I. F., Van Der Vliet, J., Simonneaux, V., Pévet, P., & Buijs, R. M. (2000). Melatonin sees the light: blocking GABA-ergic transmission in the paraventricular nucleus induces daytime secretion of melatonin. *Eur J Neurosci*, *12*(9), 3146-3154. https://doi.org/10.1046/j.1460-9568.2000.00202.x.
Matveyenko, A. V. (2018). Consideration for Circadian Physiology in Rodent Research. *Physiology*, *33*(4), 250-251. https://doi.org/10.1152/physiol.00012.2018.
Perreau-Lenz, S., Kalsbeek, A., Pévet, P., & Buijs, R. M. (2004). Glutamatergic clock output stimulates melatonin synthesis at night. *Eur J Neurosci*, *19*(2), 318-324. https://doi.org/10.1111/j.0953-816x.2003.03132.x.
Pittendrigh, C. S. (1981). Circadian Systems: Entrainment. In J. Aschoff (Ed.), *Biological Rhythms* (pp. 95-124). Springer US. https://doi.org/10.1007/978-1-4615-6552-9_7.
Walter F, B., & Emile L, B. (2016). *Medical Physiology*, 3rd Edition. Elsevier.

Chapter 2

The Mammalian Circadian Clocks: Clock Genes and Circadian Transcriptional Mechanisms

Gözde Öztan*, PhD
Department of Medicine, Istanbul University, Istanbul, Turkiye

Abstract

The circadian clock is a way for the body to keep track of time. It uses clock genes to make physiology and behavior follow a 24-hour cycle. The central circadian clock regulates sleep, metabolism, and the immune system in mammals. The expression of these genes shows near 24-hour oscillations in both transcripts and protein products. Specifically timed circadian oscillations in cells of many tissues in mammals are the result of interactions between the proteins that regulate circadian locomotor output cycles kaput (CLOCK), brain-and-muscle arnt-like protein 1 (BMAL1), period (PER1, PER2, and PER3), and cryptochrome (CRY1 and CRY2). Our internal clock regulates a number of bodily functions, including sleep, wakefulness, eating, fasting, hormone production, and body temperature. This central circadian oscillator sends out neuronal and hormonal signals that set the body's other clocks. Circadian rhythms have been shown to be present in cyanobacteria. They also seem to be "ubiquitous in eukaryotes." A transcription-translation feedback-loop model is used to explain how the clocks of Drosophila, Neurospora, humans, and cyanobacteria work. Mammalian circadian clocks use the heterodimeric transcription factor CLOCK: BMAL1 to regulate gene expression and optimize biological activities. Post-translational modifications are an essential component of the process that underpins

* Corresponding Author's Email: gozdeoztan@yahoo.com

In: Human Health is a Matter of Timing
Editors: Sumeyya Deniz Aybek, Gonca Gulbay and Mucahit Secme
ISBN: 979-8-89113-467-6

the development of circadian rhythms. The phosphorylation of clock parts has been studied a lot because it affects where clock parts are in the cell, how active transcription is, and how clock parts are shaped during the circadian day. This chapter focuses on the molecular mechanisms affecting the circadian clock, circadian genes, the evidence for their regulation, and recent developments.

Keywords: circadian clock, genetic regulation, molecular mechanism, clock genes

Introduction

Homeostasis in mammals depends a lot on the ability of the organism to adapt to changing conditions, such as the day-night cycle. The circadian clock is a 24-hour oscillator that is built into all cells and can be synchronized with external signals. The master circadian clock of the body is in the suprachiasmatic nucleus (SCN) of the hypothalamus. This clock is reset by light and may maintain a steady rhythm even in the darkest places. Peripheral tissues also have circadian clocks. Therefore, the SCN clock acts as a finely calibrated time-keeping mechanism that helps organisms adapt to environmental and solar cycle variations (Kinouchi & Sassone-Corsi, 2020).

The circadian rhythms of mammals are controlled by a negative feedback loop made up of the transcriptional activator genes CLOCK and BMAL1, as well as the five repressor genes period and cryptochrome. Two transcription factors, CLOCK and BMAL1, are responsible for turning on the PER and CRY genes, respectively. After a delay, the PER and CRY proteins suppress CLOCK/BMAL1-mediated transcription. The circadian clock of a mammal is controlled by a complex network of feedback loops and auxiliary circuits. A positive feedback loop between the suppression of REV-ERBα and the expression of CRY1 has been shown in previous research. Several nuclear receptors show expression patterns similar to those of the circadian clock. This suggests that they may be involved in the circadian clock through more feedback loops (Wang et al., 2017).

When it comes to the circadian timing system seen in mammals, BMAL1 is the only clock gene necessary for the production of genes in a rhythmic pattern. Targeting BMAL1 expression genetically has been done to study its role in the circadian clock and figure out how changing the clock affects behavior. People with mental disorders also experience changes in the circadian clock. Because of this, mice whose clock genes have been changed may be useful for studying depression (Haque et al., 2019).

The circadian clock regulates the body's sleep-wake cycle, which is one of the cognitive processes of the brain. The SCN circadian clock specifically controls the timing of the sleep and wake cycles. Physiological, psychological, and electrophysiological signs can be used to divide the sleep-wake cycle of a person into separate phases. There are primarily two different categories of sleep. Both rapid eye movement sleep (also known as REM sleep) and non-REM sleep, often known as deep sleep, are two different stages of sleep. A good night's sleep includes a deep series of recurring alternating bouts of non-REM and REM every 90 minutes over a protracted rest period. The average of these values, the duration of each sleep phase, the consistency of sleep activity, and the time a person goes to sleep and wakes up establish a person's sleep pattern (Piggins, 2002).

Environmental cues entrained the circadian clock of the plant, which regulates daily biological activities and growth. The transcriptional feedback loops that make up the circadian oscillator are caused by the successive activation of core clock genes that act as mutual transcriptional repressors at different times of the day. Microarray investigations show that around 30% of the genes in Arabidopsis thaliana show circadian oscillation via this regulatory mechanism. Posttranscriptional regulation of core clock genes adds complexity to the circadian-controlled gene network (Yang et al., 2020). Chalcone Synthase (CHS) expression is essential for flavonoids, which protect plants from the sun. CHS transcription is controlled by both the way cells are programmed from the inside and by how they react to signals from the outside. Evidence that the circadian clock regulates the CHS promoter comes from transgenic Arabidopsis plants with luciferase reporter gene fusions in their roots and shoots. CHS expression follows a separate circadian clock from chlorophyll a/b-binding protein (CAB) gene expression (Thain et al., 2002).

The biological clock of a Drosophila needs coordinated behavioral and physiological responses to changing environmental signals for the neuronal circuitry to work. The daily synaptic changes in the central pacemaker neurons are evidence of the circadian circuit's neuronal plasticity. Both the Drosophila central clock and the human central clock are based on transcriptional activators called CYCLE (CYC) and dCLOCK, respectively. CYC is constitutively expressed in fruit flies (Jarabo & Martin, 2017). Drosophila's 24-hour clock controls how they come out of their pupal case, move around, eat, smell, and even some parts of their sexual behavior. The molecular oscillator in Drosophila has been studied a lot, but it is still not clear how it is related to biological processes that are controlled by a clock. In the past, researchers have tried to determine how widespread circadian transcriptional regulation really is and have narrowed it down to a small set of clock-controlled "output" genes (Ceriani et al., 2002).

The ubiquitin-proteasome system (UPS), a way for proteins to break down, is related to both eukaryotes and archaea. The UPS is important for the proper functioning of many cellular processes, such as the breakdown of proteins in response to environmental signals, endocytosis, the progression of the cell cycle, growth, proliferation, and cellular senescence. The UPS also helps control the circadian clock by breaking down proteins that are important to the clock (Ukita et al., 2022). PER and/or CRY are targets for many different kinases, and both proteins can be phosphorylated in different places. They speed or delay proteasome transport. Ubiquitin "marks" degradable proteins. Timekeeping of the molecular loop throughout a 24-hour period relies on clock proteins, which are regulated post-transcriptionally to guarantee proper intracellular traffic and degradation of clock proteins (Charrier et al., 2017).

Mammalian cells have circadian rhythms because of transcriptional-translational feedback loops (TTLs) that control when master clock genes are turned on and off. CLOCK, NPAS2, and BMAL1 are transcriptional activators that bind to DNA's E-box regulatory regions; CRY1/2 and PER1/2/3 are transcriptional repressors that control their own rhythmic expression by providing negative feedback to CLOCK and BMAL1; and together these five proteins make up the core TTL (Landgraf et al., 2014).

The Molecular Clock

Halberg invented the term "circadian rhythm" to describe animals' almost 24-hour endogenous biological oscillations linked to the Earth's daily rotation. Endogenous rhythms in photosynthetic prokaryotes and higher eukaryotes show that they have a built-in circadian clock that coordinates and adjusts the internal environment to changes in the external environment. Specifically, the daily light-dark cycle is the principal external synchronizer of circadian rhythms. Mammalian eyes are equipped with a retinohypothalamic tract that transmits visual information to the hypothalamus SCN, the primary pacemaker of the body (Fagiani et al., 2022).

The phasic expression of genes shows how an organism's daily rhythms show up in its physiology and behavior. Circadian clocks are responsible for regulating about 50% of mammalian protein-coding genes in at least one tissue. An intracellular transcriptional and translational feedback loop regulates gene expression rhythmically (TTFL). Transcription factors, which make up the "forward" part of the loop, increase the expression of genes in the "negative" parts of the loop. Negative arm levels increase over the course of the day until they reach a certain point, at which point they may cross into the nucleus and stop positive arm activity. After they have broken down, the positive axis is free to begin the cycle again. The action of this feedback loop results in a nearly 24-hour-long oscillation in gene expression (Andreani et al., 2015).

The biological circadian system controls all levels of behavior (gene, cell, tissue, organ, behavior, etc.) to adapt to the environment. Only a few of the numerous genetic components that changing the circadian network may affect are mRNA, noncoding RNAs, chromatin structures, and epigenetic regulatory factors. Nevertheless, it is not totally obvious what role these elements play in the regulation of rhythmically expressed genes. More studies are needed to fill in the details of these correlations. Metabolic activities, development, aging, and sleep are all controlled by biological rhythmic regulation mechanisms. Circadian gene alterations are connected to cancer and severe depressive disorder. Hence, circadian gene research may shed light on the correlation between disruptions in the body's clock and significant diseases, including sleep disorders (Figure 1) (Sun et al., 2020).

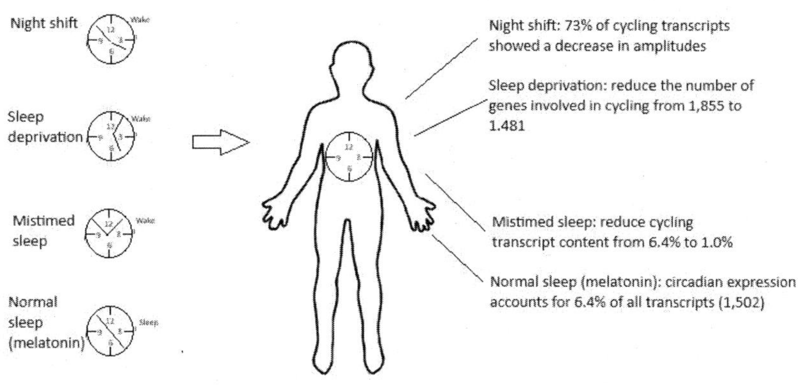

Figure 1. Human blood circadian system.

The circadian transcriptome of human blood and its response to four different sleep-wake schedules. Shift employment, mistimed sleep, and sleep deprivation may alter circadian transcriptomes. Alterations to the sleep/wake state are shown in the right-hand boxes, while the clock on the left indicates the current state. Data source: Night shift; Sleep deprivation; Mistimed sleep; Normal sleep (melatonin) (Sun et al., 2020).

As predicted, the suprachiasmatic nuclei express the mammalian Per genes, CLOCK, and BMAL, but the PER gene is rhythmic, peaking in the middle of the day and being repressed later in the cycle. The premise is that as in Drosophila, the inactivation is a result of the negative feedback of PER proteins counteracting the positive drive of CLOCK and BMAL. Double-time, the most recent fly gene to be found, is thought to code for a kinase enzyme that phosphorylates the PER protein. Flies with double-time mutations have faster clocks because PER protein degradation in the cytoplasm is reduced without phosphorylation. This speeds up the rise in PER levels, which in turn shortens the time between genes being turned on and heterodimer proteins being brought into the nucleus (Hastings, 1998).

Circadian Clock Genes

When Jeffery C. Hall, Michael Rosbash, and Michael Young at Brandeis University and Michael Young at Rockefeller University independently cloned and rescued the Drosophila period in 1984, this led to the discovery of the first clock gene known as PER. Nevertheless, the cloning of period did not immediately disclose its molecular mechanism for the circadian clock, and the years before 1988 were characterized by misunderstanding over the role of its protein product, PER. In 1988, the Drosophila single-minded gene was discovered; it produces a nuclear protein that is quite similar in sequence to the product of the period gene. This provided the first clue that PER may function as a transcription factor. The nucleus entry of the PER protein to operate as a transcription factor is unknown. In the 1990s, Young discovered the second clock gene, TIMELESS (TIM), which answered the question. The TIM mutant inhibits the rhythm of per mRNA levels and eliminates rhythmic pupal eclosion and locomotor activity, which was discovered by the group led by Young (Huang, 2018).

Konopka and Benzer found the first circadian mutant, called PERIOD, in fruit flies. Because of their efforts, mice are now subjected to genetic behavioral screens. The circadian mutant mouse found on this screen led to the cloning of the first mammalian circadian gene, called CLOCK. As research into how circadian rhythms work in mammalian exploded, scientists eventually added a few more genes to the clock core loop (Figure 2) (Rijo-Ferreira & Takahashi, 2019).

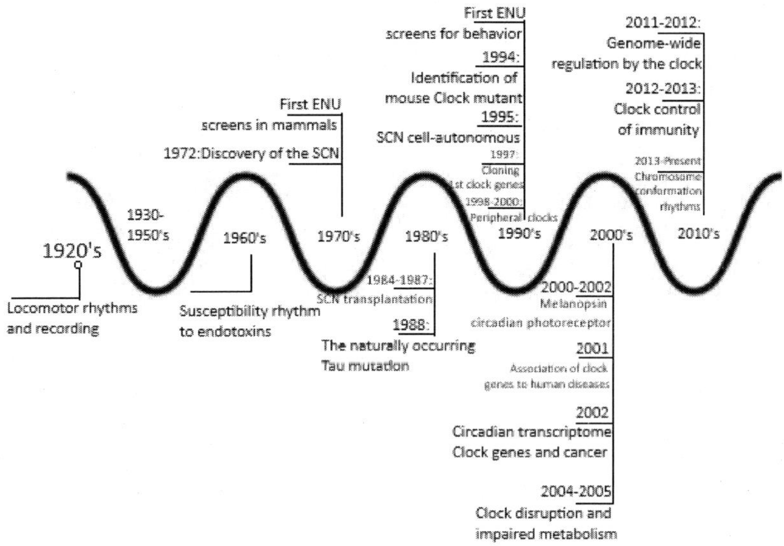

Figure 2. History of mammalian circadian clocks.

Major discoveries about mammalian circadian clocks in time. There have been long-term records of locomotor rhythms in rats since the 1920s. The first symposium on biological clocks was held in Cold Spring Harbor in 1960. The first reports of a diurnal variation in endotoxin sensitivity. Through lesion experiments, scientists found in 1972 that the SCN in the hypothalamus was in charge of both the circadian rhythms of adrenal corticosterone and alcohol consumption. The first ENU screens for identifying new genes in mammals were carried out in the late 1970s and 1980s. Between 1984 and 1990, transplantation techniques were used to find out that the SCN was a master regulator. A circadian rhythm that first appeared in 1988 Hamsters was found to have a mutation called tau. The first mammalian clock gene, CLOCK, was discovered through the use of ENU screens for behavior in the 1990s. In 1995, it was shown that the circadian rhythms of mammals are cell-autonomous because they stay the same in SCN neurons that are electrically separate. To prove that the CLOCK gene is a member of the bHLH-PAS family of transcription factors, it was cloned in 1997. In the years 1998-2000, the

CLOCK partner BMAL1/MOP3 was identified, and CRY suppression and the Per1/2-Cry1/2 feedback loop were discovered in CLOCK:BMAL1. Melanopsin, a retinal photoreceptor that detects light at night, was discovered in the 2000s. In 2001, the first mutation was found in the human CLOCK gene. In 2002, the first circadian transcriptomes uncovered a sizable cohort of genes whose expression cycles over a duration of 24 hours. A study that was conducted in 2004 and 2005 found that mutations in the CLOCK genes are related to slower metabolism. Peroxiredoxin cycles were shown to be transcription-independent in 2011. In-depth descriptions of time-dependent genome-wide regulation in 2011 and 2012. Major breakthroughs in the knowledge of the circadian regulation of immunity occurred in 2012-2013. Today, a new genome-related layer of circadian chromosomal structure is regulating the clock broadly (ENU, N-ethyl-N-nitrosourea) (Rijo-Ferreira & Takahashi, 2019).

From what we know, all eukaryotic organisms have circadian clocks at the level of their cells. For this reason, mechanistic studies may benefit from cell biology methods. Even though it has been shown that many "clock genes" are important to the circadian physiology of an organism, the mechanism of the mammalian cellular clock is still not fully understood. The phrase "clock gene" does not have a clear meaning, but it usually refers to a gene whose expression helps the body keep track of time and whose gene product turns off its own activity after a long time, causing gene expression to change over time. It has been thought that the molecular basis of the circadian rhythm in animals, plants, and fungi is a delayed negative feedback loop in gene expression. This is true even though the clock protein transcription factors in each eukaryotic kingdom are different (Putker & O'Neill, 2016).

Homologs for the genes CLOCK, BMAL1, PER, and CRY have been found in humans. CLOCK, the only circadian rhythm gene that has been cloned, is situated on chromosome 4 (Charrier et al., 2017). BMAL1, a crucial component of the molecular clock, controls the circadian clock in mammals. Human chromosome 11p15.2 is the location of the gene encoding BMAL1 (Woon et al., 2007). The transcription of the BMAL1 gene is also regulated by the retinoic acid receptor-related orphan receptor (ROR-A) and ROR-B, REV-ERF, CK1ε, and CK1δ genes. Through the albumin-D-site-binding protein (DBP), the circadian clock also controls the transcription of a number of metabolic enzymes and transcription factors (Charrier et al., 2017). Like its related PER1 and PER3 genes, the PER2 gene is highly expressed in all parts of the CNS, including the SCN and nerves in the extremities of the body. In 1971, Konopka and Benzer found the PER gene by putting Drosophila melanogaster through a test for mutations. According to the genes on the X chromosome, a short-period mutant, a long-period mutant compared to the normal period length, and an arrhythmic mutant were found (Kim et al., 2018).

CRY and PER transcription is activated throughout the day in the SCN by heterodimers of CLOCK/NPAS2 and BMAL1. These heterodimers bind to particular circadian E-box sites on the promoters of their targets. The PER and CRY proteins form complexes and translocate into the nucleus when their levels reach a crucial level in the late afternoon. They generate a negative feedback loop with CLOCK/NPAS2/BMAL1 by suppressing their gene transcription. Posttranscriptional changes give the TTL more accuracy and stability. They also play a pivotal role in how the clock oscillates. Casein kinases phosphorylate PER proteins at conserved sites, which causes them to break down and slows their entry into the nucleus. The transcription of genes such as BMAL1 and NPAS2 that contain ROR elements on their promoters is regulated by REV-ERBα and RORα, respectively (Landgraf et al., 2012). The CLOCK genes regulate the expression of the cell cycle gene, which contributes to tumor formation. In response to ionizing radiation, overexpression of PER1 triggers c-MYC and inhibits p21. PER1 also reduces cancer cell growth by inhibiting WEE1, CyclinB1, CyclinD1, and CDK1. The rhythmic profile of WEE1 is altered, and the transcript levels of p53, p21, CHK1, and CHK2 are increased when the CLOCK gene is knocked down. Moreover, the CLOCK gene directly affects the response to DNA damage. This is because it is concentrated in the spots where ionizing radiation has caused DNA to split in two (Li, 2019).

There are transcriptional and translational feedback loops in the circadian clock that create proteins that silence clock genes. In the cytoplasm, Clock forms heterodimers with BMAL1. This makes a positive transcriptional loop that supports the feedback loops of the circadian clock by binding to the E-box enhancers of PER1, PER2, CRY1, and CRY2 target genes, the CLOCK and BMAL1 complex stimulates the transcription of these genes. The transcription factors CLOCK and BMAL1 control and rhythmically transcript three period genes, mPER1-3 in mice, stabilizing a negative feedback loop. As part of the negative feedback loop, PER proteins and CRY proteins build up during the day and, in the end, stop their own transcription (Ung et al., 2021).

The nucleotide sequence for CRY1 is found in 12q23.3. It goes from position 105,909,271 to position 106,011,728. CRY1 is part of the negative arm of the circadian feedback loop, which is a very important part of keeping the circadian rhythm going (Hanoun et al., 2012). Since CRY interacts directly with the CLOCK/BMAL1 heterodimers, it plays a key role in this negative feedback mechanism. The targeted disruption of BMAL1 causes the core clock regulators, PER1 and PER2, to no longer be expressed in the SCN. This is strong evidence that the transcriptional activity of BMAL1 is closely related to the expression of PER1 and PER2. Using transient-transfection tests in HEK293 cells and BMAL1-deficient fibroblasts, recent research found that BMAL1 is crucial for CLOCK protein nuclear accumulation, degradation, and phosphorylation. However, research done in CRY1/CRY2 double mutant animals showed that both PER1 and PER2 were expressed at high levels in the liver and at medium-to-high levels in the SCN (Kwon et al., 2006).

The sirtuin 1 (SIRT1) gene has been localized at 10 q21.3, and its 11 exons have been identified (Askin et al., 2020). SIRT1 deacetylates histones and a wide range of proteins, including those that control glucose and lipid metabolism, and its activity is dependent on the NAD+ level. Through interaction with CLOCK:BMAL1 to enhance BMAL1 deacetylation, SIRT1 modifies the CLOCK:BMAL1 transcriptional activity. Since both DEC1 and DEC2 are activated by CLOCK:BMAL1, it is likely that SIRT1 changes the levels of these genes indirectly through BMAL1 deacetylation. Similarly, SIRT1 deacetylates and degrades PER2. SIRT1 deacetylates and activates the transcriptional coactivator PGC-1. This increases the expression of BMAL1 through the coactivation of ROR family members (Sato et al., 2018).

The Molecular Process Underlying the Circadian Clock

Physiological, metabolic, and behavioral processes are time-organized by endogenous oscillators called circadian clocks (Vanselow et al., 2006). The circadian clock is a key system that controls how most organisms act and work on a daily basis and helps them adapt to changes in their environment. Both theoretical and experimental research into clock mechanisms has shown the existence of a dynamic network of interconnected parts. The CLOCK:BMAL1 protein complex, which is at the core of the clock system, stimulates the transcription of the clock genes PER and CRY. The cytoplasmic PER:CRY protein complex moves into the nucleus, where it blocks the transcriptional activity of CLOCK:BMAL1 and moves the heterodimer away from its promoters. The central clock mechanism also includes a negative feedback loop between CLOCK:BMAL1 and REV-ERBα (Almeida et al., 2020). The delay between the production of the PER and CRY proteins and their own self-repression is a key part of how this oscillator works. Involvement of post-translational activities such as complex building among clock proteins, nuclear import/export, controlled degradation, transcriptional activity regulation, and chromatin modification in the development of this delay has been found (Vanselow et al., 2006).

Protein levels of hPER1 fluctuated daily, and the apparent molecular mass of hPER1 altered after serum stimulation. Based on inhibitory experiments, members of the CKI family, including CKI and CKI, phosphorylated hPER1 and caused its apparent molecular mass to increase. A CKI inhibitor called CKI-7 stopped hPER1 from breaking down, slowed its entry into the nucleus, and made it stay in the nucleus longer by stopping it from getting phosphorylated (Miyazaki et al., 2004). During the movement of PER-CRY complexes from the cytoplasm to the nucleus, PER2 interacts with nucleus receptors such as REVERBa and PPARa. Moreover, PER2 has been related to CLOCK-BMAL1 heterodimer disintegration (Kim et al., 2018). Most mammalian circadian clocks are located in the suprachiasmatic nucleus of the hypothalamus. A TTFL is what controls the circadian rhythms of mammals. This loop is made up of the negative regulators PER and CRY and the positive regulators CLOCK and BMAL1. It is important to note that the SCN acts as a coordinator for TTFL-based clocks found in all of the body's main tissues (Hastings et al., 2020).

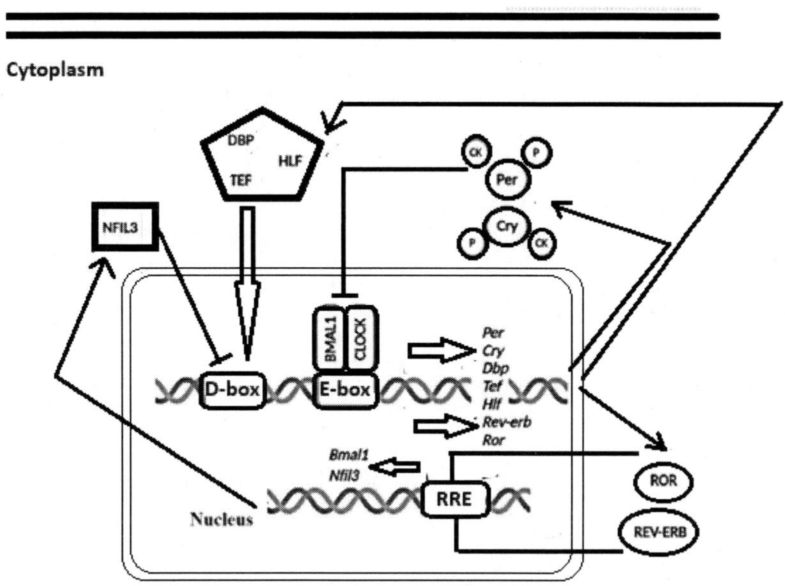

Figure 3. Circadian clock-related pathways in mammals.

A series of intricate transcriptional and translational feedback loops regulate the circadian clock (Figure 3). The genes that make up the circadian clock are controlled by a negative feedback loop in which the products of transcriptional activators act as regulators. These critical clock proteins create 24-hour circadian rhythms. The heterodimeric protein CLOCK and its binding protein BMAL1 make up the positive arm of the primary feedback loop. Two important families of transcriptional repressors, PERIOD and CRYPTOCHROME, form the negative feedback loop. When the daily CLOCK-BMAL1 cycle starts, PER and CRY are copied and built up over the course of the day (Preston et al., 2022).

CLOCK-BMAL1 heterodimers bind to E-box motifs in CCG promoter regions to produce core clock proteins. The transcriptional activity of CLOCK-BMAL1 is stopped when PER and CRY combine to form a repressor complex in the cytoplasm. Casein kinases and phosphatases facilitate the breakdown of PERs and CRYs in the cytoplasm. By binding to the retinoic acid response elements (RRE) that are found on CCGs, REV-ERBs and RORs have opposing impacts on the BMAL1 transcription process. By binding to D-box elements at regular times, the transcriptional activators DBP, TEF, and HLF, as well as the repressor NFIL3, make a third feedback loop (Preston et al., 2022).

Along with the primary CLOCK-BMAL1/PER-CRY loop, there are other feedback loops that are linked to it. The loop between REV-ERBα and RORA is particularly notable, since both are direct targets of CLOCK-BMAL1. When this loop acts as a feedback mechanism on BMAL1 transcription, it results in antiphase BMAL1 oscillations. In addition to CLOCK-BMAL1, other transcriptional targets of CLOCK-BMAL1 include the PAR-bZip family members DBP, HLF, and TEF; the bZip protein E4BP4 (NFIL3); and the bHLH proteins DEC1 and DEC2 (BHLHB2, BHLHB3) (Mohawk et al., 2012).

Circadian Transcriptional Mechanisms

The circadian clock is fundamentally based on transcriptional cycles. The condition of chromatin is crucial to the control of transcription, so knowing how it varies over time is crucial to understanding transcriptional rhythms. It is possible to change chromatin on many different levels, such as the DNA sequence, histones, and the way chromatin is structured and organized at a high level. DNA methylation is needed for animals to grow and develop, and it also affects how plants and other organisms grow and develop in response to their environment. DNA methylation pathway mutations are better tolerated by plants, and methylation mutants often display minimal symptoms. Nonetheless, aberrant genetic lesions may accumulate in plants through repeated self-pollination, so it is important to keep an eye out for them (Chen & Mas, 2019).

Now, a transcriptional feedback loop containing at least 10 genes is considered necessary to regulate the molecular clock in mammalian cells. CLOCK and BMAL1 produce bHLH-PAS (basic helix-loop-helix; Per-Arnt-Single-minded) proteins for the positive feedback circuit. The transcription process begins when the CLOCK:BMAL1 heterodimer binds to E-boxes (5′-CACGTG-3′) and E′-boxes (5′-CACGTT-3′) at the promoters of target genes. The PER and CRY genes are examples of those on the "negative limb" of the feedback loop that also function. Restarting the cycle from a low level of transcriptional activity is made possible by the PER and CRY proteins that are produced as a result. When they form dimers, they prevent CLOCK:BMAL1 from doing any more transcriptional work. The periodic acetylation and deacetylation of histones in various clock target genes demonstrate that clock-specific and ubiquitous histone-modifying proteins remodel chromatin for cyclic transcriptional activity (Buhr & Takahashi, 2013). In addition to CLOCK/BMAL1, REVERBs/RORs, and DBP, which are the main outputs of the core circadian clock, PER1 and CRY1/2 seem to affect genes outside of the core regulatory feedback loop. CLOCK and BMAL1 work in tandem with other histone-modifying enzymes and transcriptional coactivators, including Sirtuin 1 and CBP/p300, to increase gene expression and the periodic recruitment of RNA polymerase (Cox & Takahashi, 2019).

Changes in mRNA after transcription occur in all areas of biology, even when scientists look at circadian rhythms. The fundamental clock genes seem to be rhythmically transcribed; however, not all rhythmically transcribed genes are de novo. It has also been shown that changes made after transcription may have an effect on the clock frequency. In one study, selective N6-methylation of denosine (m6A) was studied in numerous gene transcripts, including clock gene transcripts such as Period, CLOCK, BMAL1, CK1δ, and REV-ERBα, was studied. Compared to unmodified PER2 transcripts, those without a 3' UTR or an endogenous PER2' 3' UTR substituted with an SV40 late poly(A) tail had a longer half-life. This finding suggests that the 3' UTR contributes to the stability and degradation of clock gene transcripts (Yi et al., 2022).

Conclusion

Humans have biological clocks, which are marked by the regular occurrence of a wide range of physiological and biochemical processes and behaviors (like heart rate, temperature, blood pressure, muscle strength, emotional and cognitive states, etc.). Several physiological and biochemical activities in the human body follow circadian rhythms, which scientists have studied for decades and now understand quite well. The human body's internal clock, or biological clock, is crucial to our well-being. Circadian rhythm disturbances have been linked to insomnia, fatigue, depression, a weaker immune system, and even cancer. Mutations in the genes responsible for controlling the circadian clock may also cause circadian rhythm disturbances. Individuals are able to increase their productivity at work, have better rest, and improve their physical and mental health by arranging their daily activities in accordance with the periodic changes that occur in their physiological and biochemical activity (Yu, 2018).

The circadian clock is the result of a long-term process of evolution. It synchronizes physiological and behavioral processes, such as the metabolism of substances, eating cycles, and the sleep-wake cycle, so that organisms can adapt to changes in light and temperature. A molecule oscillator controls transcription-translation feedback loops, which produce circadian rhythms at the molecular level. The expression of these genes, which are called "circadian clock genes," changes about once every 24 hours. The mammalian core clock genes identified by genetic analysis are CLOCK, ARNTL, PER1, PER2, PER3, CRY1, and CRY2 (L. L. Zhang et al., 2021).

BMAL1 and CLOCK heterodimerize and induce the expression of core clock genes or output genes by binding to enhancer boxes on target promoters. There has been much investigation into the connection of the clock system to energy metabolism in peripheral organs. While the SCN clock does play a role in circadian changes in glucose homeostasis through glucose absorption and insulin release, peripheral clocks may also play a role in the regulation of these processes, adding an additional layer of control (Sato & Sassone-Corsi, 2022). The PER and CRY proteins are nuclear imports at certain times throughout their development. There, they stop transcription by inhibiting the activity of the CLOCK-BMAL1 heterodimer. The BMAL1 gene is regulated by a feedback loop formed by the REV-ERBα/β and RORα proteins, which, respectively, inhibit and promote transcription of the gene. Recent research suggests that rhythmicity is maintained by proteasomal degradation, epigenetic control of gene expression, and post-translational changes in mRNA. This has led to some rethinking of the traditional paradigm, which was based on transcription (Stangherlin & Reddy, 2013).

The circadian clock regulates many physiological systems in mammals that undergo diurnal (day to night) changes. The suprachiasmatic nucleus of the hypothalamus is where the main clock of the circadian system is located. Other clocks can be found in different parts of the brain and in a few other organs. Some of the external environmental cues that have been shown to change clock phases are light and dark cycles, diet, stress, and physical activity (Tahara et al., 2017). The presence of the circadian clock in most mammalian cells suggests its modulatory complexity. The retina of a mammal responds to light and sends a signal to the SCN. The SCN is in charge of getting information from the outside world, processing it, and putting it to use in tissues. It does this by synchronizing the signals that keep the circadian oscillations in neuronal activity strong (Z. Zhang et al., 2021).

The human body has an internal circadian clock that encourages 24-hour regularity in a variety of behavioral and physiological processes. Delayed Sleep Phase Disorder, or DSPD, is a common reason why people can't sleep. It causes sleep times to change to later times than what society expects. Patke et al. found a type of DSPD that runs in families and is linked to a dominant coding variant in the central circadian clock gene CRY1, which makes a transcriptional inhibitor that binds to CLOCK and BMAL1 more strongly. This gain-of-function CRY1 mutation reduces the expression of important transcriptional targets and slows circadian molecular rhythms, both of which are linked to symptoms of DSPD (Patke et al., 2017).

The association between mutations in clock genes and diurnal variability in human behaviors was discovered by genetic investigations of circadian rhythm sleep disorders (CRSD), including familial advanced sleep phase syndrome (ASPS) and delayed sleep phase syndrome (DSPS), and morningness-eveningness. Different versions of the CLOCK gene, such as the T3111C variant, have been thought to play a role in morningness and eveningness. The S662G mutation in the PER2 gene and the T44A mutation in the CK1δ gene both generate two families with familial ASPS (FASPS) but are not present in any additional FASPS families. In particular, it has been shown that a missense variant in the PER3 gene makes people more likely to get DSPS, while a similar mutation in the CK1ε gene is likely to protect people from getting DSPS (Ebisawa, 2007).

Environmental and dietary factors also have an impact on how mammals coordinate their circadian time with their internal clock. Okada Y and Okada M examined how several clock genes and genes related to aging were expressed in both young and old fibroblast cells to determine what was going on. Quercetin made SIRT1 work better in older fibroblast cells, and cafeic acid made SIRT6 work better in older cells, which suggests an anti-aging effect. Resveratrol decreased clock gene expression. Quercetin and cafeic acid both upregulated clock-controlled genes (SIRT1, NR1D1) more than resveratrol in young fibroblast cells. In primary cultures of primary fibroblasts from young adults, where researchers were looking for PER1 upregulation, only cafeic acid was found to have an activating effect on NR1D1 (Okada & Okada, 2020).

Both the circadian clock and the sleep-wake cycle are complex, interrelated processes that have far-reaching effects on brain function and neurodegeneration. Although we have made considerable progress in understanding the underlying processes driving the circadian clock and sleep neural circuitry, our knowledge of how these systems are affected in the brain during aging and neurodegenerative diseases is still quite shallow. More research needs to be done to find out how the circadian and sleep systems affect aging and neurodegeneration, as well as how these two things are linked (Musiek & Holtzman, 2016). To keep daily circadian oscillations at about 24 hours, the negative feedback loop of the clock network needs a long time between activating transcription and stopping it. This is done through post-translational modifications (PTMs). Mitogen-activated protein kinases and glycogen synthase kinase-3b phosphorylate the transcription activator BMAL1, and the clock has intrinsic histone acetyltransferase activity, linking the clock mechanism with chromatin remodeling. Core clock proteins regulate clock gene transcription by PTMs such as phosphorylation, ubiquitylation, sumoylation, acetylation, and epigenetic alterations (Wang & Li, 2021).

How the circadian system controls the cellular, systemic, and behavioral functions of genes, the effective molecular mechanisms in this system, and the regulation of genes that play a role in the circadian clock are discussed in this chapter. Unique to circadian biology is the fact that the rhythm of gene transcription almost exactly matches the pattern of behavior. Gene transcription and translation make up this basic oscillatory mechanism. Tracking clock gene oscillation in real time throughout the genome, the cell, the tissue, the brain, and the whole organism may help answer the question of where and how the time signal is first made and how it enters higher levels of life. The study of biological clocks provides a link between individual genes and the organism as a whole, opening up the exciting possibility of investigating the integrational process of "time" in a vertical structure.

References

Almeida, S., Chaves, M., & Delaunay, F. (2020). Transcription-based circadian mechanism controls the duration of molecular clock states in response to signaling inputs. *J Theor Biol*, *484*, 110015. https://doi.org/10.1016/j.jtbi.2019.110015.

Andreani, T. S., Itoh, T. Q., Yildirim, E., Hwangbo, D. S., & Allada, R. (2015). Genetics of Circadian Rhythms. *Sleep Med Clin*, *10*(4), 413-421. https://doi.org/10.1016/j.jsmc.2015.08.007.

Askin, L., Tibilli, H., Tanriverdi, O., & Turkmen, S. (2020). The relationship between coronary artery disease and SIRT1 protein. *North Clin Istanb*, *7*(6), 631-635. https://doi.org/10.14744/nci.2020.31391 .

Buhr, E. D., & Takahashi, J. S. (2013). Molecular components of the Mammalian circadian clock. *Handb Exp Pharmacol*(217), 3-27. https://doi.org/10.1007/978-3-642-25950-0_1.

Ceriani, M. F., Hogenesch, J. B., Yanovsky, M., Panda, S., Straume, M., & Kay, S. A. (2002). Genome-wide expression analysis in Drosophila reveals genes controlling circadian behavior. *J Neurosci*, *22*(21), 9305-9319. https://doi.org/10.1523/JNEUROSCI.22-21-09305.2002

Charrier, A., Olliac, B., Roubertoux, P., & Tordjman, S. (2017). Clock Genes and Altered Sleep-Wake Rhythms: Their Role in the Development of Psychiatric Disorders. *Int J Mol Sci*, *18*(5). https://doi.org/10.3390/ijms18050938 .

Chen, Z. J., & Mas, P. (2019). Interactive roles of chromatin regulation and circadian clock function in plants. *Genome Biol*, *20*(1), 62. https://doi.org/10.1186/s13059-019-1672-9.

Cox, K. H., & Takahashi, J. S. (2019). Circadian clock genes and the transcriptional architecture of the clock mechanism. *J Mol Endocrinol*, *63*(4), R93-R102. https://doi.org/10.1530/JME-19-0153.

Ebisawa, T. (2007). Circadian rhythms in the CNS and peripheral clock disorders: human sleep disorders and clock genes. *J Pharmacol Sci*, *103*(2), 150-154. https://doi.org/10.1254/jphs.fmj06003x5.

Fagiani, F., Di Marino, D., Romagnoli, A., Travelli, C., Voltan, D., Di Cesare Mannelli, L., Racchi, M., Govoni, S., & Lanni, C. (2022). Molecular regulations of circadian rhythm and implications for physiology and diseases. *Signal Transduct Target Ther*, *7*(1), 41. https://doi.org/10.1038/s41392-022-00899-y.

Hanoun, M., Eisele, L., Suzuki, M., Greally, J. M., Huttmann, A., Aydin, S., Scholtysik, R., Klein-Hitpass, L., Duhrsen, U., & Durig, J. (2012). Epigenetic silencing of the circadian clock gene CRY1 is associated with an indolent clinical course in chronic lymphocytic leukemia. *PLoS One*, *7*(3), e34347. https://doi.org/10.1371/journal.pone.0034347.

Haque, S. N., Booreddy, S. R., & Welsh, D. K. (2019). Effects of BMAL1 Manipulation on the Brain's Master Circadian Clock and Behavior. *Yale J Biol Med*, *92*(2), 251-258. https://www.ncbi.nlm.nih.gov/pubmed/31249486.

Hastings, M. (1998). The brain, circadian rhythms, and clock genes. *BMJ*, *317*(7174), 1704-1707. https://doi.org/10.1136/bmj.317.7174.1704.

Hastings, M. H., Smyllie, N. J., & Patton, A. P. (2020). Molecular-genetic Manipulation of the Suprachiasmatic Nucleus Circadian Clock. *J Mol Biol*, *432*(12), 3639-3660. https://doi.org/10.1016/j.jmb.2020.01.019.

Huang, R. C. (2018). The discoveries of molecular mechanisms for the circadian rhythm: The 2017 Nobel Prize in Physiology or Medicine. *Biomed J*, *41*(1), 5-8. https://doi.org/10.1016/j.bj.2018.02.003.

Jarabo, P., & Martin, F. A. (2017). Neurogenetics of Drosophila circadian clock: expect the unexpected. *J Neurogenet*, *31*(4), 250-265. https://doi.org/10.1080/01677063.2017.1370466.

Kim, M., de la Pena, J. B., Cheong, J. H., & Kim, H. J. (2018). Neurobiological Functions of the Period Circadian Clock 2 Gene, Per2. *Biomol Ther (Seoul)*, *26*(4), 358-367. https://doi.org/10.4062/biomolther.2017.131.

Kinouchi, K., & Sassone-Corsi, P. (2020). Metabolic rivalry: circadian homeostasis and tumorigenesis. *Nat Rev Cancer*, *20*(11), 645-661. https://doi.org/10.1038/s41568-020-0291-9.

Kwon, I., Lee, J., Chang, S. H., Jung, N. C., Lee, B. J., Son, G. H., Kim, K., & Lee, K. H. (2006). BMAL1 shuttling controls transactivation and degradation of the CLOCK/BMAL1 heterodimer. *Mol Cell Biol*, *26*(19), 7318-7330. https://doi.org/10.1128/MCB.00337-06.

Landgraf, D., McCarthy, M. J., & Welsh, D. K. (2014). The role of the circadian clock in animal models of mood disorders. *Behav Neurosci*, *128*(3), 344-359. https://doi.org/10.1037/a0036029.

Landgraf, D., Shostak, A., & Oster, H. (2012). Clock genes and sleep. *Pflugers Arch*, *463*(1), 3-14. https://doi.org/10.1007/s00424-011-1003-9.

Li, H. X. (2019). The role of circadian clock genes in tumors. *Onco Targets Ther*, *12*, 3645-3660. https://doi.org/10.2147/OTT.S203144.

Miyazaki, K., Nagase, T., Mesaki, M., Narukawa, J., Ohara, O., & Ishida, N. (2004). Phosphorylation of clock protein PER1 regulates its circadian degradation in normal human fibroblasts. *Biochem J*, *380*(Pt 1), 95-103. https://doi.org/10.1042/BJ20031308.

Mohawk, J. A., Green, C. B., & Takahashi, J. S. (2012). Central and peripheral circadian clocks in mammals. *Annu Rev Neurosci*, *35*, 445-462. https://doi.org/10.1146/annurev-neuro-060909-153128.

Musiek, E. S., & Holtzman, D. M. (2016). Mechanisms linking circadian clocks, sleep, and neurodegeneration. *Science*, *354*(6315), 1004-1008. https://doi.org/10.1126/science.aah4968.

Okada, Y., & Okada, M. (2020). Quercetin, caffeic acid and resveratrol regulate circadian clock genes and aging-related genes in young and old human lung fibroblast cells. *Mol Biol Rep*, *47*(2), 1021-1032. https://doi.org/10.1007/s11033-019-05194-8.

Patke, A., Murphy, P. J., Onat, O. E., Krieger, A. C., Ozcelik, T., Campbell, S. S., & Young, M. W. (2017). Mutation of the Human Circadian Clock Gene CRY1 in Familial Delayed Sleep Phase Disorder. *Cell*, *169*(2), 203-215 e213. https://doi.org/10.1016/j.cell.2017.03.027.

Piggins, H. D. (2002). Human clock genes. *Ann Med*, *34*(5), 394-400. https://doi.org/10.1080/078538902320772142.

Preston, R., Meng, Q. J., & Lennon, R. (2022). The dynamic kidney matrisome - is the circadian clock in control? *Matrix Biol*, *114*, 138-155. https://doi.org/10.1016/j.matbio.2022.05.005.

Putker, M., & O'Neill, J. S. (2016). Reciprocal Control of the Circadian Clock and Cellular Redox State - a Critical Appraisal. *Mol Cells*, *39*(1), 6-19. https://doi.org/10.14348/molcells.2016.2323.

Rijo-Ferreira, F., & Takahashi, J. S. (2019). Genomics of circadian rhythms in health and disease. *Genome Med*, *11*(1), 82. https://doi.org/10.1186/s13073-019-0704-0.

Sato, F., Kohsaka, A., Bhawal, U. K., & Muragaki, Y. (2018). Potential Roles of Dec and Bmal1 Genes in Interconnecting Circadian Clock and Energy Metabolism. *Int J Mol Sci*, *19*(3). https://doi.org/10.3390/ijms19030781.

Sato, T., & Sassone-Corsi, P. (2022). Nutrition, metabolism, and epigenetics: pathways of circadian reprogramming. *EMBO Rep*, *23*(5), e52412. https://doi.org/10.15252/embr.202152412.

Stangherlin, A., & Reddy, A. B. (2013). Regulation of circadian clocks by redox homeostasis. *J Biol Chem*, *288*(37), 26505-26511. https://doi.org/10.1074/jbc.R113.457564.

Sun, L., Ma, L., Turck, C. W., Xu, P., & Wang, G. Z. (2020). Genome-wide circadian regulation: A unique system for computational biology. *Comput Struct Biotechnol J*, *18*, 1914-1924. https://doi.org/10.1016/j.csbj.2020.07.002.

Tahara, Y., Aoyama, S., & Shibata, S. (2017). The mammalian circadian clock and its entrainment by stress and exercise. *J Physiol Sci*, *67*(1), 1-10. https://doi.org/10.1007/s12576-016-0450-7.

Thain, S. C., Murtas, G., Lynn, J. R., McGrath, R. B., & Millar, A. J. (2002). The circadian clock that controls gene expression in Arabidopsis is tissue specific. *Plant Physiol*, *130*(1), 102-110. https://doi.org/10.1104/pp.005405.

Ukita, Y., Okumura, M., & Chihara, T. (2022). Ubiquitin proteasome system in circadian rhythm and sleep homeostasis: Lessons from Drosophila. *Genes Cells*, *27*(6), 381-391. https://doi.org/10.1111/gtc.12935.

Ung, W., Vivarelli, S., Falzone, L., Libra, M., & Bonavida, B. (2021). Regulation of the c-myc Oncogene by the Circadian Clock and Oncogenesis. *Crit Rev Oncog*, *26*(4), 55-66. https://doi.org/10.1615/CritRevOncog.2022042689.

Vanselow, K., Vanselow, J. T., Westermark, P. O., Reischl, S., Maier, B., Korte, T., Herrmann, A., Herzel, H., Schlosser, A., & Kramer, A. (2006). Differential effects of PER2 phosphorylation: molecular basis for the human familial advanced sleep phase syndrome (FASPS). *Genes Dev*, *20*(19), 2660-2672. https://doi.org/10.1101/gad.397006.

Wang, X. L., & Li, L. (2021). Circadian Clock Regulates Inflammation and the Development of Neurodegeneration. *Front Cell Infect Microbiol*, *11*, 696554. https://doi.org/10.3389/fcimb.2021.696554.

Wang, Y., Ni, X., Yan, J., & Yang, L. (2017). Modeling transcriptional co-regulation of mammalian circadian clock. *Math Biosci Eng*, *14*(5-6), 1447-1462. https://doi.org/10.3934/mbe.2017075.

Woon, P. Y., Kaisaki, P. J., Braganc, J., Thérèse Bihoreau, M., Levy, J. C., Farrall, M., & Gauguier, D. (2007). Aryl hydrocarbon receptor nuclear translocator-like (BMAL1) is associated with susceptibility to hypertension and type 2 diabetes. *Proceedings of the National Academy of Sciences*, *104*(36), 14412–14417. https://doi.org/10.1073/pnas.0703247104.

Yang, Y., Li, Y., Sancar, A., & Oztas, O. (2020). The circadian clock shapes the Arabidopsis transcriptome by regulating alternative splicing and alternative polyadenylation. *J Biol Chem*, *295*(22), 7608-7619. https://doi.org/10.1074/jbc.RA120.013513.

Yi, J. S., Diaz, N. M., D'Souza, S., & Buhr, E. D. (2022). The molecular clockwork of mammalian cells. *Semin Cell Dev Biol*, *126*, 87-96. https://doi.org/10.1016/j.semcdb.2021.03.012.

Yu, Q. (2018). Biological clock: the oscillator of gene expression. *Sci China Life Sci*, *61*(1), 128-130. https://doi.org/10.1007/s11427-017-9239-6.

Zhang, L. L., He, Q. K., Lv, Y. N., Zhang, Z. J., & Xiang, Y. K. (2021). Expression pattern and prognostic value of circadian clock genes in pancreatic adenocarcinoma. *Chronobiol Int*, *38*(5), 681-693. https://doi.org/10.1080/07420528.2021.1890760.

Zhang, Z., Zeng, P., Gao, W., Zhou, Q., Feng, T., & Tian, X. (2021). Circadian clock: a regulator of the immunity in cancer. *Cell Commun Signal*, *19*(1), 37. https://doi.org/10.1186/s12964-021-00721-2.

Chapter 3

Hormonal Rhythm

Gül Akar[1,*], PhD
and Fatma Şengül[2], PhD
[1]Department of Medical Services and Techniques, Kütahya Health Sciences University, Kütahya, Turkiye
[2]Department of Biochemistry, Adıyaman University, Adıyaman, Turkiye

Abstract

The circadian (daily) system consists of a central clock located in the suprachiasmatic nucleus (SCN) of the hypothalamus and a series of peripheral clocks located in other body tissues such as the liver, pancreas, gastrointestinal tract, skeletal muscle, and adipose tissue. The central clock synchronizes the body to light or the sun and primarily uses the light and dark cycles for this purpose, while the peripheral clock uses signals from the SCN and autonomic rhythm responses to stimuli from external factors such as light, nutrition, physical activity, and sleep. In hormonal homeostasis, apart from hormones with circadian fluctuations such as melatonin, glucocorticoids, prolactin, FGF21, thyroid hormone, and growth hormone; insulin, leptin, ghrelin, and adiponectin, which are regulated by environmental stimuli such as feeding time and light-dark cycles, are also released in circadian rhythm. The presence of melatonin receptors in almost all tissues leads to the view that melatonin is a key clock cycle molecule in the whole body. The circadian activity of pineal melatonin secretion is regulated by the main biological clock found in mammals within the SCN of the anterior hypothalamus. In this chapter,

* Corresponding Author's Email: akargul@windowslive.com.

In: Human Health is a Matter of Timing
Editors: Sumeyya Deniz Aybek, Gonca Gulbay and Mucahit Secme
ISBN: 979-8-89113-467-6

information is presented from the current literature on hormones that fluctuate depending on the circadian clock.

Keywords: circadian system, melatonin, suprachiasmatic nucleus, hormonal homeostasis

Introduction

The circadian clock is a system that expresses molecular, behavioral, and physiological changes over a period of approximately 24 hours. There are two types of circadian clocks: the central pacemaker (central clock) located in the suprachiasmatic nucleus (SCN) in the anterior hypothalamus region of the brain, which is sensitive to light, and peripheral oscillators (peripheral clocks) located in various tissues of the body (liver, heart, adipose tissue, pancreas, etc.) (Richards & Gumz, 2012). These clocks produce self-sustained oscillations over a period of about 24 hours, referred to as 'circadian rhythms.' The SCN, which consists of single-cell circadian oscillators, is activated by a neural network called the retinohypothalamic pathway. The activated SCN contributes to physiological events by stimulating other brain regions and regulating the circadian clock. Although the main stimulating factor for the SCN is known to be light, it is stated that stimuli such as hormones, food, sleep-wake state, temperature, physical activity, etc. may also play a role. The main regulatory factor is the sleep-wake state. Recently, due to increased interaction with electronic devices, the sleep cycle has started to be negatively affected, and there have been changes in the circadian clock (Froy, 2010; Serin & Tek, 2019).

The circadian clock is regulated by a transcriptional and translational feedback loop (TTFL) with positively regulated clock genes such as Clock (circadian locomotor output cycles kaput), Bmal1 (brain and muscle antlike protein-1) and NPAS2 (neuronal PAS domain protein 2) and negatively regulated clock genes such as Period (Per1, Per2, and Per3) and Cryptochrome (Cry1/Cry2). There are also several post-translational and non-transcriptional mechanisms (Tiwari et al., 2023).

The endocrine system is one of the main mechanisms that coordinate physiological systems according to the circadian clock. Both central and peripheral clocks affect the endocrine system, while hormonal signals regulate the circadian clock through a feedback mechanism (Tsang et al., 2016).

Hormones

Melatonin (N-acetyl-5-methoxytryptamine)

Melatonin hormone, an indole compound synthesized from tryptophan, an essential amino acid, mainly in the pineal gland, is best known for its regulation of circadian rhythm. Melatonin, which is an active hormone as a biological clock in the regulation of the sleep/wake cycle, is also a hormone that helps to establish biological rhythms. Whether diurnal or nocturnal, melatonin is synthesized and released at night in all mammals and is therefore also called the night hormone (Pevet & Challet, 2011). Studies conducted since the discovery of melatonin have shown that melatonin plays an important role in the synchronization of many physiological functions from adiposity to aggression, hibernation to circadian rhythm, tissue regeneration, regulation of seasonal reproductivc activity, facilitation of sleep physiology, elimination of free radicals, promotion of immune response, suppression of carcinogenesis, promotion of stem cell proliferation, anti-inflammation and modulation of aging (Chowdhury et al., 2008; Majidinia et al., 2018).

Melatonin regulates various physiological and neuroendocrine functions in mammals through the activation of two types of G-protein mediated receptors identified as Melatonin receptor 1 (MT_1) and Melatonin receptor 2 (MT_2). Apart from MT_1 and MT_2 receptors, melatonin also interacts with intracellular proteins such as quinone reductase 2, and calmodulin. Melatonin exerts its circadian and reproductive effects through the MT1 receptor. The MT2 receptor is associated with dopaminergic functions in the brain and retina. It has been found that MT1 and MT2 receptors have more effects on circadian rhythm than intracellular proteins. When melatonin diffuses into the cell due to its lipophilic structure, it elicits transcriptional effects through nuclear receptors from the retinoid Z receptor and the retinoid acid receptor-related orphan receptor family (Chowdhury et al., 2008). In humans, melatonin can suppress cortisol production by modulating adrenal glucocorticoid production via the MT1 receptor. The secretion of many hormones such as and gonadotropin-releasing hormone (GnRH), luteinizing hormone (LH), and follicle stimulating hormone (FSH) is similarly under the control of melatonin (Pandi-Perumal et al., 2006). In the body, melatonin receptors are found in the retina, brain, pituitary, and most peripheral tissues such as the spleen, erythrocytes, leukocytes, thyroid gland, skin, thymus, placenta, endometrium, and gastrointestinal tract, where they modulate other physiological functions through paracrine signaling. The presence of melatonin receptors in almost all tissues leads to the view of melatonin as a key clock cycle molecule in the whole body (Tordjman et al., 2017).

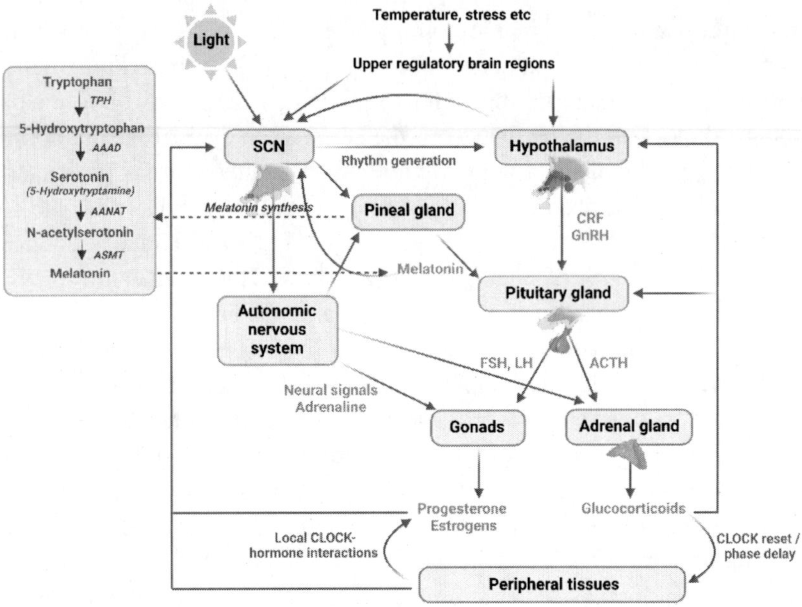

SCN, Suprachiasmatic Nucleus;
CRF, Corticotropin Releasing Factor;
GnRH, Gonadotropin-Releasing Hormone;
FSH, Follicle Stimulating Hormone;
LH, Luteinizing Hormone;
ACTH, Adrenocorticotropic Hormone;
TPH, Tryptophan hydroxylase;
AAAD, Aromatic L-amino acid decarboxylase;
AANAT, arylalkylamine N-acetyltransferase;
ASMT, N-acetylserotonin O-methyltransferase.

Figure 1. Regulation of peripheral clocks by the supraciasmatic nucleus.

The secretion of melatonin is regulated by different neurotransmitters and nerve conduction systems. Apart from the pineal gland, there are also studies showing that this hormone is synthesized in neuroendocrine cells in the retina, gastrointestinal tract, and pancreas. The circadian activity of pineal melatonin secretion is regulated by the master central clock found in mammals within the SCN of the anterior hypothalamus. The SCN is located on both sides of the third ventricle of the brain, just above the optic chiasm. The retinal ganglion transmits the signals from the photoreceptors to the SCN via the optic nerves, and then reaches the epiphysis via the superior cervical ganglion. Melatonin is a hormone that acts as the body's timer with stimuli from the SCN; it informs all cells with secretion changes depending on years, seasons, days, and hours. In this way, it contributes to the harmonious functioning of all body cells and tissues. For melatonin biosynthesis, circulating tryptophan is hydrolyzed by tryptophan hydroxylase to form 5-hydroxytryptophan, which is then decarboxylated by aromatic amino acid decarboxylase (AAAD) to from serotonin. Serotonin, which is converted to N-acetylserotonin by the arylalkylamine-N-acetyltransferase (AANAT) enzyme, is metabolized to N-acetyl-5-methoxytryptamine, namely melatonin, by the N-acetylserotonin hydroxyindole-O-methyltransferase (ASMT) enzyme (Figure 1) (Amaral & Cipolla-Neto, 2018; Doghramji, 2007).

Thanks to its lipophilic properties, melatonin is able to reach all organelles of the cell and the cell nucleus and cross the blood-brain barrier. Most of the synthesized melatonin diffuses into the cerebrospinal fluid from the third ventricle of the brain, while the rest is released into the bloodstream and distributed to all tissues. The production and release of melatonin are stimulated by darkness and suppressed by light. Although the SCN is stimulated by many rhythm transmitters, the most important rhythm transmitter is light. Light from the retina stimulates the SCN via the retinohypothalamic pathway and regulates biological activities related to circadian rhythm such as body temperature, cortisol, and thyroid hormones (Cermakian & Boivin, 2003). In daylight, retinal photoreceptor cells hyperpolarize and inhibit the release of norepinephrine. This leads to suppression of the retinohypothalamopineal system and very little melatonin release. In the dark, this suppression disappears, and melatonin production and release increases. In humans, the increase in melatonin levels starts immediately after the disappearance of daylight and reaches its highest concentration between 02:00 and 04:00 in the morning, after which it decreases. Melatonin secretion also shows seasonal differences. In summer, secretion occurs later, while in winter, secretion starts earlier. It has been found that prolonged melatonin secretion is seen on short days and short-term melatonin secretion is seen on long days. Melatonin concentration also varies with age; secretion is very low in newborns, increases shortly after birth, peaks between 1-3 years of age, and then decreases again. During puberty and adolescence, secretion becomes circadian. After the twenties, the rate of synthesis and secretion of melatonin decreases, reaching even lower levels in the 60s (Beyer et al., 1998).

Oxidative stress reactions triggered by free radicals, which are chemical products formed during cellular metabolism in the body or by exogenous agents, can lead to DNA damage with a tendency to cancer. Melatonin, which has a strong antioxidant activity, can prevent these DNA damages and prevent a possible cancer development. One of the antioxidant effects of melatonin is its direct radical scavenging effect by providing electrons to the oxidant substance (free radical, reactive oxygen derivative, etc.) independently of the receptor, and the other is its indirect effect by activating endogenous antioxidant mechanisms in a receptor-dependent manner. With its direct scavenging effect, it has been shown to render radical and reactive substances such as superoxide, hydrogen peroxide, hydroxyl radical, and peroxynitrites harmless. As an indirect effect, it has been shown that it increases the expression of antioxidant enzymes such as superoxide dismutase, glutathione peroxidase, catalase, and glutathione reductase at the DNA level and inhibits the inducible nitric oxide synthase enzyme that can cause an increase in peroxynitrites. Melatonin is different from classical antioxidants (vitamin E, vitamin C, β-carotene, etc.) in several ways. After classical antioxidants exert their effects, they turn into prooxidant substances, that is, only less harmful substances than the oxidant substances they scavenge. However, after melatonin acts on oxidant substances, in the intermediate stages, the resulting products are again antioxidant effective, and due to this feature, it is considered a suicidal antioxidant (García et al., 2014).

Glucocorticoids

Glucocorticoids are steroid hormones secreted from the adrenal cortex, have a strong circadian rhythm, exert immunosuppressive and anti-inflammatory effects, and regulate many physiological functions including glucose, lipid, and protein metabolism. In humans, the main glucocorticoid is cortisol. Glucocorticoids are released in an ultradian and circadian rhythmic pattern. Ultradian (also known as pulsatile) glucocorticoid rhythms are controlled by a negative feedback loop through a neuroendocrine pathway, the hypothalamus-pituitary-adrenal (HPA) axis, where it suppresses the production of Adrenocorticotropic Hormone (ACTH). Circadian glucocorticoid rhythms are regulated by three main factors: the endocrine hypothalamic-pituitary-adrenal (HPA) axis, local adrenocortical circadian clocks, and SCN-controlled autonomic innervation. The circadian rhythm of glucocorticoid secretion results in maximal production in the early morning (dawn) for the diurnal phase and in the early evening (dusk) for the nocturnal phase. Glucocorticoids are thought to exhibit a strong circadian rhythm that peaks at the end of the sleep phase because they prepare the body for energetically demanding processes during the active phase (Nicolaides et al., 2014; Scherholz et al., 2019).

The circadian clock of glucocorticoids is realized by signals from the SCN stimulating the paraventricular nucleus of the hypothalamus and the release of corticotropin-releasing hormone (CRH). ACTH is released from the pituitary gland stimulated the circadian rhythm or by CRH in response to stress. ACTH secretion is mediated by stimulation of CRH and arginine vasopressin (AVP). CRH has a strong effect, and AVP has a weak effect. CRH and AVP are secreted from the hypothalamus. When ACTH reaches the adrenal cortex, the major low-density lipoprotein (LDL)-cholesterol is removed from the circulation, and the cellular processes involved in the production and release of cortisol are initiated. Cortisol, a hormone with 19 carbon atoms synthesized from cholesterol by cytochrome P450 enzymatic chain, is the hormone with the strongest glucocorticoid activity. Since cortisol, which has a steroid structure, cannot be stored in the cell, it is rapidly produced in the adrenal cortex and released outside the cell when needed. The regulation of cortisol synthesis is controlled by a negative feedback mechanism involving corticosteroid receptors in the hypothalamus and anterior pituitary, whereby high serum cortisol levels to suppress the release of AVP, CRH, and ACTH. In humans, cortisol production increases during the night and peaks in the morning (07:00-08:00), thereby adjusting the endocrine balance for stress to be connected with awakening (Spencer et al., 2018).

Growth hormone (GH)

The peptide growth hormone secreted from the anterior pituitary, and also known as somatotropin, peaks at night (between 02.00-04.00). Human growth hormone interacts with special receptors on the surfaces of cells in protein, carbohydrate, and lipid metabolism in the control of physiological activities including growth and metabolism. It is essential to pay attention to the fact that especially children in the growth period are sleeping during the release times of this hormone, which has many important functions, including growth and development in metabolism. If the balance between the circadian clock and growth hormone is disrupted due to reasons such as sleep disorders, the hormone cannot be released at normal levels (Serin & Tek, 2019). GH, which has anti-insulin activity, stimulates glucose biosynthesis by suppressing insulin uptake into peripheral tissues stimulated by insulin and enhances the mineralization of bones by stimulating calcium (Ca) retention in the body. In addition to the known growth-promoting effect of GH, it is also involved in the absorption of amino acids from the intestines and their use in protein synthesis in the liver and muscles, stimulation of lipolysis through the stimulation of beta-adrenergic receptors in adipocytes, which are adipose tissue cells, amino acid transport in the blood, conversion of preadipocytes into adipocytes, and the use of fatty acids released by the breakdown of fat stores in protein biosynthesis in muscles, The effects of ghrelin on abdominal fat transport to the periphery, lowering blood cholesterol levels through regulation of hepatic LDL receptors, stimulation of glucose metabolism, stimulation of gonadal insulin-like growth factor-1 (IGF-1) production, stimulation of luteal progesterone synthesis through gonodotropins and parathormone are also known. Hypothalamic growth hormone-releasing hormone and gastric ghrelin stimulate GH release, while hypothalamic somatostatin inhibits it. There are other regulators of GH release. IGF1, which is responsible for the peripheral effects of GH, inhibits GH release. Fasting, malnutrition, and intravenous administration of amino acids also stimulate GH release. Hyperglycemia and leptin inhibit the release of GH (Caputo et al., 2021; Kim & Park, 2017).

GH secretion is involved in a circadian and diurnal rhythm that follows a sleep pattern, and the peak in GH secretion occurs during sleep in the dark phase of the diurnal cycle (Linkowski et al., 1994). Studies have found that human GH RNA expression oscillates over a 24-hour period, different from that of mice (Vakili et al., 2016). In another study, it was found that circadian clock dysfunction severely affects the biological activity of GH and that the circadian clock is involved in the signaling process of GH. In the same study, it was found that circadian clock deficiency leads to GH resistance, GH signaling is reduced in circadian clock deficiency in a mouse model, and circadian clock deficiency increases the expression of negative signaling proteins (Lyu et al., 2021).

Prolactin (PRL)

Prolactin is a polypeptide hormone of 199 amino acids synthesized from the anterior pituitary and is a lactogenic hormone closely related to growth hormone. The PRL receptor (PRLR) is widely expressed in the brain, and its synthesis increases during pregnancy and lactation. Primarily responsible for lactation, PRL also acts as a neurotransmitter, growth factor, and immunoregulator. At high concentrations, PRL inhibits ovulation by reducing the sensitivity of LH and FSH receptors in the gonads. PRLR is a member of the type 1 cytokine/hematopoietic receptor superfamily and is expressed by many immune system cells such as T-lymphocytes, macrophages, and B-lymphocytes. Therefore, released prolactin plays a proinflammatory role by binding to PRLR. PRL production and release are stimulated by the hypothalamic peptides thyroid releasing hormone and vasoactive intestinal peptide. Prolactin levels reach high levels in the second half of the night and early in the morning (Egli et al., 2010; Saleem et al., 2018).

There are studies examining the relationship between circadian rhythm and prolactin. In these studies, factors that play a role in the circadian regulation of prolactin levels (Stangerup & Hannibal, 2020), the relationship between prolactin and sleep disorders, and circadian rhythm (Mills & Kuohung, 2019) have been investigated. Furthermore, one study reported that the circadian rhythm of prolactin was altered in patients with polycystic ovary syndrome (Wang et al., 2021).

Insulin

Insulin is a peptide hormone secreted by beta (β) cells in the pancreatic islets of Langerhans in our body, which plays an important role in the regulation of blood glucose levels. Insulin, which has anabolic effects, regulates the utilization of energy by tissues. Released during satiety, insulin prevents an excessive increase in blood glucose concentration by activating the glucose utilization, glycogenesis, and lipogenesis metabolic pathways of tissues (Campbell & Newgard, 2021). Insulin concentrations show circadian changes depending on the SCN and decrease especially between 03:00-05:00 hours. Peripheral clocks in beta cells in the islets of Langerhans act as a gating mechanism for insulin release. With positive regulation of the peripheral clock, hypoinsulinemia is observed due to impaired insulin secretion because of deletion of tissue-specific Clock or Bmal1, while with negative regulation of the clock, hyperinsulinemia occurs because of deletion of tissue-specific Per or Cry (Barclay et al., 2013).

Leptin

Leptin hormone release is dependent on the circadian rhythm and serum leptin levels are low in the midday and afternoon hours and reach the highest levels at night. The main neuronal targets of leptin, a hormone secreted from adipose tissue and composed of 167 amino acids, are located in specific regions of the hypothalamus. There is a satiety center in the ventromedial hypothalamic nuclei and a hunger center in the lateral hypothalamic nuclei. Leptin regulates appetite and metabolism by inhibiting the synthesis and release of neuropeptide-Y and agouti-related protein (AgRP), which are mainly involved in the regulation of many pituitary hormones and whose main effect is to increase appetite. Leptin suppresses appetite by increasing the transcription of Proopiomelanocortin (POMC), a hormone that suppresses food cravings. In conclusion, leptin modulates the activity of POMC and NPY/AgRP neurons and maintains homeostasis (Picó et al., 2022).

Once synthesized in adipocytes, some leptin is released into the bloodstream, and the rest is stored in fat cells. Leptin expression, which varies daily according to nutritional status, is also regulated by various hormones such as insulin, catecholamines, and glucocorticoids. Prolonged elevation of the insulin hormone, which is the regulator of leptin production, causes an increase in the plasma concentration of leptin. Catecholamines inhibit leptin synthesis by binding to β2- and β3-adrenergic receptors. This is indicative of the presence of negative feedback between adipose tissue and the brain. It is also thought that leptin synthesis is decreased by thyroid hormones, while tumor necrosis factor-α and corticosteroids stimulate leptin synthesis. It is mainly involved in the regulation of energy metabolism through lipid synthesis, control of lipid sources, lipid mobilization and oxidation, activation of the sympathetic nervous system, stimulation of thyroid hormones, and stimulation of thermogenesis. The uncoupling protein (UCP) involved in thermogenesis inhibits ATP synthesis in mitochondria, allowing energy to be used as heat. The hormone leptin leads to increased UCP production by increasing sympathetic nervous system activation and thyroid hormone levels. Increased amounts of UCP also allow energy to be used as heat (Picó et al., 2022; Tsujino & Sakurai, 2012).

Leptin directly modulates the conduction properties of SCN neurons through leptin receptors in the SCN, contributing to the mechanism by which metabolic processes influence the circadian clock. Physiologically, leptin is known to have a circadian rhythm with the highest concentration during the night and the lowest concentration during the day. Leptin is largely secreted after mealtime, and thus the postprandial leptin elevation may provide post-feeding time cues to the central or peripheral clocks. These data demonstrate the contribution of rhythmic leptin to the regulation of circadian rhythmicity as a time transmitter closely related to glucose metabolism.

Adiponectin

Adiponectin is a 244 amino acid protein with anti-inflammatory, anti-atherogenic effects and reduces insulin resistance. Adiponectin is secreted from adipose tissue and controls body weight and metabolic rate by increasing insulin sensitivity, thermogenesis, and fatty acid oxidation. Women have higher levels of plasma adiponectin because they are more sensitive to insulin than men. It has been observed that adiponectin peaks between 12.00-14.00 in humans. Plasma adiponectin concentrations are inversely correlated with leptin, plasma triglyceride levels, body fat percentage, fasting insulin concentration, and body mass index, and are directly correlated with plasma high-density lipoprotein levels. Circulating levels decrease with high weight gain and increase with weight loss. Adiponectin receptor 1 (AdipoR1), one of the 2 receptors defined as adiponectin receptors, is mainly expressed in striated muscle, while Adiponectin receptor 2 (AdipoR2) is expressed mainly in the liver. AdipoR1 functions by activating mitogen activated protein kinase (MAPK), AMP-activated protein kinase (AMPK), and AdipoR2 by activating PPAR-α signaling molecules.Adiponectin is involved in the regulation of inflammatory responses through different pathways in different cell types (Ghoshal & Bhattacharyya, 2015).

According to a study on glucose and lipid metabolism in adinopectin knockout mice, gluconeogenesis activity and blood glucose levels were higher in adinopectin knockout mice compared to the control group throughout the day, and the circadian rhythm of the liver and serum lipid levels were altered. In conclusion, adinopectin regulates the circadian rhythm of liver metabolism. While its levels decrease in disorders of energy metabolism such as obesity, decreasing levels alter the circadian rhythm of metabolism. The disturbed circadian rhythm exacerbates metabolic disorders, leading to further decreases in adinopectin levels (Wada et al., 2022). In the study investigating adinopectin and circadian rhythm disorder in Alzheimer's disease, adinopectin deficiency increased circadian rhythm disorder, inhibited glycogen synthase kinase 3β activity and caused abnormal expression of Bmal1 mRNA/protein induced by amyloid-β protein 31-35 in HT22 hippocampal neurons (Yuan et al., 2021). In a study conducted by Gómez-Abellán et al. in morbidly obese patients, adinopectin and its receptors were found to show a 24-hour rhythm in adipose tissue (Gómez-Abellán et al., 2010).

Ghrelin

The ghrelin hormone, consisting of 28 amino acids, which is synthesized at low levels in the placenta, pancreas, kidneys, and intestines, although it is mostly secreted from the oxyntic glands in the stomach, was discovered in 1999 as a growth hormone secretagogue. A fatty acid (octanoyl) modification of the third serine amino acid in ghrelin is required for binding to GHS-R1a (growth hormone secretagogue receptor 1a). When ghrelin binds to this receptor, it exerts its effect through calcium (Ca2+), inositol triphosphate (IP_3) and phospholipase C. The Ghrelin-GHS-R1a axis increases intracellular Ca2+ concentrations through IP_3. Calcium activates calmodulin-dependent protein kinase b, leading to AMPK activation by AMP (adenosine mono-phosphate). Ghrelin-induced AMPK activation suppresses acetyl-CoA carboxylase activity, decreases malonyl-CoA levels, and activates carnitine palmitoyl transferase 1a (CPT1a), allowing the transport of long-chain fatty acids into mitochondria. Fatty acids entering the mitochondria undergo β-oxidation. Ghrelin can be found in the bloodstream in different forms depending on the type of acyl modification, such as des-acylated, octanoylated, hexanoylated, and decanoylated ghrelin. This peptide hormone is secreted in the stomach during hunger and transmits hunger signals to the central nervous system. Having gastric protective and intestinal inflammation-regulating effects, ghrelin affects gastric acid secretion, increases gastrointestinal motility, and accelerates gastric emptying. Ghrelin directly stimulates glucose output from hepatocytes. Ghrelin acts as a potential feedback signal for the SCN on the circadian system and acts directly in the SCN to modulate circadian system activity by inducing phase advances in the circadian rhythm (Qian et al., 2019; Yanagi et al., 2018). Ghrelin levels were found to peak at 13.00 h in fasting and at 02.00-04.30 h in satiety. Plasma ghrelin concentration, which increases during fasting, decreases after food intake.

Thyroid Stimulating Hormone (TSH)

TSH, synthesized by the anterior pituitary gland, is a non-covalently linked heterodimer glycoprotein composed of α and β subunits. Thyroid hormone secretion is closely regulated by the hypothalamic-pituitary-thyroid axis, which is controlled by the circadian rhythm. Thyrotropin-releasing hormone (TRH) is released from the hypothalamus and stimulates the synthesis and secretion of TSH. TSH, in turn, controls the synthesis and secretion of the thyroid hormones, thyroxine (T4) and triiodothyronine (T3). More than 99.5% of T4 and T3 are bound to protein in serum and therefore metabolically inactive. A small percentage of free T4 and T3 act on metabolic functions and control the release of both TRH and TSH using a negative feedback system. TSH responds quickly to changes in the environment aimed at maintaining homeostasis in the human body. TSH levels are affected by drugs, acute and chronic diseases, malnutrition, the biological clock, seasonality, pregnancy, and other hormones such as cortisol. Plasma concentrations begin to increase before sleep begins or in the early evening and reach maximum levels in the early night. TSH reaches the highest levels between 2:00-4:00 and the lowest levels between 16:00-20:00 (Ikegami et al., 2019).

Fibroblast Growth Factor 21 (FGF21)

FGF21, first isolated in 2000, is an endocrine fibroblast growth factor consisting of 208 amino acids. FGF21 has attracted attention in recent years due to its pleiotropic effects in response to various pathological and physiological stresses. Thanks to the intramolecular disulfide bond it contains, it increases its stability in the plasma and functions as a hormone. FGF21 is produced in many organs, such as the liver, adipose tissue, the pancreas, and the heart. The expression and secretion of FGF21 are regulated by several proteins (Badman et al., 2007). As a stress-induced factor, the circadian rhythm of FGF21 is closely related to various biological events, such as dietary intervention, exercise, and exposure to cold. FGF21 stimulates glucose uptake in adipocytes through the induction of glucose transporter-1 independent of insulin. FGF21 decreases hepatic glucose production by suppressing glucagon secretion and increases insulin sensitivity. Studies have shown that the circulating FGF21 level begins to rise at midnight, reaches the highest concentration in the early morning hours, and decreases to the basal concentration in the afternoon. It was determined that the basal concentration was higher in obese individuals, but the magnitude of the nocturnal increase was suppressed. Furthermore, the release pattern of FGF21 is similar to free fatty acid and cortisol; shown to be opposite to insulin and glucose (Yu et al., 2011).

The relationship between the hormones described in this chapter and the circadian rhythm is summarized in Figure 2.

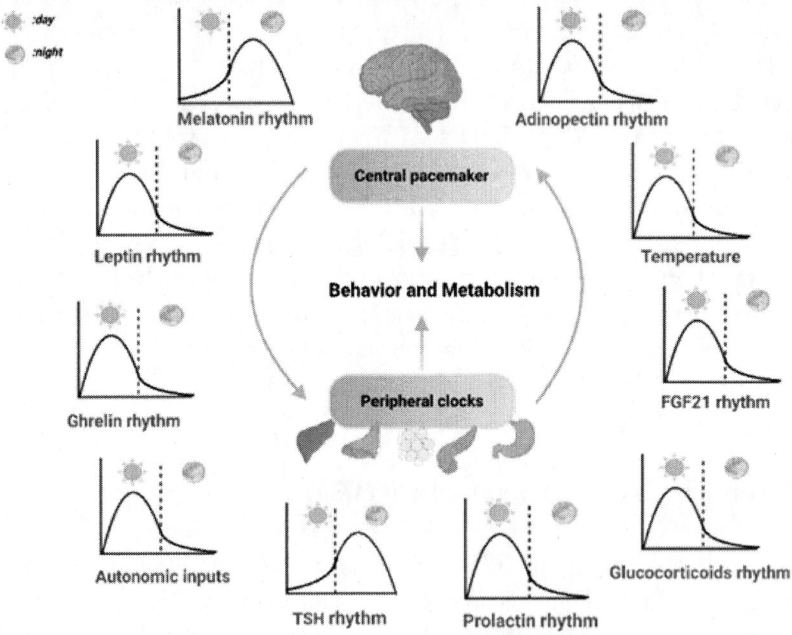

Figure 2. Circadian rhythms for various hormones and the relationship between central and peripheral clocks. *FGF21, Fibroblast Growth Factor 21; TSH, Thyroid Stimulating Hormone (Created with Biorender.com).*

Conclusion

The importance of hormonal homeostasis of the circadian clock in humans is nowadays highly salient, with circadian rhythm disturbances common in modern life.

Circadian rhythms consist of a complex and highly integrated network of clocks distributed throughout the organism, including the endocrine glands.

As shown in Figure 2, the central clock in the SCN and the peripheral clocks in the circadian of the tissues influence nearly all aspects of physiology and behavior, including the rest-wake cycle, cardiovascular activity, hormone secretion, body temperature, and metabolism. The central clock in the SCN not only synchronizes peripheral clocks, but also influences multiple processes that affect the physiological daily rhythms in sleep-wake behavior, food intake, hormone secretion, the daily rhythm in glucose metabolism, including insulin.

Melatonin provides homeostasis as an endogenous regulator. With stimuli from the SCN, it informs all cells of daily, monthly, and yearly secretion differences. This hormone epigenetically controls clock genes in cells. Additionally, melatonin increases the nocturnal temperature drop and facilitates falling asleep. The effects and functions of melatonin can be listed as regulation of endocrine rhythm, sleep regulator, chronobiological regulator, antioxidant, immune supporter, anti-cancer, blood pressure regulator, antigonadotropic effects, protective effect on the nervous system, and regulator of reproductive functions.

The hormones cortisol and melatonin, body temperature, and the sleep-wake cycle are the most important indicators of the human circadian rhythm. Chronic circadian disruption caused by shift work, traveling across time zones, or irregular sleep-wake cycles has long-term consequences for health, including weight gain, type 2 diabetes mellitus, cardiovascular disease, and the likelihood of developing various types of cancer. The circadian clock is the most important factor in the synthesis of antioxidants and metabolic proteins that make up the daily antioxidative defense system. The circadian clock can be affected by factors such as light, sleep, nutrition, environmental factors, working hours and conditions, hormones, temperature, age, gender, diseases, or medications.

As a result, it was clearly observed that hormonal homeostasis exhibits periodic fluctuations; endocrine rhythms and circadian rhythms are tightly interconnected, and the central clock interacts deeply with environmental factors to maintain internal balance.

References

Amaral, F. G. D., & Cipolla-Neto, J. (2018). A brief review about melatonin, a pineal hormone. *Arch Endocrinol Metab*, *62*(4), 472-479. https://doi.org/10.20945/2359-3997000000066.

Badman, M. K., Pissios, P., Kennedy, A. R., Koukos, G., Flier, J. S., & Maratos-Flier, E. (2007). Hepatic fibroblast .growth factor 21 is regulated by PPARalpha and is a key mediator of hepatic lipid metabolism in ketotic states. *Cell Metab*, *5*(6), 426-437. https://doi.org/10.1016/j.cmet.2007.05.002.

Barclay, J. L., Shostak, A., Leliavski, A., Tsang, A. H., Jöhren, O., Müller-Fielitz, H., Landgraf, D., Naujokat, N., van der Horst, G. T., & Oster, H. (2013). High-fat diet-induced hyperinsulinemia and tissue-specific insulin resistance in Cry-deficient mice. *American journal of physiology-endocrinology and metabolism*, *304*(10), E1053-E1063. https://doi.org/doi:10.1152/ajpendo.00512.2012.

Beyer, C. E., Steketee, J. D., & Saphier, D. (1998). Antioxidant properties of melatonin—an emerging mystery. *Biochemical pharmacology*, *56*(10), 1265-1272. https://doi.org/10.1016/s0006-2952(98)00180-4.

Campbell, J. E., & Newgard, C. B. (2021). Mechanisms controlling pancreatic islet cell function in insulin secretion. *Nature reviews Molecular cell biology*, *22*(2), 142-158. https://doi.org/10.1038/s41580-020-00317-7.

Caputo, M., Pigni, S., Agosti, E., Daffara, T., Ferrero, A., Filigheddu, N., & Prodam, F. (2021). Regulation of GH and GH Signaling by Nutrients. *Cells*, *10*(6), 1376. https://doi.org/10.3390/cells10061376.

Cermakian, N., & Boivin, D. B. (2003). A molecular perspective of human circadian rhythm disorders. *Brain Research Reviews*, *42*(3), 204-220. https://doi.org/10.1016/s0165-0173(03)00171-1.

Chowdhury, I., Sengupta, A., & Maitra, S. K. (2008). Melatonin: fifty years of scientific journey from the discovery in bovine pineal gland to delineation of functions in human. *Indian J Biochem Biophys*, *45*(5), 289-304.

Doghramji, K. (2007). Melatonin and its receptors: a new class of sleep-promoting agents. *J Clin Sleep Med*, *3*(5 Suppl), S17-23.

Egli, M., Leeners, B., & Kruger, T. H. (2010). Prolactin secretion patterns: basic mechanisms and clinical implications for reproduction. *Reproduction*, *140*(5), 643-654. https://doi.org/10.1530/rep-10-0033.

Froy, O. (2010). Metabolism and circadian rhythms—implications for obesity. *Endocrine reviews*, *31*(1), 1-24. https://doi.org/10.1210/er.2009-0014.

García, J. J., López-Pingarrón, L., Almeida-Souza, P., Tres, A., Escudero, P., García-Gil, F. A., Tan, D. X., Reiter, R. J., Ramírez, J. M., & Bernal-Pérez, M. (2014). Protective effects of melatonin in reducing oxidative stress and in preserving the fluidity of biological membranes: a review. *J Pineal Res*, *56*(3), 225-237. https://doi.org/10.1111/jpi.12128.

Ghoshal, K., & Bhattacharyya, M. (2015). Adiponectin: Probe of the molecular paradigm associating diabetes and obesity. *World journal of diabetes*, *6*(1), 151. https://doi.org/10.4239%2Fwjd.v6.i1.151.

Gómez-Abellán, P., Gómez-Santos, C., Madrid, J. A., Milagro, F. I., Campion, J., Martínez, J. A., Ordovás, J. M., & Garaulet, M. (2010). Circadian expression of adiponectin and its receptors in human adipose tissue. *Endocrinology*, *151*(1), 115-122. https://doi.org/10.1210/en.2009-0647.

Ikegami, K., Refetoff, S., Van Cauter, E., & Yoshimura, T. (2019). Interconnection between circadian clocks and thyroid function. *Nature Reviews Endocrinology*, *15*(10), 590-600. https://doi.org/10.1038/s41574-019-0237-z.

Kim, S. H., & Park, M. J. (2017). Effects of growth hormone on glucose metabolism and insulin resistance in human. *Ann Pediatr Endocrinol Metab*, *22*(3), 145-152. https://doi.org/10.6065/apem.2017.22.3.145.

Linkowski, P., Kerkhofs, M., Van Onderbergen, A., Hubain, P., Copinschi, G., L'Hermite-Balériaux, M., Leclercq, R., Brasseur, M., Mendlewicz, J., & Van Cauter, E. (1994). The 24-hour profiles of cortisol, prolactin, and growth hormone secretion in mania. *Arch Gen Psychiatry*, *51*(8), 616-624. https://doi.org/10.1001/archpsyc.1994.0395 0080028004.

Lyu, X., Wang, G., Pi, Z., & Wu, L. (2021). Circadian clock disruption attenuated growth hormone(GH)-mediated signalling. *Gen Comp Endocrinol*, *302*, 113670. https://doi.org/10.1016/j.ygcen.2020.113670.

Majidinia, M., Reiter, R. J., Shakouri, S. K., & Yousefi, B. (2018). The role of melatonin, a multitasking molecule, in retarding the processes of ageing. *Ageing Research Reviews*, *47*, 198-213. https://doi.org/10.1016/j.arr.2018.07.010.

Mills, J., & Kuohung, W. (2019). Impact of circadian rhythms on female reproduction and infertility treatment success. *Curr Opin Endocrinol Diabetes Obes*, *26*(6), 317-321. https://doi.org/10.1097/med.0000000000000511.

Nicolaides, N. C., Charmandari, E., Chrousos, G. P., & Kino, T. (2014). Circadian endocrine rhythms: the hypothalamic-pituitary-adrenal axis and its actions. *Ann N Y Acad Sci*, *1318*, 71-80. https://doi.org/10.1111/nyas.12464.

Pandi-Perumal, S. R., Srinivasan, V., Maestroni, G., Cardinali, D., Poeggeler, B., & Hardeland, R. (2006). Melatonin: Nature's most versatile biological signal? *The FEBS journal*, *273*(13), 2813-2838. https://doi.org/10.1111/j.1742-4658.2006.05322.x.

Pevet, P., & Challet, E. (2011). Melatonin: both master clock output and internal time-giver in the circadian clocks network. *Journal of Physiology-Paris*, *105*(4-6), 170-182. https://doi.org/10.1016/j.jphysparis.2011.07.001.

Picó, C., Palou, M., Pomar, C. A., Rodríguez, A. M., & Palou, A. (2022). Leptin as a key regulator of the adipose organ. *Reviews in Endocrine and Metabolic Disorders*, *23*(1), 13-30. https://doi.org/10.1007/s11154-021-09687-5

Qian, J., Morris, C. J., Caputo, R., Garaulet, M., & Scheer, F. A. (2019). Ghrelin is impacted by the endogenous circadian system and by circadian misalignment in humans. *International Journal of Obesity*, *43*(8), 1644-1649. https://doi.org/10.1038/s41366-018-0208-9.

Richards, J., & Gumz, M. L. (2012). Advances in understanding the peripheral circadian clocks. *The FASEB Journal*, *26*(9), 3602-3613. https://doi.org/10.1096/fj.12-203554.

Saleem, M., Martin, H., & Coates, P. (2018). Prolactin biology and laboratory measurement: an update on physiology and current analytical issues. *The Clinical Biochemist Reviews*, *39*(1), 3.

Scherholz, M. L., Schlesinger, N., & Androulakis, I. P. (2019). Chronopharmacology of glucocorticoids. *Advanced Drug Delivery Reviews*, *151-152*, 245-261. https://doi.org/ https://doi.org/10.1016/j.addr.2019.02.004.

Serin, Y., & Tek, N. A. (2019). Effect of circadian rhythm on metabolic processes and the regulation of energy balance. *Annals of Nutrition and Metabolism*, *74*(4), 322-330. https://doi.org/10.1159/000500071.

Spencer, R. L., Chun, L. E., Hartsock, M. J., & Woodruff, E. R. (2018). Glucocorticoid hormones are both a major circadian signal and major stress signal: How this shared signal contributes to a dynamic relationship between the circadian and stress systems. *Frontiers in neuroendocrinology*, *49*, 52-71. https://doi.org/10.1016/j.yfrne.2017.12.005.

Stangerup, I., & Hannibal, J. (2020). Localization of Vasoactive Intestinal Polypeptide Receptor 1 (VPAC1) in Hypothalamic Neuroendocrine Oxytocin Neurons; A Potential Role in Circadian Prolactin Secretion. *Front Neuroanat*, *14*, 579466. https://doi.org/10.3389/fnana.2020.579466.

Tiwari, A., Rathor, P., Trivedi, P. K., & Ch, R. (2023). Multi-Omics Reveal Interplay between Circadian Dysfunction and Type2 Diabetes. *Biology*, *12*(2), 301. https://doi.org/10.3390/biology12020301.

Tordjman, S., Chokron, S., Delorme, R., Charrier, A., Bellissant, E., Jaafari, N., & Fougerou, C. (2017). Melatonin: pharmacology, functions and therapeutic benefits. *Current neuropharmacology*, *15*(3), 434-443. https://doi.org/10.2174%2F1570159X14666161228122115.

Tsang, A. H., Astiz, M., Friedrichs, M., & Oster, H. (2016). Endocrine regulation of circadian physiology. *J endocrinol*, *230*(1), R1-R11. https://doi.org/10.1530/joe-16-0051

Tsujino, N., & Sakurai, T. (2012). Circadian rhythm of leptin, orexin and ghrelin. *Nihon rinsho. Japanese journal of clinical medicine*, *70*(7), 1121-1125.

Vakili, H., Jin, Y., & Cattini, P. A. (2016). Evidence for a Circadian Effect on the Reduction of Human Growth Hormone Gene Expression in Response to Excess Caloric Intake. *J Biol Chem*, *291*(26), 13823-13833. https://doi.org/10.1074/jbc.M116.722744.

Wada, T., Yamamoto, Y., Takasugi, Y., Ishii, H., Uchiyama, T., Saitoh, K., Suzuki, M., Uchiyama, M., Yoshitane, H., Fukada, Y., & Shimba, S. (2022). Adiponectin regulates the circadian rhythm of glucose and lipid metabolism. *Journal of Endocrinology*, *254*(2), 121-133. https://doi.org/10.1530/joe-22-0006.

Wang, F., Xie, N., Wu, Y., Zhang, Q., Zhu, Y., Dai, M., Zhou, J., Pan, J., Tang, M., Cheng, Q., Shi, B., Guo, Q., Li, X., Xie, L., Wang, B., Yang, D., Weng, Q., Guo, L., Ye, J., Pan, M., Zhang, S., Zhou, H., Zhen, C., Liu, P., Ning, K., Brackenridge, L., Hardiman, P. J., & Qu, F. (2021). Association between circadian rhythm disruption and polycystic ovary syndrome. *Fertil Steril*, *115*(3), 771-781. https://doi.org/10.1016/j.fertnstert.2020.08.1425.

Yanagi, S., Sato, T., Kangawa, K., & Nakazato, M. (2018). The Homeostatic Force of Ghrelin. *Cell Metabolism*, *27*(4), 786-804. https://doi.org/https://doi.org/10.1016/j.cmet.2018.02.008.

Yu, H., Xia, F., Lam, K. S., Wang, Y., Bao, Y., Zhang, J., Gu, Y., Zhou, P., Lu, J., & Jia, W. (2011). Circadian rhythm of circulating fibroblast growth factor 21 is related to diurnal changes in fatty acids in humans. *Clinical chemistry*, *57*(5), 691-700. https://doi.org/10.1373/clinchem.2010.155184.

Yuan, Y., Li, C., Guo, S., Sun, C., Ning, N., Hao, H., Wang, L., Bian, Y., Liu, H., & Wang, X. (2021). Adiponectin improves amyloid-β 31-35-induced circadian rhythm disorder in mice. *Journal of Cellular and Molecular Medicine*, *25*(20), 9851-9862. https://doi.org/10.1111/jcmm.16932.

Chapter 4

The Circadian Regulation and DNA Damage

Saime Sezer Sondas*, **PhD**
Department of Medicine Malatya Turgut Ozal University, Malatya, Turkiye

Abstract

The circadian clock is a cycle that lasts approximately 24 hours, controlling the everyday rhythms of the behavior, physiology, and biochemistry of organisms. The circadian system can be divided into two parts that are thought to be interconnected. These systems are 1) the central clock (located in the superior chiasmatic nucleus of the hypothalamus (SCN, suprachiasmatic nucleus); 2) the peripheral clock (liver, pancreas, intestines, and skeleton in other body tissues such as muscle and adipose tissue takes place). In recent years, there have been studies suggesting that the circadian clock plays a significant role in systems such as repair, checkpoints, and cell death. DNA synthesis and repair, circadian clocks, and biological events can be an important example of regulation. DNA repair increases when oxidative stress is high, and DNA synthesis may decrease during sleep. From this, therefore, the circadian clock is correctly processing, as cells associated with these clocks keep the risk of mutation at a minimum. The purpose of this chapter is to examine the circadian system its functioning and to understand how pathways involved in DNA repair affect the circadian rhythm.

Keywords: circadian clock, DNA damage, repair

* Corresponding Author's Email: saime.sondas@ozal.edu.tr.

In: Human Health is a Matter of Timing
Editors: Sumeyya Deniz Aybek, Gonca Gulbay and Mucahit Secme
ISBN: 979-8-89113-467-6

Introduction

The circadian clock is a cycle that lasts about 24 hours, regulating many behaviors and physiological activities in living organisms, allowing them to anticipate and prepare for daily changes. changing environments for many organisms, from bacteria to humans, to adapt predict limits, and control activities with the circadian clock. In humans and other mammals, the circadian clock governs many important functions. These are nutrition, metabolism, hormonal secretions, sleep, and wakefulness (Lazar, 2012). The circadian rhythm can also be defined as a basic system of cyclical oscillations produced by the internal circadian clock. In fact, overall mammals have developed a circadian clock to synchronize with the communal and psycho-social abilities of organisms. The hypothalamus (SCN) regulates this circadian rhythm, the control center that produces various physiological functions is located in the suprachiasmatic nucleus (Wang & Chen, 2022). Current epidemiological, biochemical, and molecular data reveal a strong interaction between the circadian clock and the genome. Moreover, current studies say that changes in the circadian clock impair genome stability, alter DNA replication, and affect DNA damage and DNA repair (Sancar et al., 2015; Kolinjivadi et al., 2021). The circadian clock and DNA damage response control many aspects of cell psychosocial and the cell's adaptation to the external perimeter. However, the two systems can both work independently of each other and under psychosocial conditions, the two systems interact with each other. In other words, a signal affects other systems to the extent of the systems it affects (Sancar et al., 2010). In the cellular regulation, such as the replication of DNA in the S phase in the cell cycle and, the segregation of chromosomes, there are very important molecular events (Kolinjivadi et al., 2021). It is now known that the circadian clock affects many genes both in the cell cycle and in their responses to DNA damage. Moreover, the circadian clock marks the entry of cells into the S-phase, where DNA replicates itself and provides the transition between G2-phase and M-phase. It can also be said that it allows the cell to divide mitotically. With this cell cycle control, it can be said that it is the center of prevention of effects related to cancer formation. By arresting the cell cycle, both the possible correction of DNA damage and cell death harmful effects can be destroyed (Mustafa et al., 2021).

Molecular Mechanism and Genes of the Circadian Clock

Mechanisms related to the circadian clock cell cycle, DNA damage response, and tumor suppression are extremely important. At the molecular level, circadian clocks are transcription-translational "clock genes" regulated in the regulatory system, some clock genes encode transcriptional activators, while others encode proteins that can inhibit expression codes. Molecular rhythms are regulated by post-transcriptional regulation, post-transcriptional changes, chromatin rearrangement, intracellular location, and precisely clock proteins. In other words, clock genes are necessary for the creation and regulation of circadian rhythms in all cells of the organism. The basic molecular behind the circadian rhythm mechanisms consists of these clock genes. These genes are two gene families; they consist of the *period genes* (*Per1, 2*, and *3*) and the *Cryptochrome* (*Cry1* and *Cry2*) genes. These are activated from CLOCK (hood from circadian locomotor output loops) and BMAL1 (brain and muscle arly hydrocarbon receptor nuclear antigen 1) proteins. Thus, they heterodimerize the expression of other clock genes (such as *Per1, 2, 3,* and *Cr 1, Cry2*). The PER proteins contain two PAS cascade regions and can interact with each other and with other proteins through these regions. PER and CRY proteins are synthesized in the cytoplasm and are known to associate before entering the nucleus. Once in the nucleus, CRYs suppress CLOCK and BMAL1 activities. Therefore, it affects their own expressions negatively. *PER3* is clock-controlled but is not required for rhythm generation. Here, CLOCK-BMAL1 activity thus inhibits its expression (negative feedback). Likewise, PER proteins positively act on the promoter transcription of BMAL1. BMAL1, CLOCK-BMAL1 heterodimerization enables the cycle to start again (Beckett & Roden, 2009; Rana & Mahmood, 2010; Özbayer & Değirmenci 2011).

Cell Cycle in the Circadian Clock

There are current studies showing that the circadian clock regulates cell cycle checkpoints. It can be said that these checkpoints of the cell cycle are the G1/S and G2/M checkpoints. The cell cycle is coordinately synchronized. The circadian clock also controls the expression of cell cycle regulators such as Wee1, c-Myc, p20, p21, and Cyclin D1. Moreover, it can be said that *PER1* and *PER2* suppressors are important circadian clock regulators in cell cycle control. (Masri et al., 2015). The circadian clock, like all other biochemical pathways, is related to cell cycle-related genes or proteins. In particular, the p21, p27 proteins, CDK4/6, and CyclinB1/CDKs at cell cycle checkpoints are controlled by the nuclear circadian transcription-translation feedback loop (TTFL). TIMELESS is involved in the circadian clock by interacting with CRYs and interacting with cell cycle control kinases. It also participates in the intra-S checkpoint and replication protection chain. (Yang et al., 2021). Additionally, Temozolomide (TMZ) is known to be a chemotherapeutic alkylating agent. TMZ and radiation therapy regulate cellular proliferation. It is known to do this by inhibiting DNA replication. When DNA is damaged, cell cycle checkpoints are affected, and the cycle is disrupted. The mechanisms responsible for DNA repair detect this and try to repair the error. Its response to DNA damage (DDR) contributes to chemotherapy while at the same time trying to preserve genomic integrity. In other words, checkpoints in the cell cycle are very important and prevent uncontrolled proliferation (Wang & Chen, 2022).

DNA Damage

Environmental factors such as ultraviolet rays and chemical compounds that cause DNA damage constantly threaten the integrity of human genomic DNA (Jackson and Bartek, 2009). The structure of DNA can be damaged by base loss caused by the alkylation and hydrolysis of bases. Thus, it can cause breaks, insertions, deletions, basic domains and DNA-protein cross-linking in the single and double helix of DNA (Onur et al., 2009). During events such as DNA replication and recombination, endogenous agents such as free radicals produced as a byproduct of cellular metabolism also cause DNA damage (Clancy, 2008).

DNA packaged in chromatin must be loosened so that repair factors can bind to damaged DNA Mammalian PIKK kinases involved in DNA signaling are ATR, ATX/SMG-1, ATM, and DNA-PKcs (Valerie & Povirk, 2003). Checkpoint kinase ATM relaxes the heterochromatin structure by phosphorylating and activates the repair of double helix breaks. These proteins (350-450 kDa) perform their functions by phosphorylating many substrates from the amino acids glutamine, and then serine and threonine residues. ATM and DNA PKcs have a dominant role in the response to DNA double-strand breaks, while ATR signaling is actively involved in single-strand breaks induced by ionizing radiation (Valerie & Povirk, 2003).

Single-stranded DNA-binding replication protein A (RPA) wraps the single-stranded regions and assembles the ATR and central ATRIPs when the double strand is cleaved by the helicase during replication. ATM cell transport is stopped, responding to DNA machinery and double helix strands by initiating signaling cascades that cause apoptosis. At the same time, ATM works by phosphorylating numerous proteins at checkpoints of cell life such as CHK1, CHK2, p53, and FANCD2. In undamaged cells, the ATM protein is inactive as an ATM dimer. The inactive kinase region of the ATM protein is blocked by the FAT (FRAP/ATM/TRRAP) region of another ATM molecule. When the cell is exposed to ionizing radiation, it stimulates autophosphorylation from ser1981 localized in the FAT region and separates the inactive form ATM dimers from each other and converts them into an enzymatically active monomer and thus, ATM activation occurs (Ditch & Paull, 2012). Activation of ATM occurs very quickly after ionizing radiation. Although the mechanism for activating ATM is not clearly known, the functional MRN complex is thought to play a role in the activation of ATM. Activated ATM protein responds to DNA damage by phosphorylating many substrates involved in cell cycle, apoptosis, and repair. Proteins involved in the recognition of double chain breaks, such as histone H2AX and RAD17, components of the MRN complex, are target proteins phosphorylated by ATM. The phosphorylation of CHK1 and CHK2 kinases by the ATM protein causes these kinases to be involved in cell cycle pathways and DNA repair (Jackson & Bartek, 2009; Lovejoy & Cortez, 2009). Activated ATM stops the cell cycle at three important points. The pause in the G1-S phase provides sufficient time for DNA damage to be repaired before replication occurs. ATM-dependent G1-S checkpoint inhibition is dependent on TP53 and CHK2 and also requires activation of p21, a cyclin-dependent kinase inhibitor. Additionally, S and G2-M checkpoints are also monitored by the ATM. DNA-dependent protein kinases or ATM proteins that perform H2AX phosphorylation are important in ATR and ATM-dependent signaling pathways. The formation of the alpha-H2AX locus is important for the MRN complex and mediator proteins such as BRCA1 to remain at the break site (Jackson & Bartek, 2009; Czornak et al., 2008; Vassin et al., 2009). All these DNA damage proteins can activate DNA repair mechanisms, depending on the type of damage that has occurred. In doing so, they inhibit cell cycle progression. For example, repairing alkylated bases with enzymes such as O-6-methylguanine-DNA methyltransferase (MGMT); Nucleotide excision repair (NER) of DNA nucleotide insertions; It can be said that single-stranded DNA breaks are repaired by excision repair, and smaller nucleotide mutations are repaired by Mismatch Repair. Double-strand breaks are repaired by Homologous Recombination (HR) and Non-Homologous End-joining (NHEJ). If the damage to the repair mechanisms is not repaired, apoptotic pathways are triggered. Recently, the relationship between mammalian DNA repair systems and the circadian clock *PER1*, CLOCK, and CRY1, whose core clock factors can be said, can be directly involved in DNA protection mechanisms (Palombo et al., 2015).

DNA Damage and Circadian Rhythm

Circadian control of DNA damage; It is related to proteins without controlling the response to genotoxic stress at the cellular and organism levels in the cell proliferation process. These proteins are important circadian proteins. The DNA damage triggers cellular response mechanisms that can result in cell cycle arrest, DNA repair, or apoptosis. Thus, p53 (tumor suppressor protein) is activated in response to damage. It then either arrests the cell cycle or leads to the activation of cellular stress response pathways, including ATM/ATR and CHK1/2, leading to apoptosis (Rana and Mahmood; 2010). Similarly, the presence of DNA damage in a cell that is preparing to divide, or the inability to repair the DNA damage sufficiently, causes the cell cycle to stop, the extent of the damage is determined, the damage is attempted to be repaired, and/or the cell is directed to apoptosis (Chakarov et al., 2014). So far, two examples have focused on showing the relationship between DNA damage and the circadian rhythm. In response to DNA damage; it can be said that there is a direct relationship between ATR-mediated DNA damage checkpoint and circadian clock genes. Moreover, it can be said that PER is associated with ATM and Chk2, one of the circadian genes, ATM-mediated DNA checkpoint. (Gaddameedhi et al., 2012). It can be said that the first evidence of the relationship between DNA damage checkpoints and the circadian clock comes from studies of TIM protein (Sancar et al., 2015). Subsequently, Unsal-Kacmaz et al. in a study conducted by TIM protein, it was determined that they play an important role in DNA damage control points. They said that the TIM protein interacts with Chk1 and the ATR-ATRIP complex and Cry2 (Unsal-Kacmaz et al., 2005). Moreover, it has been found that *PER2,* a circadian clock gene, causes a decrease in protein levels when the regulation of TIM protein by siRNA is decreased. In this case, it caused a disruption of the circadian rhythm in the SCN region. Additionally, a decrease in the phosphorylation of the Chk1 protein has been observed due to reasons such as collapse of the replication fork or early mitosis, which cause damage to the S - M phase checkpoint (Unsal- Kacmaz et al., 2005; Sancar et al., 2015). Considering all these conditions, TIM was evaluated as both a circadian rhythm protein and a cell cycle control protein. That is, the decrease in TIM regulation disrupts the ATR→Chk1 DNA damage pathway and the circadian clock. (Sancar et al., 2010; Sancar et al., 2015). It can be said that the second proof of the relationship between DNA damage and circadian rhythm is obtained from studies on the ATM-Chk2 signaling pathway. As with the TIM protein, *PER1* is a circadian protein that can be said to directly participate in ATM → Chk2 signaling with ATM and Chk2 (Sancar et al., 2015). *PER1* functions as a tumor suppressor. It does this by regulating control proteins and cell cycle genes that are activated by DNA damage. For example, *PER1* is highly expressed in cancer cells. It can also be said that the inhibition of PER in the treated cells suppressed apoptosis and induced apoptosis induced by ionizing radiation (Rana & Mahmood, 2010). When the expression of PER is decreased, ATM proteins have been found to alter the ionizing radiation-induced phosphorylation of Chk2 (Gery et al., 2006). It can also be said that ionizing radiation causes suppression of p21, induction of c-Myc expression, and nuclear translocation of *PER1*. Furthermore, *PER1* interacts directly with the kinases ATM and CHK2, which are activated by double-strand breaks in DNA. All these can be considered as an indication that *PER1* acts as a tumor suppressor (Rana & Mahmood, 2010). It also suggests that *PER1* may be both a circadian rhythm protein and a checkpoint protein. In addition, it has been reported that overexpression of *PER1* sensitizes cancer cells to DNA damage-induced apoptosis, and its downregulation decreases the level of apoptosis with the effect of agents that cause double-strand breaks (Gery et al., 2006). Lee and Sancar conducted a study showing that loss of Cry1 and Cry2, which are nuclear circadian clock proteins, can sensitize tumor cells to DNA damage-induced apoptosis. This is associated with cells that have lost p53, which is mutated in most cancers. It demonstrates the important roles of circadian rhythm in regulating the DNA damage response and points to a potential avenue for the treatment of resistant p53-deficient cancers (Ramsey et al., 2011; Lee & Sancar, 2011).

Clock Control of DNA Repair

DNA repair can be defined as a collection of enzymes that remove DNA damage, which can be explained as a difference or change in DNA structure.

There are several mechanisms of DNA repair, including direct repair, nucleotide excision repair, double strand break/crosslink repair, and base excision repair. Current evidence suggests that of these repair mechanisms, only nucleotide excision repair is controlled by the circadian clock. (Sancar et al., 2010; Sancar et al., 2015). Additionally, it can be said that mismatch repair is indirectly affected by the circadian clock in the replicated tissues. It depends on clock-controlled reproduction. Similarly, the double-strand break/crosslink repair mode is clock-influenced by homologous recombination. The double-stranded break repair mode occurs in the S and G2 phases of the interphase in the cell cycle. Double-stranded break repair by non-homologous splicing occurs throughout the cell cycle (Sancar et al., 2015). (UV) radiation consists of three different wavelengths. These; They are UVA, UVB and UVC (Wavelengths respectively; 315–400 nm, 280–315 nm, and 100–280 nm). Those with shorter wavelengths produce more DNA lesions. These photolesions can interfere with important DNA metabolisms, including transcription. If this condition is not immediately repaired by repair systems, it can accumulate mutations. Moreover, it can trigger genomic instability, which is a hallmark of both cancer and aging (Kang, 2021). True UV-induced DNA photolesions in mammals are Nucleotide excision repair (NER). There are two different subpaths of NER. These are called transcription-dependent repair (TCR) and global genome repair (GGR). The genomic location of the photolesion, these two different sub-pathways can optionally operate. Repair of transcription-dependent repair DNA where damage has occurred in the transcription chain is initiated by RNA polymerase II arrest with the ability to detect transcript elongation arrest. (Kang, 2021). Since the double-strand break/cross-link repair mode is also affected by the homologous recombination clock, it can be said that the double-strand break repair mode is limited to the S and G2 phases of the cell cycle (Sancar et al., 2015).

Conclusion

The circadian clock and DNA damage are mechanisms that play a critical role in the cellular physiological pathways that establish our biological rhythm and control adaptation to the environment at the cellular and organismal levels. Although these two mechanisms can work independently of each other, it can be said that a signal that affects one also affects the other. Circadian clock gene products also interact with the cell cycle and apoptosis. It can be said that important biological pathways such as the cell cycle, response to DNA damage, and tumor suppression are also under circadian control. Disruption of the circadian system can cause disorders in the expression levels and systems of genes involved in the cell cycle. It can be said that these disturbances in the circadian system increase the risk of various diseases such as cancer, insulin resistance, obesity, digestive system diseases, cardiovascular diseases, and neurodegenerative diseases. It is important to pay attention to the biological clock system in the regulation of the treatment programs for diseases and the repair of DNA damage. It is thought that such circadian clock treatments will ensure that the targeted effect is achieved accurately. Therefore, the identification, diagnosis, and treatment methods of the disease can be arranged according to circadian rhythms, and thus the effect of treatment can be optimized. In other words, it is of great importance to pay attention to the biological clock system of the body and to regulate it accordingly in the regulation of treatment programs. By finding the right time to achieve the targeted effect, new treatment methods can be developed, and undesirable negative effects can be minimized.

References

Beckett, M., Roden, L. C. (2009) Mechanisms by which circadian rhythm disruption may lead to cancer. *South African J Sci*;10: 415-20. https://doi.org/.

Clancy, S. (2008) DNA damage & repair: mechanisms for maintaining DNA integrity. *Nature Education* 1(1):103.

Czornak, K., Chughtai, S. and Chrzanowska, K. H. (2008). Mystery of DNA repair: the role of the MRN complex and ATM kinase in DNA damage repair. *Journal of Applied Genetics*, 49(4):383-96. https://doi.org/.

Ditch, S. and Paull, T. T. (2012). The ATM protein kinase and cellular redox signaling: beyond the DNA damage response. *Trends Biochem Sci.*; 37(1):15-22. https://doi.org/.

Gaddameedhi, S., Reardon, J. T., Ye, R., Ozturk, N., and Sancar, A. (2012). Effect of circadian clock mutations on DNA damage response in mammalian cells. *Cell Cycle*, 11(18), 3481-349. http://dx.doi.org/10.4161/cc.21771.

Gery, S., Komatsu, N., Baldjyan, L., Yu, A., Koo, D., Koeffler, H. P. (2006). The Circadian Gene Per1 Plays an Important Role in Cell Growth and DNA Damage Control in Human Cancer Cells. *Molecular Cell*, 22 (3), 375-382. https://doi.org/10.1016/j.molcel.2006.03.038.

Jackson, S. P and Bartek, J. (2009). The DNA-damage response in human biology and disease. *Nature*, volume 461, pages1071–1078. https://doi.org/.

Kang, T. H. (2021). Circadian Rhythm of NER and ATR Pathways. *Biomolecules*, 11, 715. https://doi.org/10.3390/biom11050715.

Kolinjivadi A. M., Chong, S. T., and Ngeow, J. (2021). Molecular connections between circadian rhythm and genome maintenance pathways. *Endocr Relat Cancer*, Feb;28(2): R55-R66. https://doi.org/.

Lee, J. H., Sancar, A. (2011) Circadian clock disruption improves the efficacy of chemotherapy through p73-mediated apoptosis. *Proc Natl Acad Sci USA,* 108:10668–10672. 108(26):10668-72. https://doi.org/.

Lovejoy, C. A. and Cortez, D. (2009). Common mechanisms of PIKK regulation. *DNA Repair* (Amst). 2;8(9):1004-8. https://doi.org/.

Masri, S., Kinouchi, K, and Sassone-Corsi, P. (2015) Circadian clocks, epigenetics, and cancer. *Curr Opin Oncol,* 27(1): 50–56. https://doi.org/.

Mustafa, E., Luukkonen J., Makkonen J., Naarala J. (2021). The duration of exposure to 50 Hz magnetic fields: Influence on circadian genes and DNA damage responses in murine hematopoietic FDC-P1 cells. *Mutation Research-Fundamental and Molecular Mechanisms of Mutagenesis* 823; 111756. https://doi.org/10.1016/j.mrfmmm.2021.111756.

Onur, E., Tuğrul, B. and Bozyiğit, F. (2009). DNA Damage and Repair Mechanisms. Turkish Journal of Clinical Biochemistry, 7(2): 61-70.

Özbayer, C. and Değirmenci, İ. (2011). Circadian clock, cell cycle and cancer. *Dicle Medical Journal*, 38 (4): 514-518. https://doi.org/.

Palombo, P, Moreno-Villanueva, M., Mangerich, A. (2015). Day and night variations in the repair of ionizing-radiation-induced DNA damage in mouse splenocytes. DNA Repair (Amst). 28:37-47. https://doi.org/

Ramsey, M. R., and Ellisen, L. W. (2011). Circadian function in cancer: Regulating the DNA damage response. PNAS, June 28, vol. 108; no. 26 pp:10379–10380. *Proc Natl Acad Sci U S A*. 28;108(26):10379-80. https://doi.org/.

Rana, S. and Mahmood, S. (2010). Circadian rhythm and its role in malignancy. *J Circadian Rhythms,* 8:3. https://doi.org/.

Sancar, A., Lindsey-Boltz L. A., Kang T-H., Reardon, J. T., Lee J. H., and Ozturk, N. (2010). Circadian Clock Control of the Cellular Response to DNA Damage. *FEBS Lett*, 18;584(12):2618-25. https://doi.org/.

Sancar, A., Lindsey-Boltz, L. A., Gaddameedhi, S., Selby, C. P., Ye R, Chiou, Y., Kemp, M. G., Hu, J., Lee, J. H., and Ozturk, N. (2015). Circadian Clock, Cancer, and Chemotherapy. *Biochemistry*, 54(2):110-23. https://doi.org/.

Unsal-Kacmaz, K., Mullen, T. E., Kaufmann, W. K., and Sancar, A. (2005). Coupling of Human Circadian and Cell Cycles by the Timeless Protein. *Molecular and Cellular Biology*, 25 (8), 3109-3116. https://doi.org/10.1128/MCB.25.8.3109-3116.2005.

Valerie, K. and Povirk, L. F. (2003). Regulation and mechanisms of mammalian double-strand break repair. *Oncogene.* 1;22(37):5792-812. https://doi.org/.

Vassin, V. M. and Anantha, R. W. (2009). Human RPA phosphorylation by ATR stimulates DNA synthesis and prevents ssDNA accumulation during DNA-replication stress. *J Cell Sci*, 122 (22): 4070–4080. https://doi.org/.

Wang, Z., Chen, G. (2022). Insights about circadian clock in glioma: From molecular pathways to therapeutic drugs. *CNS Neurosci Ther.* 28(12):1930-1941. https://doi.org/.

Yang, Y., Lindsey-Boltz, L. A., Vaughn, C. M., Selby, C. P., Cao, X., Liu, Z., Hsu, D. S., and Sancar, A. (2021). Circadian clock, carcinogenesis, chronochemotherapy connections. *J. Biol. Chem*. 297(3) 101068. https://doi.org/.

Chapter 5

The Human Circadian Clock: Sleep Homeostasis and Sleep Disorders

Meryem Pelin*, PhD
and Havva Sert, PhD
Department of Nursing, Sakarya University Sakarya, Turkiye

Abstract

Circadian rhythms repeat on average every 24 hours and are governed by the suprachiasmatic nucleus of the hypothalamus. The most well-known is the sleep-wake cycle, but also the heart rate, blood pressure, body temperature, blood sugar, etc. Many physiological, biochemical, and behavioral processes such as these are managed from this center and show circadian rhythmicity. Many genetic, socio-cultural, and environmental factors affect the circadian rhythm. Many factors, such as the development of electric and artificial lights that modern life has made traditional, electromagnetic waves, shift work, and irregular nutrition, affect the biological processes by changing the rhythm of melatonin, which has an important role in the circadian rhythm. Disruptions in the circadian rhythm due to these effects are also called circadian disruption, which can cause symptoms and diseases ranging from daytime sleepiness to serious health problems such as depression, delirium, and cancer. As a result of the disruption of the circadian rhythm, one of the most obvious effects is in sleep, and the quality of sleep is also affected by the change in sleep habits. It is emphasized that quality sleep is necessary both for the optimal functioning of life and for survival. When the individual is sleep deprived or does not sleep in sufficient quality when they have problems such as being unable to fall asleep for various reasons and sleep

---

* Corresponding Author's Email: meryemilmek@sakarya.edu.tr.

In: Human Health is a Matter of Timing
Editors: Sumeyya Deniz Aybek, Gonca Gulbay and Mucahit Secme
ISBN: 979-8-89113-467-6

disruption, their health may be adversely affected due to insomnia, and even the healing process may be prolonged. Therefore, to maintain circadian rhythms in a healthy way, it is important to define biological rhythms, including circadian rhythm, and to know the relationship between sleep and sleep stages, and circadian rhythm. This chapter presents the progression of the sleep stages, circadian regulations of the human sleep–wake cycle, and sleep-wake cycle disorders.

Keywords: circadian clocks, biological clocks, circadian rhythm, sleep, circadian rhythm sleep disorder, sleep-wake cycle disorder

Introduction

The central circadian clock is located in the brain's hypothalamus and consists of a protein cluster known as the suprachiasmatic nucleus (SCN) (Sleep Foundation, 2023). In mammals, the circadian rhythm is regulated by the SCN located in the anterior hypothalamus. The central circadian clock in the SCN regulates the innate physiological circadian rhythms according to the light-dark cycle in the environment to harmonize and revive the internal temporal order with the environment (Zisapel, 2018). This clock resets or "entrains" every 24 hours in a healthy adult based on light and dark cycles (Sleep Foundation, 2023). The body temperature rhythm, hormones such as cortisol, melatonin, and growth hormone, and the sleep-wake cycle are controlled by the central circadian clock in the SCN. This center enables the organism to work in harmony with the external environment and maintain its functions under different conditions (Akinci and Orhan, 2016). SCN; It synchronizes physiological and behavioral circadian rhythms, including sleep and wakefulness, temperature, neuroendocrine and autonomic effects, and nutrition, in 24-hour periods in harmony with the light-dark cycle of the environment. In this way, an optimized internal temporal order is controlled. Light is the most basic stimulus that adjusts the rhythm period and phase of the SCN according to the external environment. However, due to the direct connections of the SCN with other hypothalamic nuclei, environmental signals such as food, ambient temperature, and social interactions appear as other stimuli that are effective in regulating rhythm. In this way, the organism can gain flexibility and adapt to daily activities according to its rhythm (Zisapel, 2018).

The sleep-wake cycle is the most obvious circadian rhythm. Sleep is important in regenerating brain energy, shutting down external inputs, and offline processing of information acquired while awake, consolidating, and erasing memory (Zisapel, 2018). Therefore, adequate and quality sleep should be provided. It has been shown in studies that the circadian rhythm, one of the biological rhythms, is effective in providing sufficient and quality sleep (Lou et al., 2021; Wang et al., 2022).

Biological Rhythms and Circadian Rhythm

The definition of biological rhythms has contributed significantly to disease diagnosis and treatment stages. The first foundations of chronobiology were laid with the description of the term zeitgeber by Askhuf in the 1990s. The developments in this field continued with Franz Halberg's establishment of the chronobiology laboratory, and brought the term circadian to the literature (Çalışkan and Akan, 2019). The biochemical, physiological, and cyclical responses of living things to repetitive physical factors in the outside world are called biological rhythms (Roenneberg and Merrow, 2016; Cohen, 2020). Biological rhythms according to cycle times; they are called ultradian, circadian, infradian, and circannual. Rhythms with a cycle time of less than 24 hours are called ultradian, rhythms with a cycle of 24 hours are called circadian, rhythms lasting longer than 24 hours are called infradian, and rhythms of about one year are called circannual rhythms (Çalışkan and Akan, 2019).

The term circadian, which is a combination of the Latin words circa (about) and dies (day), is used to express approximately one day (Amanpour et al., 2021; Hartsock et al., 2021). The circadian rhythm refers to the changes in the organism's biological, physiological, chemical, and behavioral processes for approximately one day, or 24 hours. The circadian rhythm is created by oscillators, and pacemakers called endogenous clocks and synchronized by environmental stimuli called zeitgebers (Selvi et al., 2011; Krishnan and Lyons, 2015). The most basic rhythm-regulating factor is light. Light is sensed by the light-sensitive melanopsin-containing ganglion cells in the retina and transferred to the SCN through the retinohypothalamic pathway. The light stimulus reaches the pineal gland through the paraventricular nucleus, the most important neural pathway in the SCN. Thus, the synthesis of melatonin, a pineal hormone known as the sleep hormone, is suppressed by the effect of light.

The light and dark cycles in the external environment are important in regulating the circadian rhythm. Melatonin synthesis is stimulated in the dark and suppressed in the daytime by the effect of light. Melatonin synthesis begins to increase approximately two hours before an individual's bedtime. However, exposure to light at night causes a decrease in plasma melatonin levels. In addition to its chronobiological effect, the hormone melatonin also has a hypnotic effect. The hormone melatonin suppresses neural stimuli in the SCN, causing a sleep-inducing and sustaining effect. In other words, external oral melatonin supplementation causes a hypnotic effect. Phase shifts in the endogenous rhythm can be achieved with melatonin supplementation and light exposure. For example, while the phase is delayed in an individual exposed to light in the evening, the phase shifts earlier in a person exposed in the morning. Based on this, the phase changes in circadian rhythm disorders can be regulated by exposure to bright light and melatonin supplementation at appropriate times (Selvi et al., 2011; Akinci and Orhan, 2016; Haspel et al., 2020).

The most basic and decisive circadian rhythm in humans; is the sleep-wake cycle (Akinci and Orhan, 2016). After birth, circadian rhythms develop when the baby is about two to three months old. As a result of this, sleep stages begin to occur (Patel et al., 2022).

Sleep

Sleep is a fundamental physiological process that affects various biological activities. It is known that sleep supports many essential and vital functions in the central nervous system, such as learning, memory, cognitive and sensory regulation, and cardiovascular, metabolic, and immunological activity. Sleep, a physiological, periodic, multidimensional, and indispensable life activity, covers one-third of human life. Sleep, which is one of the important elements of quality of life, is affected by psychological, physical, and environmental factors (Tramontano et al., 2021). Sleep can be defined both behaviorally and physiologically. Behaviorally, it consists of a species-specific body posture and a typical sleep zone, with an increased arousal threshold and a prolonged period of inactivity. Physiologically, sleep is defined by EEG, which measures the electrical activity of the cortex. Sleep consists of two phases called Rapid Eye Movement (REM) and Non-Rapid Eye Movement (NREM) sleep, which can be featured by changes in the EEG (Fisk et al., 2018). Each phase and stage of sleep includes variations in brain wave patterns, eye movements, and muscle tone. While NREM sleep consists of synchronized, rhythmic EEG activities that occur in the cortex and reflect changes during the firing of cortical neurons, REM sleep is characterized by a low-amplitude, mixed-frequency EEG similar to the waking state (Fisk et al., 2018). The human body goes through all these stages approximately 4 to 6 times a night (Saygın and Özgüner, 2020). Sleep, wakefulness (W), N1, N2, N3, and REM occur in five stages. Stages N1 to N3 are considered non-rapid eye movement (NREM) sleep. The REM stage is the stage that accounts for 25% of sleep with rapid eye movements. The sleep cycle takes about 90-110 minutes. The sleep cycle stages are described below (Patel et al., 2022).

NREM Phase

About 75% of sleep is spent in the NREM stages. The NREM stage occurs in three stages, N1, N2, and N3. With each stage, sleep becomes deeper and deeper. The majority of the NREM phase is spent in the N2 phase (Patel et al., 2022).

N1 (Stage 1, %5)

It is the lightest stage of sleep. Sleep begins with this stage. It constitutes 5% of the total sleep time and takes about 1-5 minutes. Skeletal muscle has muscle tone, and breathing tends to be regular. In this period, the awakening threshold is low, so the individual can be awakened easily (Patel et al., 2022).

N2 (Stage 2, %45)

After the N1 stage, the individual moves to the N2 stage. In this phase, which lasts about 15-20 minutes, a more intense stimulus than N1 is needed to wake up the person (Ersoy et al., 2016). During this stage, sleep becomes progressively deeper as heart rate and body temperature decrease. Stage 2 sleep lasts about 25 minutes in the first cycle and lengthens with each successive cycle, eventually accounting for about 45% of total sleep (Patel et al., 2022).

N3 (Stage 3, %25)

This stage, also called slow-wave sleep (SWS), is considered the deepest stage of sleep. This is the stage where it is most difficult to awaken the person. In fact, at this stage, a more intense stimulus is needed compared to the previous stages for the person to awaken. Some people cannot be awakened at this stage, even by loud sounds above 100 dBA. With age, the duration of the N3 stage tends to shorten, while the duration of the N2 stage tends to lengthen. In this stage, which has the highest arousal threshold, if the person awakens, they experience a temporary blurring of consciousness called sleep inertia. Cognitive tests also show that individuals awakened at this stage experience reduced mental performance between 30 minutes and one hour. During this sleep phase, the body is involved in tissue repair, bone, and muscle formation, and strengthening immunity. At the same time, sleepwalking, night terrors, and bed-wetting occur at this stage (Patel et al., 2022).

REM Phase

REM sleep occurs after slow-wave sleep. It becomes more difficult to wake up the person than during the NREM period. At this stage, the skeletal muscles are atonic and immobile, vital signs increase, and adrenaline begins to be secreted from the body. Heart rate and breathing are often irregular. In this phase, where the brain waves are very active, the eyes move abruptly and quickly. This stage is associated with dreams and is not considered a restful stage of sleep. (Patel et al., 2022).

The first REM sleep accounts for 20-25% of all sleep and is quite short. Each of the REM cycles, which begins with a duration of about 1-5 minutes, is extended throughout the night, and the final period reaches about an hour. Although the ratio of REM sleep to NREM sleep changes with each cycle, the duration, and weight of REM sleep increase towards the morning. While NREM stage 3 sleep is observed at the beginning of the night, that is, in the first 1/3 part of sleep, REM sleep is observed in the last 1-3 parts (Saygın and Özgüner, 2020; Ersoy et al., 2016). Healthy sleep can be achieved when its stages' order, time, and duration are fully realized. Healthy sleep is necessary for the regular performance of many functions in the body. Recent studies have shown that the circadian rhythm is effective in sleep. Studies investigating the relationship between sleep and circadian rhythm are increasing day by day.

Circadian Rhythm and Sleep

Sleep with phase, timing, and duration is periodic in nature. The sleep cycle is driven by the circadian clock, which is influenced by recurrent environmental events as well as genetic factors. It is stated that even the most minor functional disorders of the circadian clock can significantly affect the sleep process and the physiological functions of the body (Zaki et al., 2020).

Circadian disruption is a biological timing disorder ranging from the temporal disruption of molecular rhythms to the misalignment of behavioral cycles, such as the sleep-wake cycle, with the influence of environmental factors. Circadian disruption can cause circadian phase shifts, suppression of melatonin production, and displacement of sleep relative to the SCN. Evening or nighttime exposure to light stimuli that cause melanopsin stimulation causes further suppression of melatonin. This causes circadian phase shifts. Slow wave activity also decreases in the first NREM-REM sleep cycle with phase shifts following light exposure (Chellappa, 2021).

With the collapse of systemic homeostasis as a result of circadian disruption, people may experience many negative conditions such as depression, cancer, cardiovascular diseases, and metabolic syndrome (Su et al., 2022). For example, shift workers are often awake at night, and their eating and exercise times have often changed. With their exposure to light at night, as well as asynchronous signals of changing meal and exercise times, they mislead the internal clock. This appears as circadian disharmony. This resulting inconsistency manifests itself as metabolic disorders, psychiatric disorders, an increased risk of cardiovascular events, serious health problems such as cancer, and sleep disorders (Healy et al., 2021). As a result of the disruption of the circadian rhythm, the quality of sleep is also affected by changes in sleep habits (Engwall et al., 2015). It is emphasized that quality sleep is necessary both for the optimal functioning of life and for survival. Sleep quality consists of quantitative and subjective aspects such as night waking frequency, sleep latency, sleep duration, and depth of sleep, as well as feeling ready for a new day and feeling fit and fit. Sleep quality is affected by many psychological, physiological, and environmental factors (Palacıoğlu Açalan, 2016). When the individual is sleep deprived or does not sleep in sufficient quality, when they have problems such as not being able to fall asleep for various reasons, and sleep disruption, their health may be adversely affected due to insomnia, and even the recovery period may be prolonged (Zisapel, 2018). Sleep disorders, which cause these problems and become one of the most important problems of modern society, are called insomnia, sleep-related breathing disorders, major diseases with hypersomnia, circadian rhythm sleep-wake disorders, parasomnias, sleep-related movement disorders, and other sleep disorders. are classified. Among these sleep disorders, circadian rhythm sleep disorders are among the most common sleep disorders, and their importance has been increasing in recent years.

Circadian Rhythm Sleep Disorders

Circadian rhythm sleep disorders, also known as sleep-wake cycle disorders, are problems that occur when the body's internal clock (circadian clock), which tells it when it is time to sleep or wake up, is out of sync with the environment. This condition is continuous or repetitive. The resulting circadian sleep disorder may cause insomnia, excessive sleepiness, or both, resulting in functional loss (Akinci and Orhan, 2016).

Circadian rhythm sleep disorders are classified under seven headings according to the ICSD-3 criteria, the International Classification of Sleep Disorders. These are delayed sleep-wake phase disorder, advanced sleep-wake phase disorder, irregular sleep-wake rhythm disorder, non-24-hour sleep-wake rhythm disorder, shift work, jetlag type, and unclassifiable circadian rhythm sleep disorder. According to the DSM-5, the Diagnostic and Statistical Manual of Mental Disorders of the American Psychiatric Association, it is explained under the title of 'Sleep-Wake Disorders Related to the Twenty-Four Hour (Circadian) Scheme' and is not included in the jetlag type classification (Sateia, 2014; Akinci and Orhan 2016).

Delayed Sleep-Wake Phase Disorder

Delayed sleep-wake phase disorder; is defined as the delay of sleep hours between two and six hours according to the desired or socially accepted sleep times. People with this type of sleep disorder have difficulty falling asleep and waking up in the morning. There is a permanent sleep-wake rhythm in the form of late falling asleep and late waking up. These people are tired when they wake up earlier than when they wake up spontaneously. When they have to get up early for social reasons, they complain of daytime sleepiness and fatigue due to the shortening of their total sleep time. At the same time, functional and cognitive losses, deteriorations, decreased quality of life, and irritability can be seen as a result. Delayed sleep-wake phase disorder can mimic insomnia. One of the main differences between these two sleep disorders is that individuals with insomnia cannot sleep at standard sleep times due to ruminative thinking, while the other group of patients typically does not feel sleepy before 02:00 to 06:00 hours. Another difference, individuals with insomnia have difficulty falling asleep when they go to bed, while individuals in the other group do not have trouble falling asleep when they go to bed late (Akinci and Orhan, 2016; Brown et al., 2020; Pavlova and Latreille, 2019).

Delayed sleep-wake phase disorder is the most common of the circadian rhythm sleep disorders. Its incidence in the general population varies between 0.2% and 10%. A detailed sleep history should be taken for diagnosis. A sleep diary, at least seven days, preferably 14 days of actigraphy, is recommended for diagnosis. Additionally, circadian markers such as the dim light onset of melatonin (DLMO) and chronotype determination scales can be used in the diagnosis. The patient's compliance with sleep hygiene education is essential in the treatment. Chronotherapy, morning bright light applications, and pharmacotherapy can be used. The most common method is the timed application of bright light in the morning to shift the circadian phase earlier. Melatonin application is one of the successful options used in treatment. The application of melatonin in the evening allows the phase to move earlier. Melatonin can be administered 0.3-3 mg 2-5 hours before bedtime (Akinci and Orhan, 2016; Brown et al., 2020; Pavlova and Latreille, 2019).

Early Sleep-Wake Phase Disorder

It is characterized by sleeping before the usual or desired bedtime and waking up before the socially accepted wake-up time. Sleep is two hours or more ahead of the average expected sleep time. That is, sleep occurs systematically earlier than necessary. Although individuals wake up very early, they are usually rested. It is less common than delayed sleep-wake phase disorder. Although the mechanisms that cause this problem are not fully known, it is thought that late or early sleep may be caused by behavioral, occupational, or social reasons. Factors that may cause sleepiness, such as depression, should be excluded before diagnosis. Chronotherapy, bright light applications, and hypnotics can be tried in the treatment (Keskin and Okay, 2018).

Irregular Sleep-Wake Rhythm Disorder

Irregular sleep-wake rhythm disorder (ISWRD) is a sleep disorder with many cycles characterized by arithmetic sleep during the day. In the later stages of this disorder, sleep and wakefulness are randomly distributed throughout the day and night. Its most prominent symptoms are chronic insomnia and excessive sleepiness. It can be associated with traumatic brain injury, schizophrenia, and developmental disorders, especially neurological disorders. It is thought that it may also occur due to the scarcity of environmental stimuli called Zeitgeber, damage to the SCN, and the formation of irregular behavior patterns. In its treatment, bright light and exogenous melatonin can reshape and strengthen the circadian rhythm (Goldfarb and Sharkey, 2020; Bjorvatn and Pallesen, 2023).

Non-24-Hour Sleep-Wake Rhythm Disorder

Individuals with this type of sleep disorder sleep 1-2 hours later than the previous day and wake up later. Non-24-hour circadian rhythm disturbance occurs in more than half of visually impaired individuals. Up to 80% of this population complains of sleep disorders (Pavlova and Latreille, 2019). It is thought to occur due to the deterioration of the rhythm-regulating function of light in people with total visual impairment. A sleep diary and a recording of the actigraphy for at least two weeks are helpful in the diagnosis process. Intermittent melatonin measurements are also considered an option in diagnosis. Behavioral approaches and melatonin can be used in its treatment. It is important to establish a regular sleep-wake program and sleep hygiene and provide social and physical activities (Akinci and Orhan, 2016; Pavlova and Latreille, 2019).

Shift Work Type Sleep Phase Disorder

It is a circadian rhythm disorder that does not comply with social sleep-wake hours due to occupation, which can cause insomnia, excessive sleepiness, as well as loss of functionality, which occurs as a result of shift-style work. Shift workers need to get used to the light and dark cycles of the new shift when they switch from the day shift to the night shift or vice versa. This habituation process, in situations such as working or driving in social life, it can last for several days with the danger of excessive sleepiness. The retraining time to transition from day shift to night shift differs from night shift to day shift. At low light intensity, these times can be quite long. The high light intensity can significantly reduce the relapse time after certain transitions between shifts (Diekman and Bose, 2022). Actigraphy and at least one week of a sleep diary can be helpful in describing the disturbed sleep structure. The treatment aims to increase the individual's sleep and quality of life. In this way, both the work performance is increased, and the risk of accident is reduced. Behavioral and pharmacological approaches are often preferred simultaneously in treatment (Akinci and Orhan, 2016).

JetLag Type Sleep Phase Disorder

Jetlag, due to time zone changes, often develops after long-haul flights. Rapid relocation between regions with significant time differences causes a mismatch between the endogenous circadian rhythm and environmental conditions. The body cannot adapt to the new, rapidly changing time zone. As the body's endogenous rhythm continues to maintain its accustomed rhythm in the period in the destination region, temporary disruptions occur in bodily functions and sleep patterns. Because the endogenous circadian rhythm is a little longer than 24 hours, it is easier to delay the sleep phases than to delay it. In daily life, it is more difficult to adapt the endogenous circadian rhythm to the destination region when traveling east than west. In traveling to the east, the sleep phase should be taken earlier to adapt to daily life since there is a phase delay in the endogenous rhythm of the individual according to the time reached (Akinci and Orhan, 2016).

Unclassifiable Circadian Rhythm Sleep Disorder

Since individuals experience frequent symptoms such as excessive daytime sleepiness or insomnia, it resembles other circadian rhythm sleep disorders, but individuals do not meet the diagnostic criteria for sleep disorders in the other group. For this reason, it is defined as an unclassifiable circadian rhythm sleep disorder. It often develops due to underlying health conditions (Sleep Foundation, 2023).

Conclusion

Sleep is the most prominent and fundamental circadian cycle in human biology. Sleep has an important role in many areas, from the regeneration of brain energy to processes such as recording and erasing memory. For this reason, creating a healthy sleep cycle with an average of 90-minute cycles consisting of NREM and REM periods is essential. As a result of technological developments, an increase in artificial light, circadian disturbances, and phase shifts are among the most important problems today. Because even the slightest disturbance in the circadian rhythm causes suppression of melatonin synthesis and can significantly affect sleep with circadian phase shifts. When a person is sleep deprived or does not have enough quality sleep, their health can be adversely affected, and even the healing process of diseases can have adverse effects. Therefore, it is essential to maintain the circadian rhythm to ensure a healthy sleep cycle. Sleep quality and circadian rhythm are mechanisms that affect each other bidirectionally. For this reason, it is necessary to ensure healthy sleep by maintaining the circadian rhythm, paying attention to sleep duration, and light exposure during sleep.

References

Akinci, E., & Orhan, F. Ö. (2016). Sirkadiyen Ritim Uyku Bozuklukları [Circadian rhythm sleep disorders]. *Psikiyatride Guncel Yaklasimlar*, 8(2), 178-189. https://doi.org/10.18863/pgy.81775.

Amanpour, A., Kahraman, S., Çınar, B., & Çelik, F. (2021). Mavi ışık maruziyetinin sirkadiyen ritim ve beslenme üzerindeki etkisi [Blue light exposure effect on circadian rhythm and nutrition]. *Celal Bayar Üniversitesi Sağlık Bilimleri Enstitüsü Dergisi*, 8(3), 566-573. https://doi.org/10.34087/cbusbed.891351.

Bjorvatn, B., & Pallesen, S. (2023). Irregular sleep–wake rhythm disorder. In: C. A. Kushida (Ed). *Encyclopedia of sleep and circadian rhythms* (2. Edition, pp.617-623). Academic Press. https://doi.org/10.1016/B978-0-12-822963-7.00114-6.

Brown, G. M., Pandı-Perumal, S. R., & Cardınalı, D. P. (2020). Circadian rhythm sleep disorders. In: A. Chopra, P. Das, & K. Doghramji (Eds.). *Management of Sleep Disorders in Psychiatry* (pp. 172-193). Oxford University Press.

Chellappa, S. L. (2021). Individual differences in light sensitivity affect sleep and circadian rhythms. *Sleep*, 44(2), 1-10. https://doi.org/10.1093/sleep/zsaa214.

Cohen S.E. (2020) Circadian Clocks in Cyanobacteria. In: Q. Wang (Ed). *Microbial Photosynthesis (p. 169-180)*. Springer, Singapore. https://doi.org/10.1007/978-981-15-3110-1_9.

Çalışkan, G., & Akan, L. S. (2019). Sirkadiyen ritim, uyku ve beslenmenin obezite üzerine etkileri [Effects of circadian rhythm, sleep and nutrition on obesity]. *Atlas Journal*, *5*(17), 131-139. https://doi.org/10.31568/atlas.297.

Diekman, C. O., & Bose, A. (2022). Beyond the limits of circadian entrainment: Non-24-h sleep-wake disorder, shift work, and social jet lag. *Journal of Theoretical Biology*, 545, 111148. https://doi.org/10.1016/j.jtbi.2022.111148.

Engwall, M., Fridh, I., Johansson, L., Bergbom, I., & Lindahl, B. (2015). Lighting, sleep and circadian rhythm: An intervention study in the intensive care unit. *Intensive and Critical Care Nursing*, 31(6), 325-335. https://doi.org/10.1016/j.iccn.2015.07.001.

Ersoy, E. O., Demir, A. U., & Topeli, A. (2016). Yoğun bakımda uyku: var mı, yok mu? [Sleep in intensive care: is there or not?]. *Turkish Journal of Medical & Surgical Intensive Care Medicine/Dahili ve Cerrahi Bilimler Yogun Bakim Dergisi*, 7(1), 28-33. https://doi.org/10.5152/dcbybd.2016.1125.

Fisk, A. S., Tam, S. K., Brown, L. A., Vyazovskiy, V. V., Bannerman, D. M., & Peirson, S. N. (2018). Light and cognition: roles for circadian rhythms, sleep, and arousal. *Frontiers in Neurology*, 9, 1-18. https://doi.org/10.3389/fneur.2018.00056.

Goldfarb, D., Sharkey, K.M. (2020). Irregular sleep-wake rhythm disorder. In: R. R. Auger (Ed). *Circadian Rhythm Sleep-Wake Disorders* (p. 137-148). Springer, Cham. https://doi.org/10.1007/978-3-030-43803-6_10.

Hartsock, M. J., Strnad, H. K., & Spencer, R. L. (2022). Iterative metaplasticity across timescales: how circadian, ultradian, and ınfradian rhythms modulate memory mechanisms. *Journal of Biological Rhythms*,37 (1),February:29–42. https://doi.org/10.1177/07487304211058256.

Haspel, J. A., Anafi, R., Brown, M. K., Cermakian, N., Depner, C., Desplats, P., Gelman, A. E., Haack, M., Jelic, S., Kim, B. S., Laposky, A. D., Lee, Y. C., Mongodin, E., Prather, A. A., Prendergast, B. J., Reardon, C., Shaw, A. C., Sengupta, S., Szentirmai, E., Thakkar, M., Walker, W. E., & Solt, L. A. (2020). Perfect timing: circadian rhythms, sleep, and immunity—an NIH workshop summary. *JCI Insight*, 5(1), 1-14. https://doi.org/10.1172/jci.

Healy, K. L., Morris, A. R., & Liu, A. C. (2021). Circadian synchrony: sleep, nutrition, and physical activity. *Frontiers in Network Physiology*, 1,732243,1-22. https://doi.org/10.3389/fnetp.2021.732243.

Keskin, N., & Tamam, L. (2018). Uyku bozuklukları: sınıflama ve tedavi [Sleep disorders: classification and treatment]. *Arşiv Kaynak Tarama Dergisi*, 27(2), 241-260. https://doi.org/10.17827/aktd.346010.

Krishnan, H. C., & Lyons, L. C. (2015). Synchrony and desynchrony in circadian clocks: impacts on learning and memory. *Learning & Memory,* 22(9), 426-437. http://www.learnmem.org/cgi/doi/10.1101/lm.038877.115.

Lou, X., Wang, H., Tu, Y., Tan, W., Jiang, C., Sun, J., & Bao, Z. (2021). Alterations of sleep quality and circadian rhythm genes expression in elderly thyroid nodule patients and risks associated with thyroid malignancy. *Scientific Reports*, 11(1), 1-12. https://doi.org/10.1038/s41598-021-93106-x.

Palacıoğlu Açılan, M. (2016). Sirkadiyen Ritme Bağlı Olarak Uyku Kalite Durumunun Kan Lipid Profili Üzerine Etkisinin Belirlenmesi [Determination of relation between the blood lipid profile and circadian RHYTM depending on sleep quality status]. Master's Thesis. (Thesis Advisor: Prof. Dr. M. Emel Tüfekçi ALPHAN). Okan University Institute of Health Sciences, İstanbul.

Patel AK, Reddy V, Shumway KR, et al. Physiology, Sleep Stages. [Updated 2022 Sep 7]. In: StatPearls [Internet]. Treasure Island (FL): *StatPearls Publishing*; 2022 Jan-.

Pavlova, M. K., & Latreille, V. (2019). Sleep disorders. *The American Journal of Medicine*, 132(3), 292-299. https://doi.org/10.1016/j.amjmed.2018.09.021.

Roenneberg, T., & Merrow, M. (2016). The circadian clock and human health. *Current Biology*, 26(10), R432-R443. https://doi.org/10.1016/j.cub.2016.04.011.

Sateia, M. J. (2014). International classification of sleep disorders. *Chest,* 146(5), 1387-1394. https://doi.org/10.1378/chest.14-0970.

Saygın, M., & Özgüner, M. (2020). Uykunun Mikro Yapısı ve Mimarisi [Micro-structure and architecture of sleep]. *Uyku Bülteni*, 1(1), 19-29.

Selvi, Y., Beşiroğlu, L., & Aydın, A. (2011). Kronobiyoloji ve duygudurum bozuklukları [Chronobiology and mood disorders]. *Psikiyatride Güncel Yaklaşımlar*, 3(3), 368-386. https://doi.org/10.5455/cap.20110317.

Sleep Foundation. (2023). Circadian rhythm sleep disorders. Avaible from https://www.sleepfoundation.org/circadian-rhythm-sleep-disorders.

Su, K., Din, Z. U., Cui, B., Peng, F., Zhou, Y., Wang, C., Zhang, X., Lu, J., Luo, H., He, B., Kelley, K., & Liu, Q. (2022). A broken circadian clock: The emerging neuro-immune link connecting depression to cancer. *Brain, Behavior, & Immunity-Health*, 26, 100533. https://doi.org/10.1016/j.bbih.2022.100533.

Tramontano, M., De Angelis, S., Galeoto, G., Cucinotta, M. C., Lisi, D., Botta, R. M., D'ippolito, M., Morone G., & Buzzi, M. G. (2021). Physical therapy exercises for sleep disorders in a rehabilitation setting for neurological patients: a systematic review and meta-analysis. *Brain Sciences*, 11(9), 1176. https://doi.org/10.3390/brainsci11091176.

Wang, T., Li, J., Wang, Y., Dai, S., Shao, R., & Hao, L. (2022). Active interventions of dynamic lighting on human circadian rhythm and sleep quality in confined spaces. *Building and Environment*, 226, 109766. https://doi.org/10.1016/j.buildenv.2022.109766.

Zaki, N. F., Spence, D. W., Subramanian, P., Bharti, V. K., Karthikeyan, R., BaHammam, A. S., & Pandi-Perumal, S. R. (2020). Basic chronobiology: what do sleep physicians need to know?. *Sleep Science*, 13(4), 256. https://doi.org/10.5935/1984-0063.20200026.

Zisapel, N. (2018). New perspectives on the role of melatonin in human sleep, circadian rhythms and their regulation. *British Journal of Pharmacology*, 175(16), 3190-3199. https://doi.org/10.1111/bph.1411.6.

Chapter 6

The Metabolic Clock: Rhythmicity of Metabolic Processes, Circadian Disruption, and Diseases

Duygu Keser*, **MSc**
Department of Biology, Enka Technical School, Kocaeli, Turkiye

Abstract

Metabolism can be defined as the chemical processes that occur in a living organism to sustain life and are tightly regulated. Most evidence supports the close relationship between clocks and metabolism. Metabolism, physiology, and behavior are organized by the circadian system in a daily cycle of circadian rhythms. Circadian rhythmicity disruption has been implicated in the pathogenesis of several diseases, including metabolic disorders. Circadian systems are in a hierarchy, and the central timer is the SCN. Independently of the SCN, the rhythm continues in peripheral tissues. Circadian rhythm can be observed in living organisms, as well as in lower structures, such as systems, organs, tissues, and cells. The cell-autonomous clock machinery has several transcriptional-translational feedback loops, allowing for autonomous oscillations with a period of approximately 24 hours. The clock genes contribute to the emergence of the circadian rhythm. The relationship between the circadian rhythm and metabolism should be examined bidirectionally. Human metabolism can adapt well to daily fluctuations because of the rhythmicity of the physiology. The reciprocal coordination of circadian and metabolic pathways is very important for cellular homeostasis and the health of the organism. An imbalance in energy

* Corresponding Author's Email: dukeser@gmail.com.

In: Human Health is a Matter of Timing
Editors: Sumeyya Deniz Aybek, Gonca Gulbay and Mucahit Secme
ISBN: 979-8-89113-467-6

intake and expenditure causes the accumulation of nutrients and metabolites. Therefore, this situation contributes to metabolic diseases. Food is a non-photic stimulus that can reset the circadian rhythm and one of our peripheral clocks' external synchronizers. The increased number of proofs shows that the proper functioning of peripheral and central clocks is crucial for the well-being of the organism. A deeper understanding of the molecular clock's role in the regulation of daily physiological processes will enable the development of new treatments, more effective therapeutic delivery, and better preventive strategies for the management of diabetes, obesity, and other metabolic disorders.
This chapter aims to consecutively guide researchers through the research findings that have improved our understanding of metabolism, circadian clock, metabolism-circadian clock relations, metabolic diseases-circadian clock relations, energy homeostasis, and food intake-circadian rhythms-metabolism relations.

Keywords: circadian clock, circadian disruption, metabolism, energy, food

Introduction

Metabolism

Metabolism is a term that encompasses a variety of chemical and physical processes in tissues on which the body's heat production and growth depend and from which the energy required for muscular activity and maintaining vital activity and vital functions is obtained. Catabolism is the destructive process through which living cells convert complex substances into simpler ones, whereas anabolism refers to the constructive processes through which living cells convert simple substances into more complex ones, particularly living matter (Kopera, 1985). Metabolism in all living organisms involves catabolic and anabolic processes, and glycolysis, glycogenolysis, glycogenesis, gluconeogenesis, lipogenesis, lipolysis, protein synthesis, and proteolysis are essential metabolic processes in living organisms. In addition to these metabolic processes, are several related hormones that play an essential part (Qaid and Abdelrahman, 2016).

Metabolism is tightly regulated (Feng and Lazar, 2012). However, the imbalance between energy intake and expenditure causes nutrients and metabolites to accumulate, which ultimately causes metabolic diseases (Zakhari, 2013). A common subject in metabolic control is the transcriptional regulation of rate-limiting metabolic enzymes, generally including epigenomic mechanisms. Environmental factors, e.g., exercise, nutrition, stress, and aging, can be signaled through metabolic hormones, including leptin and insulin, and metabolites, including nicotinamide adenine dinucleotide (NAD+), acetyl-CoA, ADP, and S-adenosylmethionine (SAM). The epigenome is regulated by these signals by modulating the function of chromatin-modifying enzymes as well as the transcription factors involved in recruiting the mentioned before enzymes (Feng and Lazar, 2012). On most days, the daily order of temporal life occurs unconsciously. For this reason, unsurprisingly, a conceptual framework for research on biological timing remains outside of the area of modern medical practice. Over the past 20 years, with a change in our conception of the molecular mechanism that encodes circadian systems, novel research has started to fill the gap from molecular clocks to human biology. An insight into metabolism and circadian clocks originates directly from the finding that biological rhythms are maintained by a transcription network that is encoded genetically and acts as a molecular oscillator with a precision close to 24 hours in the majority of cell types, sustaining phase alignment in various behavioral, physiological, and biochemical processes with the environmental light cycle (Marcheva et al., 2013). A close association between metabolism and clocks is supported by most of the evidence (Shi et al., 2013). It is known that the internal circadian rhythm controls metabolism and that the cell-autonomous clock machinery has a few transcriptional-translational feedback loops, allowing for autonomous oscillation with a period of about 24 hours. The clock genes make a contribution to the emergence of the circadian rhythm (Hussain and Pan, 2009; Lowrey and Takahashi, 2004). The influence of circadian timing on human health has started to be revealed by observational population studies conducted in people exposed to sleep restriction, jet travel, and shift work, as well as experimental research demonstrating broad pathophysiological implications (Marcheva et al., 2013).

Clocks, Rhythms, Metabolism, and Diseases

Circadian Rhythm, Central Nervous System, and Metabolic Process

There is an interaction between circadian and metabolic processes at the neuroendocrine and neuroanatomic levels to regulate overall metabolic homeostasis. To assess in a better way how whole-body metabolism is regulated by the circadian clock network in the brain, it is significant to reveal the anatomical connections between brain centers that are important for circadian rhythmicity and those controlling energy expenditure and appetite (Marcheva et al., 2013). Circadian rhythmicity represents a crucial component of physiological processes, providing them with a 24-hour temporal organization and adjustment to cyclical variations in the environment (Challet, 2014). A central clock in the suprachiasmatic nucleus (SCN) of the brain, synchronizing peripheral clocks in peripheral tissues, controls the circadian clock (Zhang et al., 2020). Peripheral clocks (non-SCN brain clocks) have been determined within the brain, involving the olfactory bulb, retina, mediobasal hypothalamus, etc. The SCN coordinates peripheral clocks in behavioral, neuroendocrine, and autonomic ways (Asher and Sassone-Corsi, 2015). The suprachiasmatic nuclei synapse in a direct way with ventral and dorsal subventricular regions, cell bodies in ventral and dorsal subventricular areas, and the dorsomedial hypothalamus. Despite the interaction of the said regions with each other, neurons in the dorsal supraventricular region regulate thermogenesis more effectively. However, the ventral supraventricular region is primarily responsible for the regulation of activity and sleep-wake cycles. Furthermore, the paraventricular hypothalamus is involved in corticosteroid release, while the lateral hypothalamus plays a role in alertness and nutrition (Serin and Tek, 2019). The SCN is activated by the retinohypothalamic tract (RHT) (Hannibal et al., 2000). The subparaventricular zone (SPZ) also projects to the dorsomedial hypothalamus (DMH), a brain region that is essential for the rhythms of the sleep/wake cycle, body temperature, locomotor activity, food intake, corticosteroid secretion and projections of neurons within the DMH target neuronal centers that take part in regulating corticosteroid release (paraventricular nucleus—PVN), sleep/wake cycle (ventrolateral preoptic nucleus—VLPO), and feeding and wakefulness (lateral hypothalamus—LHA). Hence, DMH functions as a transmission center that amplifies circadian signals from the SCN to many brain regions that play a role in regulating sleep, feeding, and activity (Marcheva et al., 2013). The arcuate nucleus of the hypothalamus (ARH) is the main part of various homeostatic circuits. ARH is a particularly essential site for the central regulation of energy expenditure, food intake, and body weight. From the ARH, leptin signals are distributed via neural projections to other regions implicated in feeding control, including the paraventricular nucleus of the hypothalamus (PVH), the lateral hypothalamic area (LHA), and the dorsomedial hypothalamic nucleus (DMH) (Bouret et al., 2004). Most neurons on the ventromedial side of the arcuate nucleus that synthesize the agouti-related peptide (AGRP) and orexigenic peptides neuropeptide Y (NPY) also contain the vesicular GABA transporter (VGAT) and the GABA-synthesizing enzyme glutamic acid decarboxylase (GAD), thus supporting their GABAergic character (Meister, 2007). In cases of low leptin levels, the orexigenic neurons in the ARC synthesize AgRP and NPY, thus stimulating hunger and reducing energy expenditures by signaling to the LHA (Marcheva et al., 2013). Another neuron population within the ARC comprises the POMC and CART neurons, exerting a powerful anorexigenic effect—secretion of the POMC and CART neuropeptides from the above-mentioned neurons reduces body weight and food intake (Varela and Horvath, 2012).

Peripheral Clocks, Rhythms, and Metabolic Process

The circadian system regulates a wide variety of physiological and behavioral rhythms (Lowrcy and Takahashi, 2004; Reppert and Weaver, 2002). It is arranged in a hierarchy of oscillators in the mammalian circadian system. The suprachiasmatic nucleus (SCN) of the anterior hypothalamus is at the top of this hierarchy (Yamazaki et al., 2000; Yoo et al., 2004). The SCN is a central synchronizer and master oscillator. It coordinates the peripheral clocks. Circadian clocks can measure approximately and, therefore, they need to be synchronized every day to stay in resonance with geophysical time. The oscillators of the SCN neurons synchronize via photic signals primarily. Then, they transmit rhythmic information to organs by neuronal and endocrine signals (Nagoshi et al., 2004; Dibner et al., 2010). The rhythm continues in peripheral tissues independently of the SCN. In lung, liver, kidney, pancreas, spleen, stomach, heart, cornea, skeletal muscle, thyroid, and adrenal gland tissue cultures, gene expressions depending on the circadian clock continue strongly (Balsalobre et al., 1998; Nagoshi et al., 2004; Izumo et al., 2006). In short, circadian rhythm can be observed in living organisms as well as in lower structures such as systems, organs, tissues, and cells (Kondratov et al., 2007). Research conducted in the 2000s has demonstrated that there are autonomic circadian oscillators in peripheral tissues and organs, e.g., the intestine, heart, liver, and retina, and contribute to metabolic processes by cellular clock genes in the said tissues/organs (Serin and Tek, 2019). Moreover, subsequent molecular analyses have shown that the clock network is expressed not only in the SCN but in the majority of mammalian tissues involving tissues crucial for cardiometabolic function, e.g., the pancreas, liver, heart, and muscle (Marcheva et al., 2013).

The clock represents an intracellular mechanism that shares the same molecular components in SCN neurons and peripheral cells in mammals, and the molecular mechanism for the production of circadian rhythms depends on the concerted coexpression of specific clock genes. Transcriptional-translational feedback loops are located exactly at the heart of the core clock mechanism. Furthermore, many clock gene products act as transcription factors that contain PAS (PER, ARNT, and SIM) and basic helix-loop-helix domains that participate in protein-protein and protein-DNA interactions, respectively. The expression of the factors in question is finally activated or repressed by them. Hence, the factors mentioned above are a self-sustained transcriptional feedback loop. Alterations in concentration, posttranslational modifications (acetylation, phosphorylation, deacetylation, and SUMOylation), subcellular localization, and delays between transcription and translation cause a cycle of about 24 hours (Froy, 2010).

For instance, the circadian system coordinates the timing of numerous physiological processes, including glucose metabolism (Mason et al., 2020). The daily rhythm of glucose metabolism is managed via the circadian clock, comprising cell-autonomous clock machinery present in almost each body tissue (Nakao et al., 2018). The suprachiasmatic nuclei play an important role in the regulation of glucose metabolism. For example, rats with lesions in the SCN have impaired insulin sensitivity and glucose uptake. The disrupted circadian clock may cause an impairment in insulin secretion and hypoinsulinemia. The CLOCK and BMAL1 proteins related to the circadian rhythm take part in the production and release of insulin. The proteins mentioned above bind to the pancreatic β-cells' distal regions, regulating the circadian rhythm in these events. Insulin is insufficient or absent in both type 1 and 2 diabetes because of β-cell damage. Thus, the function of circadian rhythm in diabetes etiology should not be ignored concerning β-cell damage (Serin and Tek, 2019). It is known that insulin action and glucose tolerance change during the day since oral glucose tolerance is disrupted in the evening hours in comparison with the morning hours because of the combined impacts of decreased insulin sensitivity and insulin secretion at night. Additionally, glucose levels alone demonstrate circadian oscillations and reach the highest level prior to the onset of the active period. Therefore, it is essential to better understand the molecular mechanisms that underlie the circadian control of glucose homeostasis and other physiological processes for the purpose of enabling temporal assessment in the diagnosis and treatment of metabolic disorders (Marcheva et al., 2013). Moreover, daily blood glucose homeostasis includes control by the hypothalamic clock in the SCN and peripheral clocks, for example, in the pancreas, liver, white adipose tissue, and muscle (Kalsbeek et al., 2014).

Rhythmicity of Metabolic Processes

The fasting/feeding and sleep/wake cycles represent the most obvious mammalian clock's outputs. However, the circadian clock also affects homeostasis in various processes, including glucose and lipid metabolism, endocrine hormone secretion, body temperature, and cardiovascular health (Marcheva et al., 2013).

There is a tight interconnection at the molecular level between cellular metabolism and circadian clocks. Circadian rhythmicity that has been shaped as a result of evolution over millions of years creates an internal timing that controls the metabolism and sleep-wake cycles. A master hypothalamic clock, which is reset primarily by ambient light, coordinates the daily alterations between sleep/fasting/catabolism and wakefulness/feeding/anabolism. Normally, the master clock synchronizes secondary clocks, including the liver and adipose tissue. However, they are also sensitive to feeding time, especially in the case of meals during the usual rest period (Challet, 2013). The fact that the circadian clock improves energetic efficiency through the temporal separation of catabolic and anabolic reactions (including glycolysis and gluconeogenesis) may be its advantage obtained as a result of evolution (Marcheva et al., 2013). The abnormal functioning of the clock results in serious dysfunctions and pathologies (Saha and Sassone-Corsi, 2007).

In most organisms, every day is arranged in two phases. The first is characterized by activity and feeding, and the other by resting and fasting. In the active period, the ingested nutrients supply substrates, e.g., lipids, glucose, and amino acids, fueling the metabolic pathways in our cells. Nevertheless, the energy and substrates stored in our body are mobilized with the objective of maintaining metabolic homeostasis during the resting period. The hypothalamus controls various changing physiological and behavioral processes, involving food and water intake, thermoregulation, sleep and arousal, and energy expenditure. A molecular mechanism present in the central clock in the SCN of the hypothalamus defines the periods of activity/feeding and resting/fasting, establishing a rhythm of about 24 hours (i.e., "circadian") (Kalsbeek et al., 2014).

The adipose tissue is a central metabolic organ that regulates whole-body energy homeostasis. The function of the white adipose tissue is the main energy reservoir for other organs. Lipids are accumulated by the brown adipose tissue for cold-induced adaptive thermogenesis. Various cytokines, hormones, and metabolites controlling systemic energy balance through the regulation of appetitive signals coming from the central nerve system and metabolic activity in peripheral tissues are secreted by adipose tissues (Choe et al., 2016). Leptin is synthesized by adipocytes, and it influences the mediobasal hypothalamus for the inhibition of food intake. Additionally, leptin represents a hormone, which takes part in the peripheral metabolism of glucose and lipids (Challet, 2015; Lammert et al., 2001). It has been shown that some characteristics of adipose-related physiology, involving adipokine release, display daily oscillations. Physical exercise has a strong effect on adipokine release and a potential reverse disruption of peripheral circadian clocks. Leptin shows circadian oscillations under normal dietary conditions. Moreover, it reaches its highest level in the early dark phase in humans and diurnal animals, increases after food intake, and decreases during fasting (Bilski et al., 2016). Both leptin and thyroid hormones may take part in the adaptive thermogenesis through mitochondrial uncoupling proteins and heat production since both triiodothyronine and thyroxine take part in the starvation-induced reduction in thermogenesis. Leptin probably has an essential role in the pathophysiology of the thyroid (Zimmermann-Belsing et al., 2003). Leptin release takes place in a circadian cycle. Serum leptin levels peak at night. Therefore, the disrupted circadian balance may impact leptin secretion, energy homeostasis, and thermogenesis in an indirect way (Serin and Tek, 2019).

Melatonin is the principal hormone of the vertebrate pineal gland. The pineal gland produces circulating melatonin under the control of the central circadian system located in the suprachiasmatic nucleus (SCN) of the hypothalamus (Gamble et al., 2014). The pineal gland always releases this lipophilic hormone at night in diurnal (active during the day) and nocturnal (active nocturnal) animals (Challet, 2015). The stimulation of melatonin synthesis and release occurs in the darkness at night. However, light suppresses it in the daytime. The secretion of melatonin reaches its maximum level, and its concentration in the blood increases 3-10-fold, particularly between 11:00 p.m. and 5:00 a.m. However, exposure to light in the nighttime lowers melatonin levels in plasma (Serin and Tek, 2019).

The orexinergic features of the ghrelin hormone are known. These features activate neurons in arcuate nuclei that contain the neuropeptide Y and the agouti-related peptide (Challet, 2015). It is an endogenous ligand for growth hormone secretagogue receptors and strongly stimulates the growth hormone release. Furthermore, it causes an increase in appetite and weight gain by increasing food intake and decreasing fat burning. Although ghrelin levels appear to vary under fasting or satiety conditions, there is a significant correlation (Natalucci et al., 2005). Ghrelin receptors take an essential part in modulating the circadian system activity by displaying a direct effect on the SCN under normal circumstances or restricted feeding schedules (Engin, 2017). Growth hormone (GH) is an important metabolic homeostatic factor secreted in a circadian pattern. Nevertheless, it is not known whether it is synthesized rhythmically (Vakili et al., 2016). The concentration of GH in the blood reaches the highest level between 2 and 4 a.m., a normal sleep period. If there is no sleep, the rhythm collapses, and GH is not secreted in a normal way (Sato et al., 2017).

The adrenal gland secretes glucocorticoids in circadian cycles in mammals, which causes temporally regulated peaks and troughs in systemic hormone levels. Although the function of the said oscillation in secretion is not fully revealed, it is considered to be essential for energy balance since feeding time and diet affect the secretion rhythm (So et al., 2009). Cortisol has a specific circadian rhythm impacted by sleep. According to normal physiology, there are lower cortisol levels at the beginning of sleep. However, an increase occurs at the end of the sleep period, peaking just minutes before a person wakes up. The rhythm mentioned above is formed in a tight relationship with the sleep-wakefulness cycle, i.e., cortisol plays an essential role in the circadian system, which influences almost every body organ and tissue, controlling particular biological cyclical functions, such as cardiovascular functions. Obvious differences in cortisol levels in the day and nighttime can assist with explaining the cortisol function in health and diseases. Furthermore, the cortisol status is an objective biological marker of the stress response, which can be associated with most cardiovascular diseases. The timing of cardiovascular events such as ventricular fibrillation and acute myocardial infarction may affect the seriousness of the disease and survival, whereas a poor prognosis is related to the occurrence in the early morning (Azmi et al., 2021). Cortisol is the main catabolic signal that acts with testosterone to maintain anabolic-catabolic homeostasis in men. The prolonged circadian misalignment reduces the overall cortisol exposure (O'Bryne et al., 2021). Many metabolic processes, such as the stimulation of glycogenolysis and lipolysis, are modulated by cortisol. It reveals a biphasic impact on the homeostasis of glucose, inducing insulin resistance chronically and acutely inhibiting the secretion of insulin. Early in the morning (~1:00 am), circulating cortisol levels peak in humans and promote fuel mobilization at the said time. The effect of corticosterone on metabolic homeostasis depends on the time of day. Thus, hydrocortisone that is infused at 1 p.m. (abnormally high) versus 5 a.m. (normally high) leads to augmented plasma glucose and insulin levels in humans. At the beginning of the active period, the diurnal rhythms of cortisol secretion and sensitivity possibly increase the availability of fuel (McGinnis and Young, 2016).

Circadian oscillations influence lipid metabolism. Studies display that many proteins associated with lipid metabolism (e.g., ApoA1, ApoB, and ApoA4), intestinal fatty acid binding protein, and intestinal microsomal triglyceride transport protein vary during the day. Additionally, research on mice has reported higher lipid and cholesterol absorption in the dark phase in comparison with the light phase. Several lipid metabolism products also display a circadian rhythm. For instance, circulating non-esterified fatty acids in humans increase in the nighttime because of the elevated lipolytic activity (Serin and Tek, 2019).

In all mammals, including humans, physiology is rhythmic in almost all respects. Therefore, the cardiovascular system (heartbeat and heart pressure), cerebral activities, renal activity (plasma flow, blood pressure, urine production, electrolyte, and water balance), endocrine system (production and secretion of hormones), metabolism, immune system, and body temperature can adapt well to daily fluctuations (Asher and Schibler, 2011; Morris et al., 2012; Firsov et al., 2012; Tsang et al., 2014). These rhythms are under stable conditions that do not receive time cues from the environment and are mostly managed by the endogenous circadian timing system (Bollinger and Schibler, 2014). In addition to their own endogenous rhythms, the circadian clock controls the rhythms of many activities, and there is a simple linear relationship between them. Although metabolic events occur according to the circadian clock, many metabolic parameters can affect the clock genes expression. Therefore, the relationship between the circadian rhythm and metabolism should be examined bidirectionally (Green et al., 2008).

Circadian Rhythm and Energy Homeostasis

It is crucial that non-SCN clocks in the brain are also synchronized with the SCN for optimal energy homeostasis. However, they may be excluded from the SCN control under some special circumstances, such as restricted nutrition. The SCN produces a circadian rhythm transmitted to the remaining body parts through other brain nuclei. DNA microarrays show that SCN controls approximately 8-10% of the transcriptome in a tissue, which shows the significance of the circadian clock in numerous processes in the body (Oosterman et al., 2015). The obtained data suggest that the mutual coordination of circadian and metabolic pathways is very important for cellular homeostasis and the health of an organism (Sancar and Brunner, 2014).

Different enzymes, hormones, and transport systems regulate energy metabolism, and their secretion, expression, and/or activation are modulated by the circadian rhythm in an effective way. The metabolic pathways ensuring energy homeostasis are coordinated through metabolites proposing changes and proactively preparing the molecular environment and acute signaling systems that respond immediately to variations in circadian clocks. Energy metabolism is regulated at the cellular level by hormone receptors, interactions between genes, and intracellular oxidation or reduction reactions. There is an important interaction between the aforesaid pathways and the biological metabolic clock. The functioning of hormone receptors (peroxisome proliferator-activated receptor [PPAR]α, REV-ERBα, and PPARγ) and a number of genes at the cellular level (SIRTUIN) can be affected by the circadian clock. Moreover, ligands and nuclear hormone receptors (PPARα, REV-ERBα, PPARγ, HNF4α, RORα, NURR1, and TRα) in metabolic tissues act as sensors combining metabolic and circadian pathways (Serin and Tek, 2019). For instance, PPARs play a crucial part in energy metabolism (Chen and Yang, 2014) and represent a connection between energy metabolism and the circadian clock. Transcriptional factors increasing lipid storage and lipogenesis are activated by PPARγ localized in adipose tissue. Ketogenesis and hepatic fatty acid oxidation are triggered by PPARα from nuclear hormone receptors as a reaction to starvation, whereas PPARδ represents the most common nuclear cell receptor in the body and can correlate daily variations in body temperature with the circadian clock (Serin and Tek, 2019).

The number of proofs that an endogenous clock that functions smoothly is very important for energy balance in organisms is increasing. External and internal clock resonance is advantageous for an organism in energetic terms. In mammals, there can be a few reasons for the advantage mentioned above, such as preventing aging and dementia pathologies through the effective removal of oxidative stress-induced DNA damage (Eckel-Mahan and Sassone-Corsi, 2009). The mammalian family of sirtuins, including SIRT1~7, take part in numerous biological processes, e.g., cell proliferation and survival, stress response, senescence, metabolism, and genome stability. According to the acquired data, sirtuins act as essential energy status sensors and ensure cell protection against metabolic stresses (Ye et al., 2017). SIRT3 and SIRT6 play a very significant part in lipid and glucose metabolism, while SIRT1 provides the regulation of insulin secretion and adiponectin production, gluconeogenesis, inflammation, circadian rhythms, and oxidative stress, which contribute as a whole to developing insulin resistance. Furthermore, the overexpression of SIRT1 and some SIRT1 activators positively impact insulin sensitivity and glucose homeostasis in diabetic animal models and humans (Kitada et al., 2013). The recent finding indicating that the activity of SIRT1, a longevity-related protein and a member of the family of NAD+-activated histone deacetylases, oscillates in a circadian manner is added to our knowledge of the interaction between metabolism and the circadian clock and also demonstrates a gap in our understanding of the molecular support for this interaction. SIRT1 (the mammalian ortholog of yeast SIR2) oscillates in activity, impinging back on the circadian clock by changing BMAL1 acetylation and CLOCK–BMAL1-induced gene transcription. During the yeast metabolic cycle, the finding of metabolite oscillations combined with the proof of circadian sirtuin activity allows for speculating on whether metabolites, e.g., NAD+ themselves, play the main role in the cellular connection between the circadian clock and metabolism (Eckel-Mahan and Sassone-Corsi, 2009). While circadian clocks, DNA repair, apoptosis, insulin secretion, inflammatory pathways, and mitochondrial biogenesis are controlled by SIRT1, AMPK (AMP-activated protein kinase) acts in coordination with SIRT1 and controls the expression of genes with a role in energy metabolism in the muscles (Lee and Kim, 2013).

The core clock genes of mammalian are well identified. Nevertheless, the exact role of central and peripheral oscillators in maintaining energy balance and metabolic homeostasis has not been comprehended completely. Studies that aim to demonstrate the molecular pathways that link the circadian clock with metabolic sensors are still an active field of research (Marcheva et al., 2013). The experiments conducted recently have suggested that cellular energy levels can affect rhythms. CLOCK and NPAS2 can bind in an efficient way to BMAL1 and, accordingly, to E-box sequences when reduced NADH and NADPH are present. The oxidized forms of the nicotinamide adenine dinucleotides (NAD^+ and $NADP^+$) inhibit the DNA binding of CLOCK:BMAL1 NPAS2:BMAL1 because the $NAD(P)^+$/NAD(P)H redox equilibrium is dependent on the cell metabolic status, the rate in question can dictate the binding of CLOCK/NPAS2:BMAL1 to E-boxes and lead to the phase-shifting of cyclic gene expression (Froy, 2010). The elevated levels of AMP (adenosine monophosphate) and intracellular NAD+ levels are low energy indicators. AMP-activating protein kinase (AMPK) acts as a food sensor and ensures the activation of intracellular energy supply pathways when intracellular ATP levels are reduced. In this way, the AMP/ATP ratio may also be a connection between energy metabolism and the circadian rhythm (Serin and Tek, 2019). CRY represses gluconeogenesis by the inhibition of protein kinase A–mediated phosphorylation of the cAMP response element–binding protein (CREB) when fasting by blocking glucagon-mediated increases in the intracellular cAMP concentration. Furthermore, gluconeogenesis is downregulated by SREBP1c via FOXO1 degradation mediated by CRY1 for the purpose of regulating hyperglycemia in db/db mice (Guan and Lazar, 2021).

The mitochondrial production of ATP is synchronized by the circadian clock for the purpose of supplying daily changes in cellular energy requirements. Liver kinase B1 activates AMP-activated protein kinase (AMPK) in the case of the increasing AMP/ATP ratio. The SIRT1-dependent deacetylation of PGC-1α and FOXO1 transcription regulators is translated. Additionally, AMPK activity shows circadian rhythms in peripheral tissues as a critical cellular energy sensor. The phosphorylation and destabilization of the CRY and PER proteins are accelerated by AMPK, which transmits energy-dependent signals to the mammalian clock, and the loss of AMPK signaling leads to the stabilization of CRYs and disruption of circadian rhythms. The AMPK-mediated phosphorylation of casein kinases and CRY ensures the regulation of the negative feedback control of the circadian clock by the proteolytic degradation of PER2 (Engin, 2017; Cantó et al., 2010). Hypothalamic metabolic sensors are essential to control nutrition and energy homeostasis. Hence, PAS kinase (PASK), mTOR, and AMPK represent crucial nutrient sensors for glucose metabolism and cellular energy requirements. The PASK function takes an essential part in maintaining nutrient action in the AMPK and mTOR/S6K1 pathways. Changes in hypothalamic AMPK activity are adequate to alter body weight and food intake. Additionally, acetyl-coenzyme A carboxylase/malonyl coenzyme A/carnitine palmitoyltransferase-1/fatty acid oxidation and mTOR signalization are putative down-regulated pathways for regulating food intake as a reaction to hypothalamic AMPK. On the contrary, defects in genes that encode leptin, or its receptor cause severe obesity and hyperphagia (Hurtado-Carneiro et al., 2014; Minokoshi et al., 2008).

All aspects of energy metabolism, from food intake to intracellular signaling pathways, are strongly impacted by circadian rhythmicity. In contrast, the suprachiasmatic clock is synchronized via ambient light, when the timing of meals represents an effective synchronizer (time-giver) for adjusting the phase of the peripheral clocks. Under particular nutritional circumstances (such as low- or high-calorie diets), the suprachiasmatic clock functioning is modulated by metabolic factors that should be identified. Animal obesity and diabetes models show circadian variations. On the other hand, lipid and glucose metabolism are dysregulated in cases of disrupted circadian rhythmicity because of the circadian clock with genetic defects or circadian desynchronization (chronic exposure to light or repeated meals at irregular times in the cycle). The metabolic effect of circadian desynchronization rationalizes the development of therapeutic or preventive strategies, which can rely on dietary interventions that combine specific compositions and timed meals (Challet, 2014).

Enabling metabolic tissues to predict the supply and demanding of energy in the body is an advantage of the metabolic rhythms in question. Moreover, they ensure the optimization of both energy storage and usage. For this reason, it is believed that uncoupling the energy supply from its demand in every metabolic organ leads to impaired body energy metabolism in mammals. For a long time, both experimental and clinical research has asserted that disturved behavioral rhythms, including hunger/feeding or sleep/wake cycles, cause defects in lipid and glucose metabolism (Sato et al., 2018).

Our body is exposed by the function of a number of organs to oscillating inputs superimposing on the time of the day. As is understood, the circadian clock rhythms in our body are not only governed by the light/dark cycle. Especially the liver has a main role in maintaining energy homeostasis during storage, usage over the diurnal cycle, and coping with considerable temporal changes in energy income. Thus, the feeding and fasting cycle represents a more powerful zeitgeber for the liver clock in comparison with the systemic signals that the SCN controls (Damiola et al., 2000; Saini et al., 2013).

Energy metabolism can also affect the circadian clock, a process named entrainment. Therefore, there is a tight interconnection between energy metabolism and the circadian clock. The said interaction and its effects on health are not well comprehended. However, it is essential to avoid any kind of desynchronization between energy metabolism and the circadian clock in order to maintain health (Kessler et al., 2014).

Impact of Dietary Intake on Circadian Rhythms

The circadian clock aligns feeding and fasting periods with cycles of sleep and wakefulness in anticipation of the Earth's rotation (Cedernaes et al., 2019). There are a few underlying mechanisms to take into account concerning the significance of chrono-nutrition for metabolic health. First, changes in circadian rhythms affect the digestion and absorption of nutrients and energy metabolism with the main clock genes (BMAL-1, CLOCK, PER1/2, and CRY1/2). Second, the timing of meals influences the clock system output. For instance, when a person skips breakfast, the risk of obesity increases, whereas eating regularly reduces the risk of obesity. Third, sleep represents a significant determining factor of the inner body clock and is capable of mediating the impact through food intake. There is an association between reduced sleep and increased food intake, excess body weight, and poor diet quality, in addition to increased risks of chronic diseases, e.g., hypertension and diabetes (Pot, 2018). The correlation between metabolism and the circadian system is bidirectional in nature. The deterioration of the circadian system causes obesity and changes in the circadian rhythms because of metabolic abnormalities (Ferrari et al., 1990). For instance, obese individuals have lacks in typical daily rhythms of glucose and insulin sensitivity. It is thought that eating causes circadian desynchronization during abnormal circadian times and therefore sleep patterns occur. The increasing risk of some diseases, such as obesity, diabetes, and cancer, is associated with this situation (Patterson et al., 2015). It is believed that the central clock organizes peripheral clocks by neuronal and humoral signals. Additionally, the time asynchrony between the clocks causes unpredictable situations such as metabolic disorders, cancer, and psychiatric disorders (Albrecht, 2012).

Owing to the coordination of the oscillators, glucose homeostasis is tightly regulated in metabolic organs (Gachon et al., 2017; Reinke and Asher, 2016). While the liver excretes glucose in the resting phase, glucose is taken up by adipose tissue, skeletal muscle, and liver cells during the feeding or activity phase (Lamia et al., 2008). The fine-tuning of the blood glucose homeostasis is completed by the rhythmic secretion of insulin and glucagon from the pancreas and the incretin hormone GLP1 from the intestines during the day. At several levels, circadian oscillators control lipid and protein metabolism (Sinturel et al., 2020), cholesterol, detoxification pathways, and inflammatory responses (Keller et al., 2009; Loboda et al., 2009; Eckel-Mahan et al., 2013).

Many pieces of evidence suggest that the time of feeding affects obesity and metabolic state. For instance, body weights of mice fed a high-fat diet, their food intake and locomotor activity during the 12-hour circadian light phase or the 12-hour dark phase were measured throughout 6 weeks. It was found that mice fed a high-fat diet during only 12 hours of the light phase gained weight more than mice fed a high-fat diet during only the 12-hour dark phase (Arble et al., 2009). Obesity is induced by diets with a high-fat content, increasing the risk of metabolic diseases. However, obesity and metabolic diseases are suppressed by time-restricted feeding with a high-fat diet without a reduction in calories. There is a tight connection between circadian clocks and energy homeostasis in animals. They are impacted by the time of feeding and food composition/components (Oike et al., 2014).

Some articles show that in rodents, food availability, light, and feeding regimens represent the dominant external events that influence especially peripheral clocks (Hatori et al., 2012; Damiola et al., 2000). Furthermore, feeding with a calorically dense high-fat diet causes molecular and behavioral circadian rhythm alterations (Hatori et al., 2012; Kohsaka et al., 2007). Changes in clock oscillations are observed in numerous metabolic conditions, including type 2 diabetes, obesity, cardiovascular disease, and metabolic syndrome (Maury et al., 2010; Ando et al., 2009). Moreover, in general terms, some studies have shown that changes in the circadian clock occur simultaneously with different human pathologies, including metabolic, cardiovascular, and immune diseases and cancer (Stenvers et al., 2019; Mannic et al., 2013; Sinturel et al., 2019; Sadowski et al., 2018; Philippe and Dibner, 2015; Ditisheim et al., 2013; Gonzalez Rodriguez et al., 2012; Wefers et al., 2018). Studies on mice have demonstrated that many environmental factors, e.g., restriction of feeding during the inactive period, wheel-running exercise only at the beginning or at the end of the active period, and psychological and physical stress, influence the peripheral clock phase but not the central clock. Additionally, these studies on mice have defined cortisol and insulin as the primary entrainment factors when the peripheral clocks are influenced by exercise, feeding, and stress (Orihara et al., 2020).

Circadian Disruption and Disease

Obesity

Obesity is defined as the increased amount of adipose tissue. It is a frequently encountered chronic condition in developed and developing countries (Dina,

2008). Obesity represents a serious public health problem because it is related to diabetes, insulin resistance, hypertension, atherosclerosis, chronic kidney disease, and elevated cardiovascular morbidity and mortality (Reaven et al., 2004; Shamseddeen et al., 2011). Excessive fat accumulation is the result of hypertrophy and hyperplasia of white adipocytes within the framework of positive energy balance in white adipose tissue (WAT) or other organs. A complex circuitry of anorexigenic and orexigenic signals and an endogenous clock setting a circadian rhythm of appetite-satiety, which is a function considerably impacted by modern life habits, control this balance at the hypothalamic level. WAT is considered an active endocrine organ synthesizing and releasing multiple adipokines with a number of autocrine and paracrine functions. As a result, obesity is the consequence of a multifactorial combination of genetic background, endocrine, metabolic, inflammatory, and circadian dysfunctions, the maintenance of which in the long term is promoted by behavioral disorders (Pagano et al., 2017). Furthermore, there is an interaction between the disrupted circadian clock system because of light conditions, a high-fat diet, and gene deletion and the disruption of the metabolic system, which causes obesity (Orihara et al., 2020). The most important phenomenon regulating circadian processes is the light-dark cycle. Human circadian physiology has developed to support activities such as moving and feeding during the day, in addition to sleeping and not feeding at night (Bass and Takahashi, 2010).

Various studies on humans have demonstrated that obesity is associated with biological rhythm disorders, e.g., those that govern food intake and sleep (Orihara et al., 2020). Nowadays, the best-known epidemiological findings indicate that shift work and sleep disturbances are significantly related to dyslipidemia, obesity, and type 2 diabetes in people (Sato et al., 2018). The desynchronization between the central and peripheral clocks takes place because of the changed timing of food intake and the composition of the diet. The above-mentioned desynchronization can cause the uncoupling of peripheral clocks from the central pacemaker and metabolic disorders. There is a correlation between metabolic dysfunction and circadian disorders at the central and peripheral levels and the final disruption of the circadian clockwork may cause obesity. PPARα increases the transcriptional level of brain and muscle ARNT-like 1 (BMAL1) in individuals with obesity when the expression levels of CLOCK are elevated with obesity induced by a high-fat diet (Engin, 2017).

Physiological and cellular processes are coordinated and synchronized with daily cycles by the biological clock of the circadian timing system.

Feeding patterns are also regulated by circadian clocks. Adipocytokines and clock genes display circadian rhythmicity. The dysfunction of the above-mentioned genes plays a role in altering the said adipokines when obesity develops (Engin, 2017). The chronic advance of the light period caused an increase in appetite and a reduction in energy expenditure and metabolism, while encouraging considerable alterations in lipid metabolism, neuropeptides, and inflammation in rats. The research conducted previously has indicated that the impacts of a high-fat diet on biological rhythm are caused by the impaired clock gene and clock-controlled gene expression rhythm, which may result from the impaired food intake rhythm. It has been displayed that feeding with a high-fat diet changes the clock gene phase and the clock-controlled gene expression rhythm in numerous peripheral organs, impairs the phosphorylation rhythms of the metabolic regulators CREB and S6, disturbs CLOCK:BMAL1 recruitment, and encourages the activation of pathways via the transcriptional regulator PPARγ (Orihara et al., 2020).

An increasing number of evidence indicates that genetic changes in circadian genes impact metabolic parameters in people. Several genome-wide association studies (GWAS) have revealed connections between polymorphisms in the CLOCK gene and susceptibility to obesity, hypertension, and metabolic syndrome. Moreover, there is a correlation between single-nucleotide polymorphisms (SNPs) in CLOCK and elevated ghrelin concentrations in plasma, changed eating behaviors, and short sleep duration, causing higher total energy intake, reduced compliance with prescribed diet plans, and, finally, resistance to weight loss. According to case-control studies, a relationship has been revealed between the severity and incidence of nonalcoholic fatty liver disease (NAFLD) and common genetic variations of CLOCK (Marcheva et al., 2013). The ablation of the PER or CRY genes in mice causes opposite phenotypes of energy expenditure, body composition, and body weight because of a differential disruption of central melanocortin signaling mediated by leptin, but not leptin expression in white adipose tissue. The disruption of the SCN clock because of chronic jet lag causes changes in energy balance in both PER and CRY mutants. However, such shifts are not observed in BMAL1-null mice insensitive to alterations in environmental light cues. The peripheral clock is disrupted in a similar way and leptin is deregulated in fat in PER- and CRY-mutant mice. However, such mice display the opposite body weight and composition phenotypes associated with their distinct patterns of POMC neuron deregulation in the arcuate nucleus (Kettner et al., 2015). While PER2 polymorphisms have also been associated with abdominal obesity, hyperglycemia, and unhealthy feeding behavior phenotypes, the PER2 mRNA expression can also be related to metabolic markers in people (Marcheva et al., 2013).

Many hormones in metabolism, including glucagon, insulin, corticosterone, adiponectin, ghrelin, and leptin, display circadian oscillations, and disrupted circadian rhythms play a role in developing cancer, obesity, and metabolic syndrome (Froy, 2007). A study found that subjects with short duration of sleep had decreased leptin and increased ghrelin levels, and the mentioned differences in ghrelin and leptin can possibly lead to increased appetite, which probably explains the increased body mass index with short duration of sleep (Taheri et al., 2004). Nutrition at an inappropriate circadian time causes adverse health effects (Mattson et al., 2014). A study showed that the time of meal consumption impacts the thermogenic response and should be taken into account in the energy balance (Romon et al., 1993).

Diabetes

Type 2 diabetes (T2D) is a health problem concerning the whole world. The prevalence of obesity and T2D is considerably higher in employees who work in shifts compared to those who work regular hours. A widely accepted hypothesis states that the elevated risk of metabolic health problems results from eating behavior with abnormal timing, i.e., eating not synchronously with the biological clock. The biological clock represents part of the internal circadian timing system. The feeding/fasting and sleep/wake cycles and numerous metabolic processes in the body, such as the timing of eating behavior and processes that take part in glucose homeostasis, are controlled by the biological clock. Research on rodents has demonstrated that desynchronization between rhythms of the central and peripheral clock systems and between rhythms of various tissue clocks (such as muscle and liver clocks) occurs because eating is not synchronous with the endogenous clock (Oosterman et al., 2020). For example, pancreas-specific BMAL1 knockout (KO) mice develop diabetes because of the disrupted insulin secretion since the circadian clock in pancreatic β cells is involved in insulin exocytosis. A study showed that glucose uptake and metabolism are controlled by the muscle clock and daily gluconeogenesis rhythms and fasting glucose levels are regulated by the hepatic clock by utilizing muscle- and liver-specific BMAL1 KO mice, respectively (Hasan et al., 2021). Epidemiological research has demonstrated that employees working in shifts are at increased risk of developing obesity and pathologies associated with obesity, such as T2D, possibly because they eat asynchronously with the endogenous biological clock. A hypothesis can be established, indicating that asynchrony between various organs plays a significant part in T2D etiology since the aforesaid circadian misalignment will lead to a mismatch of glucose and lipid fluxes between different organs. Under other conditions, the disruption of tissue clocks can probably lead to tissue-level insulin resistance. However, the precise mechanisms underlying metabolic disturbances that are caused by disrupted circadian rhythms have still not been elucidated (Oosterman et al., 2020).

Insulin secretion estimates the body's upcoming glucose metabolism in humans and peaks in the early morning hours. Thus, the central clock prepares individuals for the next activity period through two different mechanisms. These mechanisms increase the glucose concentration in plasma and make tissues more sensitive to glucose demand (Fleur et al., 2001). Glucose tolerance is observed to be lower in the evening and at night than in the morning. A study showed that the circadian system makes a significant contribution to decreased glucose tolerance in the evening in comparison with the morning. Moreover, glucose tolerance is reduced by circadian misalignment, providing a mechanism that helps to explain the elevated risk of diabetes in employees working shifts (Morris et al., 2015). Furthermore, specifically in pancreatic islet cells, the elimination of CLOCK or BMAL1 results in decreased glucose tolerance, disrupted insulin secretion, and a change in the proliferation and size of islet cells (Marcheva et al., 2010). In humans, CLOCK's genetic variants and BMAL1 are related to susceptibility to obesity and T2D, respectively (Sookoian et al., 2008). A study showed that the β-cell clock plays a role in the coordination of insulin secretion with the sleep-wake cycle and demonstrated that the diabetes mellitus onset can be triggered by the ablation of the pancreatic clock (Marcheva et al., 2010). Additionally, the timing and amplitude of the clock in different organ systems can be disturbed by metabolic disease and obesity, which further worsens the progression of the disease. There is a correlation between decreased melatonin levels and mutations and/or genetic polymorphisms of melatonin receptors and an elevated risk of T2D (Forrestel et al., 2017). Furthermore, genetic variants in BMAL1 are associated with hypertension and T2D, and SNPs at loci in or near CRY2 are related to fasting glucose concentrations. A rare variant of NAMPT1, which is a gene playing a role in a clock negative feedback loop, is related to protecting against obesity (Marcheva et al., 2013).

Light is associated with different complicated mechanisms, including the circadian system synchronization. Melatonin is regarded to be the classical phase marker for assessing the mammalian biological clock timing. Daily rhythms in concentrations of hormones, including glucagon, insulin, and corticosterone, and enzymes that take part in glucose and lipid metabolism, e.g., glucose-6-phosphate dehydrogenase, are directed by the SCN. Thus, endocrine imbalances and the incidence of obesity and T2D can manifest impaired circadian coordination, which raises a controversial question of whether exposure to abnormal light can affect metabolism by altering the timing of the circadian system. Some researchers showed the melatonin-induced inhibition of insulin secretion through cyclic adenosine monophosphate (cAMP) and cyclic guanine monophosphate (cGMP) and the existence of melatonin receptors 1 (MT1) and 2 (MT2) in pancreatic tissues of humans and rats. Additionally, acute melatonin administration in healthy females in the morning and evening has been shown to disrupt glucose tolerance. The impact of administering melatonin on lipid metabolism has been shown in experimental animals and humans (Albreiki et al., 2017). The advent of electricity and artificial lighting over the last 60 years has ensured that our behavioral cycles have become independent of external sunlight patterns, which has caused an equivalent increase in sleep deprivation of approximately 1 hour per night and circadian misalignment (i.e., living against the clock). According to evidence from experimental animals and controlled human subjects, it is possible that both circadian misalignment and sleep deprivation lead in a direct manner to metabolic dysfunction, inducing diabetes (Parameswaran and Ray, 2022). Experimental studies have demonstrated that sleep restriction reduces glucose tolerance and compromises insulin sensitivity. Sleep restriction in normal individuals causes insulin responses to hyperglycemia characteristic of insulin resistance and a prediabetic metabolic state (Gangwisch, 2009). Numerous pieces of evidence have shown that sleep disturbances, including poor sleep quality and short sleep duration, are associated with the risk of obesity and diabetes, in addition to glycemic control in patients with T2D (Reutrakul et al., 2013). Non-esterified fatty acid (NEFA) levels in plasma were determined to be considerably higher before meals in dim light in comparison with bright light. In another study on healthy individuals, elevated plasma glucose levels were observed when they were awake at night under bright light (Albreiki et al., 2017). The function of various metabolic processes, involving the synthesis and breakdown of carbohydrates, proteins, and lipids, changes during the sleep/wake cycle in mammals. For example, whereas glycogen synthesis occurs during the waking period in the muscle and liver, glycogenolysis peaks in the liver during sleep. Furthermore, an increase in the activity of lipoprotein lipase, promoting lipid absorption from the bloodstream into tissues, takes place in the state of satiety (i.e., wakefulness) (Sato et al., 2018).

An increase occurs in cardiovascular diseases, diabetes, and body weight with increasing age. There is evidence for anatomical variations in circadian pacemaker neurons in the brain and alterations in the timing of circadian gene expression in the paraventricular nucleus (PVN), which is the hypothalamus region essential for integrating metabolic signals, in addition to the output of the autonomic nervous system (Laposky et al., 2008).

Insulin Resistance

Insulin resistance represents a broad term that encompasses all conditions displaying an impaired response to the hormone insulin in its target tissues. Its prevalence increases steadily, with approximately 500 million adults affected by type 2 diabetes in the world in 2021 (Catalano et al., 2023). Insulin resistance is a key feature for coronary artery disease, type 2 diabetes, and hypertension (Kadowaki et al., 2006). Insulin resistance primarily determines the development of type 2 diabetes mellitus. It is the main reason for mortality and morbidity. The circadian timing system coordinates numerous daily processes, such as the daily rhythm in the human metabolism of glucose. Whereas whole-body insulin sensitivity, food intake, and energy expenditure are regulated by the central clock, the actions mentioned above are further fine-tuned by local peripheral clocks (Stenvers et al., 2019). Glucose homeostasis demonstrates circadian rhythmicity in healthy subjects. Prior to the feeding/active period in the morning, insulin sensitivity and fasting insulin levels are higher, and the beginning phase of insulin secretion is improved in comparison with the evening prior to the fast/inactive period. The desynchronization of central and peripheral clocks is related to an elevated incidence of insulin resistance and associated diseases (Catalano et al., 2023). In Han Chinese women, the genetic polymorphisms rs2119882 in MTNR1A and rs10830963 in MTNR1B are related to an elevated risk of gestational diabetes mellitus and insulin resistance (Li et al., 2013). Due to genetic, behavioral, or environmental factors, the misalignment between various components of the circadian timing system and the daily rhythms of sleep-wake behavior or food intake can make an essential contribution to insulin resistance (Stenvers et al., 2019).

In healthy individuals, insulin resistance is induced in multiple metabolic pathways by partial sleep deprivation during a single night. The physiological observation mentioned above may be related to changes in glucoregulation in subjects with type 1 and type 2 diabetes (Donga et al., 2010). Moreover, a connection between clock-regulated sleep and insulin resistance/type 2 diabetes is the relationship between short sleep duration (because of insomnia and/or circadian disturbance) and the risk of diabetes and obesity (Shi et al., 2013). In a controlled laboratory environment, temporary circadian misalignment, which is similar to that taking place during jet lag or chronically during working in shifts, causes reduced glucose tolerance and insulin sensitivity, increased mean arterial pressure, decreased leptin levels, decreased sleep efficiency, and the completely reversed cortisol profile. At the beginning of the sleep period, abnormally high cortisol levels have been suggested to make a contribution to insulin resistance and hyperglycemia. It has been shown that circadian misalignment influences postprandial glucose at a higher rate compared to fasting glucose levels, proposing that misalignment influences muscle/fat metabolism or the function of β-cell more in comparison with hepatic gluconeogenesis. Short-term misalignment research revealed that endogenous glucose generation that is measured with a two-step hyperinsulinemic-euglycemic clamp was unaffected. Conversely, muscle insulin sensitivity decreased through circadian misalignment, indicating that actually the glucose uptake process, not the production of glucose, was disturbed in the course of the misalignment (Oosterman et al., 2020).

The circadian system is cyclically regulated by many hormones, such as orexin, leptin, cortisol, glucagon, catecholamines, growth hormone, and melatonin, modulating glucose homeostasis, insulin secretion, and feeding (Shi et al., 2013). Adiponectin represents an adipokine with a role in lipid and glucose metabolism. It increases fatty acid oxidation and potentiates insulin inhibition of hepatic gluconeogenesis, encouraging insulin sensitivity. Additionally, peroxisome proliferator-activated receptor γ (PPARγ) and its co-activator PPARγ co-activator 1α (PGC1α), the expression of which is under the control of the circadian clock, mediate the expression of adiponectin (Barnea et al., 2015).

Furthermore, adiponectin exhibits insulin-sensitizing impacts through binding to its receptors, which activates AMPK, PPAR-α, and possibly other not known. molecular pathways Both adiponectin and adiponectin receptors are downregulated in insulin resistance (obesity-linked), causing the activation of signaling pathways taking part in the regulation of metabolism. Up-regulating adiponectin/adiponectin receptors or improving the function of adiponectin receptors may be an interesting therapeutic strategy for obesity-linked insulin resistance (Caselli, 2014).

Other Diseases

Cancer is the clonal spread of cells with impaired growth characteristics. It is the most common and complicated somatic genetic disease (Futreal et al.,

2001). Today, molecular pathways have gained great importance in cancer diagnosis and treatment. Regulatory mechanisms, including the circadian clock, have been found to affect the development of cancer (Lévi, 2001; Ishida, 2007). Biological pathways are under circadian control, such as the cell cycle, tumor suppression, and response to DNA damage (Shostak, 2017). Animal models and molecular studies have demonstrated a connection between cancer metabolism and the circadian clock (Masri and Sassone-Corsi, 2018). Gene products of the circadian clock have roles as negative regulators in cancer formation, and expressions of some clock genes alter in various cancer types (Lévi, 2001; Gery et al., 2006; Walisser and Bradfield, 2006; Beckett and Roden, 2009; Pogue-Geile et al., 2006). Epidemiologic research has demonstrated that working in shifts is related to health problems involving coronary heart disease, peptic ulcer disease, and metabolic syndrome, in addition to particular cancer types (Reutrakul et al., 2013).

It is emphasized that the elevated risk of numerous diseases, such as dysplasia, carcinoma, neurodegenerative diseases, and metabolic disorders, is related to circadian disorders. It is thought that physiological processes, e.g., cell proliferation, differentiation, inflammation, oxidative stress, cellular metabolism, and synthesis regulating the circadian clock, may be some of the responsible mechanisms (Xie et al., 2019). First, CLOCK genes make a contribution to the formation and development of tumors as a result of regulating and interfering with cell cycle-related genes, e.g., P21 and P53 (Angelousi et al., 2018). Moreover, the suppression of the core clock protein BMAL1 has been found to be closely associated with tumorigenesis (Tang et al., 2017). Additionally, other studies have shown that the levels of neurohormones that play a role in cardiovascular function, e.g., renin, angiotensin II, aldosterone, atrial natriuretic peptide, and growth hormone, are regulated by the circadian clock (Bhatnagar, 2017). The neurohormones in question can play a role in elevated blood pressure and inflammation as a reaction to circadian misalignment (Xie et al., 2019).

Time signals for activities in our bodies are provided by circadian clocks, which also ensure the synchronization of metabolic reactions with the expected activity cycles. In this way, the synchronization of metabolism and behaviors by the clock maintains the internal homeostasis and energy supply (Wang et al., 2011). Unfortunately, increased night activities, such as overtime work, shift work, eating at night, sleep disturbances, and deprivation, characterize modern life (Feng and Lazar, 2012). Insomnia resulting from shift work causes excessive sleepiness and loss of functionality, which is a kind of circadian rhythm disorder (Owens et al., 2016). Studies show that employees working in shifts are at a higher risk of metabolic diseases, such as diabetes, obesity, cardiovascular diseases, and metabolic syndromes (Wang et al., 2011).

Jet lag is the travel between different time zones. Accordingly, the discrepancy between the internal clock and the light/dark cycle at the destination may cause some problems. The person's biological clock may cause difficulties in adapting to the geographical time of the country of destination, the difference between day and night, sleep patterns, eating, and working hours. These people may experience insomnia, fatigue, anorexia, bowel disorders, impaired perception of time and distance, the prolongation of reaction time, judgment and memory defects, blurred vision, bodily pain, and sweating (Chassard et al., 2005).

Conclusion

An increasing number of proofs show that the proper functioning of the peripheral and central clocks is crucial for the well-being of the organism. A deeper understanding of the role of the molecular clock in regulating daily physiological processes will ensure the development of novel treatments, more effective therapeutic delivery, and enhanced preventive strategies for the management of obesity, diabetes, and other metabolic disorders (Marcheva et al., 2013).

References

Albrecht, U. (2012). Timing to perfection: the biology of central and peripheral circadian clocks. *Neuron.*, 74(2), 246-60. https://doi.org/10.1016/j.neuron.2012.04.006.

Albreiki, M. S., Middleton, B. & Hampton, S. M. (2017). A single night light exposure acutely alters hormonal and metabolic responses in healthy participants. *Endocrine Connections.,* 6(2), 100-10. https://doi.org/10.1530/EC-16-0097.

Ando, H., Takamura, T., Matsuzawa-Nagata, N., Shima, K. R., Eto, T., Misu, H., Shiramoto, M., Tsuru, T., Irie, S., Fujimura, A & Kaneko, S. (2009). Clock gene expression in peripheral leucocytes of patients with type 2 diabetes. *Diabetologia,* 52, 329–335. https://doi.org/10.1007/s00125-008-1194-6.

Angelousi, A., Kassi, E., Nasiri-Ansari, N., Weickert, M. O., Randeva, H. & Kaltsas, G. (2018). Clock genes alterations and endocrine disorders. *European Journal of Clinical Investigation,* 48(6), e12927. https://doi.org/10.1111/eci.12927.

Arble, D. M., Bass, J., Laposky, A. D., Vitaterna, M. H. & Turek, F. W. (2009). Circadian timing of food intake contributes to weight gain. *Obesity*, *17*(11), 2100-2102. https://doi.org/10.1038/oby.2009.264.

Asher, G. & Schibler, U. (2011). Crosstalk between components of circadian and metabolic cycles in mammals. *Cell Metab*, 13(2), 125-37. https://doi.org/10.1016/j.cmet.2011.01.006.

Asher, G. & Sassone-Corsi, P. (2015). Time for Food: The Intimate Interplay between Nutrition, Metabolism, and the Circadian Clock. *Cell*, 161(1), 84-92. https://doi.org/10.1016/j.cell.2015.03.015.

Azmi, N. A. S. M., Juliana, N., Azmani, S., Effendy, N., M., Abu, I. F., Teng, N. I. M. F & Das, S. (2021). Cortisol on Circadian Rhythm and Its Effect on Cardiovascular System. *Int. J. Environ. Res. Public Health, 18*(2), 676. https://doi.org/10.3390/ijerph18020676.

Balsalobre, A., Damiola, F. & Schibler, U. (1998). A serum shock induces circadian gene expression in mammalian tissue culture cells. *Cell*, 93(6), 929-937. https://doi.org/10.1016/S0092-8674(00)81199-X.

Barnea, M., Chapnik, N., Genzer, Y. & Froy, O. (2015). The circadian clock machinery controls adiponectin expression. *Molecular and cellular endocrinology*, *399*, 284-287. https://doi.org/10.1016/j.mce.2014.10.018.

Bass, J. & Takahashi, J.S. (2010). Circadian integration of metabolism and energetics. *Science,* 330 (6009), 1349– 54. https://doi.org/10.1126/science.1195027.

Beckett, M. & Roden, L. C. (2009). Mechanisms by which circadian rhythm disruption may lead to cancer. *South African Journal of Science*, 105(11), 415-420. https://doi.org/10.10520/EJC96860.

Bhatnagar, A. (2017). Environmental determinants of cardiovascular disease. *Circulation Research*., 121(2), 162-80. https://doi.org/10.1161/CIRCRESAHA.117.306458.

Bilski, J., Jaworek, J., Pokorsk, J., Nitecki, J., Nitecka, E., Pokorska, J., Mazur-Bialy, A. & Szklarczyk, J. (2016). Effects of time of day and the wingate test on appetite perceptions, food intake and plasma levels of adipokines. *Journal of Physiology and Pharmacology*, 67 (5), 667-676.

Bollinger, T. & Schibler, U. (2014). Circadian rhythms - from genes to physiology and disease. *Swiss Med Wkly*, 144:w13984 (2930). https://doi.org/10.4414/smw.2014.13984.

Bouret, S. G., Draper, S. J. & Simerly, R. B. (2004). Formation of Projection Pathways from the Arcuate Nucleus of the Hypothalamus to Hypothalamic Regions Implicated in the Neural Control of Feeding Behavior in Mice. *Journal of Neuroscience,* 24 (11), 2797-2805. https://doi.org/10.1523/JNEUROSCI.5369-03.2004.

Cantó, C., Jiang, L. Q., Deshmukh, A. S., Mataki, C., Coste, A., Lagouge, M., Zierath, J. R. & Auwerx, J. (2010). Interdependence of AMPK and SIRT1 for metabolic adaptation to fasting and exercise in skeletal muscle. *Cell metabolism,* 11(3), 213-9. https://doi.org/10.1016/j.cmet.2010.02.006.

Caselli, C. (2014). Role of adiponectin system in insulin resistance. *Molecular genetics and metabolism,* 113(3), 155-160. https://doi.org/10.1016/j.ymgme.2014.09.003.

Catalano, F., Vito, F. D., Cassano, V., Fiorentino, T. V., Sciacqua, A. & Hribal, M. L. (2023). Circadian Clock Desynchronization and Insulin Resistance. Int. J. Environ. Res. Public Health, 20(1), 29. https://doi.org/10.3390/ijerph20010029.

Cedernaes, J., Huang, W., Ramsey, K. M., Waldeck, N., Cheng, L., Marcheva, B., Omura, C., Kobayashi, Y., Peek, C. B., Levine, D. C., Dhir, R., Awatramani, R., Bradfield, C. A., Wang, X. A., Takahashi, J. S., Mokadem, M., Ahima, R. S. & Bassl, J. (2019). Transcriptional Basis for Rhythmic Control of Hunger and Metabolism within the AgRP Neuron. *Cell Metabolism*, 29, 1078–1091. https://doi.org/10.1016/j.cmet.2019.01.023.

Challet, E. (2013). Circadian clocks, food intake, and metabolism. In M. U. Gillette (Eds.), *Chronobiology: Biological Timing in Health and Disease* (pp 105-135). Progress in molecular biology and translational science. https://doi.org/10.1016/B978-0-12-396971-2.00005-1.

Challet, E. (2014). Circadian clocks and energy metabolism in rodents. *Biol Aujourdhui*, 208(4), 269-74. https://doi.org/10.1051/jbio/2015002.

Challet, E. (2015). Keeping circadian time with hormones. *Diabetes, Obesity and Metabolism,* 17(S1), 76-83. https://doi.org/10.1111/dom.12516.

Chassard, D., Allaouchiche, B. & Boselli, E. (2005). Timing is everything: the pendulum swings on. *The Journal of the American Society of Anesthesiologists*, *103*(3), 454-456. https://doi.org/10.1097/00000542-200509000-00004.

Chen, L. & Yang, G. (2014). PPARs Integrate the Mammalian Clock and Energy Metabolism. *PPAR Research*, 2014 (Article ID 653017). https://doi.org/10.1155/2014/653017.

Choe, S. S., Huh, J. Y., Hwang, I. J., Kim, J. I. & Kim, J. B. (2016). Adipose Tissue Remodeling: Its Role in Energy Metabolism and Metabolic Disorders. *Frontiers in endocrinology*, 7, 30. https://doi.org/10.3389/fendo.2016.00030.

Damiola, F., Le Minh, N., Preitner, N., Kornmann, B., Fleury-Olela, F. & Schibler, U. (2000). Restricted feeding uncouples circadian oscillators in peripheral tissues from the central pacemaker in the suprachiasmatic nucleus. *Genes & Dev.*, 14 (23), 2950 – 2961. https://doi.org/10.1101/gad.183500.

Dibner, C., Schibler, U. & Albrecht, U. (2010). The mammalian circadian timing system: organization and coordination of central and peripheral clocks. *Annu Rev Physiol.,* 72, 517- 549. https://doi.org/10.1146/annurev-physiol-021909-135821.

Dina, C. (2008). New insights into the genetics of body weight. *Curr Opin Clin Nutr Metab Care*, 11 (4), 378-384. https://doi.org/10.1097/MCO.0b013e328303e5e6.

Ditisheim, A. J., Dibner, C., Philippe, J. & Pechere-Bertschi, A. (2013). Biological rhythms and preeclampsia. *Front Endocrinol (Lausanne),* 4, 47. https://doi.org/10.3389/fendo.2013.00047.

Donga, E., van Dijk, M., van Dijk, J. G., Biermasz, N. R., Lammers, G-J., van Kralingen, K. W., Corssmit, E. P. M. & Romijn, J. A. (2010). A single night of partial sleep deprivation induces insulin resistance in multiple metabolic pathways in healthy subjects. *The Journal of Clinical Endocrinology & Metabolism, 95*(6), 2963-2968. https://doi.org/10.1210/jc.2009-2430.

Eckel-Mahan, K. & Sassone-Corsi, P. (2009). Metabolism control by the circadian clock and vice versa. *Nature Structural & Molecular Biology*, 16, 462–467. https://doi.org/10.1038/nsmb.1595.

Eckel-Mahan, K. L., Patel, V. R., deMateo, S., Orozco-Solis, R., Ceglia, N. J., Sahar, S., Dilag-Penilla, S. A., Dyar, K. A., Baldi, P. & Sassone-Corsi, P. (2013). Reprogramming of the circadian clock by nutritional challenge. *Cell,* 155(7), 1464 – 1478. https://doi.org/10.1016/j.cell.2013.11.034.

Engin, A. (2017). Circadian Rhythms in Diet-Induced Obesity. In A.B. Engin & A. Engin (Eds.), *Obesity and Lipotoxicity* (pp.19-52). Advances in Experimental Medicine and Biology (Springer). https://doi.org/10.1007/978-3-319-48382-5_2.

Feng, D. & Lazar, M. A. (2012). Clocks, Metabolism, and the Epigenome. *Molecular Cell*, 47 (2), 158-167. https://doi.org/10.1016/j.molcel.2012.06.026.

Ferrari, E., Fraschini, F. & Brambilla, F. (1990). Hormonal circadian rhythms in eating disorders. *Biol Psychiatry,* 27(9), 1007–1020. https://doi.org/10.1016/0006-3223(90)90037-3.

Firsov, D., Tokonami, N. & Bonny, O. (2012). Role of the renal circadian timing system in maintaining water and electrolytes homeostasis. *Mol Cell Endocrinol,* 349(1), 51-5. https://doi.org/10.1016/j.mce.2011.06.037.

Fleur, S. E. L., Kalsbeek, A., Wortel, J., Fekkes, M. L. & Buijs, R. M. (2001). A daily rhythm in glucose tolerance: a role for the suprachiasmatic nucleus. *Diabetes*, 50(6), 1237-43. https://doi.org/10.2337/diabetes.50.6.1237.

Forrestel, A. C., Miedlich, S. U., Yurcheshen, M., Wittlin, S. D. & Sellix, M. T. (2017). Chronomedicine and type 2 diabetes: shining some light on melatonin. *Diabetologia*, 60, 808–822. https://doi.org/10.1007/s00125-016-4175-1.

Froy, O. (2007). The relationship between nutrition and circadian rhythms in mammals. *Front Neuroendocrinol,* 28(2-3), 61-71. https://doi.org/10.1016/j.yfrne.2007.03.001.

Froy, O. (2010). Metabolism and Circadian Rhythms—Implications for Obesity. *Endocrine Reviews*, 31(1), 1–24. https://doi.org/10.1210/er.2009-0014.

Futreal, P. A., Kasprzyk, A., Birney, E., Mullikin, J. C., Wooster, R. & Stratton, M. (2001). Cancer and genomics. *Nature*, 409, 850-2. https://doi.org/10.1038/35057046.

Gachon, F., Loizides-Mangold, U., Petrenko, V. & Dibner, C. (2017). Glucose Homeostasis: Regulation by Peripheral Circadian Clocks in Rodents and Humans. *Endocrinology,* 158 (5), 1074-1084. https://doi.org/10.1210/en.2017-00218.

Gamble, K. L., Berry, R., Frank, S. J. & Young M. E. (2014). Circadian clock control of endocrine factors. *Nature Reviews Endocrinology,* 10 (8), 466-475. https://doi.org/10.1038/nrendo.2014.78.

Gangwisch, J. E. (2009). Epidemiological evidence for the links between sleep, circadian rhythms and metabolism. *Obesity reviews*, *10(2)*, 37-45. https://doi.org/10.1111/j.1467-789X.2009.00663.x.

Gery, S., Komatsu, N., Baldjyan, L., Yu, A., Koo, D. & Koeffler, H. P. (2006). The circadian gene per1 plays an important role in cell growth and DNA damage control in human cancer cells. *Mol Cell,* 22(3), 375-382. https://doi.org/10.1016/j.molcel.2006.03.038.

Gonzalez Rodriguez, E., Hernandez, A., Dibner, C., Koehler Ballan, B., Pechère-Bertschi, A. (2012). Arterial blood pressure circadian rhythm: significance and clinical implications. *Rev Med Suisse*, 8(353), 1709-12, 1714-5.

Green, C. B., Takahashi, J. S. & Bass, J. (2008). The meter of metabolism. Cell, 134(5), 728-42. https://doi.org/10.1016/j.cell.2008.08.022.

Guan, D. & Lazar, M. A. (2021). Interconnections between circadian clocks and metabolism. *J clin Invest,* 131(15), e148278. https://doi.org/10.1172/JCI148278.

Hannibal, J., Moller, M., Ottersen, O. P. & Fahrenkrug, J. (2000). PACAP and glutamate are co-stored in the retinohypothalamic tract. *Journal of Comparative Neurology*, 418 (2), 147-155. https://doi.org/10.1002/(SICI)1096-9861(20000306)418:2<147::AID-CNE2>3.0.CO;2-%23.

Hasan, N., Nagata, N., Morishige, J. I., Islam, Md. T., Jing, Z., Harada, K. I., Mieda, M., Ono, M., Fujiwara, H., Daikoku, T., Fujiwara, T., Maida, Y., Ota, T., Shimba, S., Kaneko, S., Fujimura, A. & Ando, H. (2021). Brown adipocyte-specific knockout of Bmal1 causes mild but significant thermogenesis impairment in mice. *Molecular metabolism,* 49, 101202. https://doi.org/10.1016/j.molmet.2021.101202.

Hatori, M., Vollmers, C., Zarrinpar, A., DiTacchio, L., Bushong, E. A., Gill, S., Leblanc, M., Chaix, A., Joens, M., Fitzpatrick, J. A. J., Ellisman, M. H. & Panda, S. (2012). Time-restricted feeding without reducing caloric intake prevents metabolic diseases in mice fed a high-fat diet. *Cell metabolism, 15*(6), 848-860. https://doi.org/10.1016/j.cmet.2012.04.019.

Hurtado-Carneiro, V., Roncero, I., Egger, S. S., Wenger, R. H., Blazquez, E., Sanz, C. & Alvarez, E. (2014). PAS kinase is a nutrient and energy sensor in hypothalamic areas required for the normal function of AMPK and mTOR/S6K1. *Molecular Neurobiology,* 50(2), 314-26. https://doi.org/10.1007/s12035-013-8630-4.

Hussain, M. M. & Pan, X. (2009). Clock genes, intestinal transport and plasma lipid homeostasis. *Trends Endocrin Met,* 20(4), 177-185. https://doi.org/10.1016/j.tem.2009.01.001.

Ishida, N. (2007). Circadian clock, cancer and lipid metabolism. *Neurosci Res.,* 57(4), 483-90. https://doi.org/10.1016/j.neures.2006.12.012.

Izumo, M., Sato, T. R., Straume, M. & Johnson, C. H. (2006). Quantitative analyses of circadian gene expression in mammalian cell cultures. *PLoS Comput Biol.*, 2(10), e136. https://doi.org/10.1371/journal.pcbi.0020136.

Kadowaki, T., Yamauchi, T., Kubota, N., Hara, K., Ueki, K. & Tobe, K. (2006). Adiponectin and adiponectin receptors in insulin resistance, diabetes, and the metabolic syndrome. *J Clin Invest.,* 116(7), 1784-1792. https://doi.org/10.1172/JCI29126.

Kalsbeek, A., Fleur, S. L. & Fliers, E. (2014). Circadian control of glucose metabolism. *Molecular Metabolism*, 3(4), 372-383. https://doi.org/10.1016/j.molmet.2014.03.002.

Keller, M., Mazuch, J., Abraham, U., Eom, G. D., Herzog, E. D., Volk, H. D., Kramer, A. & Maier, B. (2009). A Circadian clock in macrophages controls inflammatory immune responses. *Proc Natl Acad Sci USA,* 106(50), 21407–21412. https://doi.org/10.1073/pnas.0906361106.

Kessler, K., Pivovarova, O. & Pfeiffer, A. F. H. (2014). Circadian clocks and energy metabolism: implications for health. *Dtsch Med Wochenschr*, 139(14), 684-686. https://doi.org/10.1055/s-0034-1369875.

Kettner, N. M., Mayo, S. A., Hua, J., Lee, C., Moore, D. D. & Fu, L. (2015). Circadian Dysfunction Induces Leptin Resistance in Mice. *Cell Metabolism,* 22(3), 448–459. http://dx.doi.org/10.1016/j.cmet.2015.06.005.

Kitada, M., Kume, S., Kanasaki, K., Takeda-Watanabe, A. & Koya, D. (2013). Sirtuins as Possible Drug Targets in Type 2 Diabetes. *Current Drug Targets*, 14(6), 622-636. https://doi.org/10.2174/1389450111314060002.

Kohsaka, A., Laposky, A. D., Ramsey, K. M., Estrada, C., Joshu, C., Kobayashi, Y., Turek, F. W. & Bass, J. (2007). High-fat diet disrupts behavioral and molecular circadian rhythms in mice. *Cell Metab.*, 6(5), 414 – 421. https://doi.org/10.1016/j.cmet.2007.09.006.

Kondratov, R. V., Gorbacheva, V. Y. & Antoch, M. P. (2007). The role of mammalian circadian proteins in normal physiology and genotoxic stress responses. *Current topics in developmental biology*, 78, 173-216. https://doi.org/10.1016/S0070-2153(06)78005-X.

Kopera, H. (1985). The history of anabolic steroids and a review of clinical experience with anabolic steroids. *Acta Endocrinologica (Norway)*, 110(3), S11-S18. https://doi.org/10.1530/acta.0.109S00011.

Lamia, K. A., Storch, K-F., & Weitz, C. J. (2008). Physiological significance of a peripheral tissue circadian clock. *Pnas*, *105*(39), 15172-15177. https://doi.org/10.1073/pnas.0806717105.

Lammert, A., Kiess, W., Bottner, A., Glasow, A. & Kratzsch, J. (2001). Soluble leptin receptor represents the main leptin binding activity in human blood. *Biochemical and biophysical research communications,* 283(4), 982-988. https://doi.org/10.1006/bbrc.2001.4885.

Laposky, A. D., Bass, J., Kohsaka, A., & Turek, F. W. (2008). Sleep and circadian rhythms: key components in the regulation of energy metabolism. *FEBS letters*, *582*(1), 142-151. https://doi.org/10.1016/j.febslet.2007.06.079.

Lee, Y., Kim, E. K. (2013). AMP-activated protein kinase as a key molecular link between metabolism and clockwork. Experimental & Molecular Medicine. 45(7), e33-e. https://doi.org/10.1038/emm.2013.65.

Lévi, F. (2001). Circadian chronotherapy for human cancers. *Lancet Oncol.,* 2(5), 307-15. https://doi.org/10.1016/S1470-2045(00)00326-0.

Li, C., Qiao, B., Zhan, Y., Peng, W., Chen, Z. J., Sun, L., Zhang, J., Zhao, L. & Gao, Q. (2013). Association between Genetic Variations in MTNR1A and MTNR1B Genes and Gestational Diabetes Mellitus in Han Chinese Women. *Gynecol Obstet Invest,* 76 (4), 221–227. https://doi.org/10.1159/000355521.

Loboda, A., Kraft, W. K., Fine, B., Joseph, J., Nebozhyn, M., Zhang, C., He, Y., Yang, X., Wright, C., Morris, M., Chalikonda, I., Ferguson, M., Emilsson, V., Leonardson, A., Lamb, J., Dai, H., Schadt, E., Greenberg, H. E. & Lum, P. Y. (2009). Diurnal variation of the human adipose transcriptome and the link to metabolic disease. *BMC Med Genomics,* 2,7. https://doi.org/10.1186/1755-8794-2-7.

Lowrey, P. L. & Takahashi, J. S. (2004). Mammalian circadian biology: elucidating genome-wide levels of temporal organization. *Annu Rev Genomics Hum Genet,* 5, 407-441. https://doi.org/10.1146/annurev.genom.5.061903.175925.

Mannic, T., Meyer, P., Triponez, F., Pusztaszeri, M., Le Martelot, G., Mariani, O., Schmitter, D., Sage, D., Philippe, J. & Dibner, C. (2013). Circadian clock characteristics are altered in human thyroid malignant nodules. *J Clin Endocrinol Metab*, 98(11), 4446- 4456. https://doi.org/10.1210/jc.2013-2568.

Marcheva, B., Ramsey, K. M., Buhr, E. D., Kobayashi, Y., Su, H., Ko, C. H., Ivanova, G., Omura, C., Mo, S., Vitaterna, M. H., Lopez, J. P., Philipson L. H., Bradfield, C. A., Crosby, S. D., JeBailey, L., Wang, X., Takahashi, J. S. & Bass, J. (2010). Disruption of the clock components CLOCK and BMAL1 leads to hypoinsulinaemia and diabetes. *Nature*, 466, 627-31. https://doi.org/10.1038/nature09253.

Marcheva, B., Ramsey, K. M., Peek, C. B., Affinati, A., Maury, E., Bass, J. (2013). Circadian Clocks and Metabolism. In A. Kramer & M. Merrow (Eds.), *Circadian Clocks. Handbook of Experimental Pharmacology*, (pp.127-155). Springer, Berlin, Heidelberg. https://doi.org/10.1007/978-3-642-25950-0_6.

Mason, I. C., Qian, J., Adler, G. K., Scheer, F. A. J. L. (2020). Impact of circadian disruption on glucose metabolism: implications for type 2 diabetes. *Diabetologia*, 63, 462–472. https://doi.org/10.1007/s00125-019-05059-6.

Masri, S. & Sassone-Corsi, P. (2018). The emerging link between cancer, metabolism, and circadian rhythms. *Nat Med,* 24 (12), 1795–1803. https://doi.org/10.1038/s41591-018-0271-8.

Mattson, M. P., Allison, D. B., Fontana, L., Harvie, M., Longo, V. D., Malaisse, W. J., Mosley, M., Notterpek, L., Ravussin, E., Scheer, F. A. J. L., Seyfried, T. N., Varady, K. A. & Panda, S. (2014). Meal frequency and timing in health and disease. *Proc Natl Acad Sci U S A,* 111(47), 16647–16653. https://doi.org/10.1073/pnas.1413965111.

Maury, E., Ramsey, K. M. & Bass, J. (2010). Circadian rhythms and metabolic syndrome: from experimental genetics to human disease. *Circ Res,* 106(3), 447– 462. https://doi.org/10.1161/CIRCRESAHA.109.208355.

McGinnis, G. R. & Young, M. E. (2016). Circadian regulation of metabolic homeostasis: causes and consequences. *Nature and Science of Sleep*, 8, 163–180. https://doi.org/10.2147/NSS.S78946.

Meister, B. (2007). Neurotransmitters in key neurons of the hypothalamus that regulate feeding behavior and body weight. *Physiology & Behavior*, 92 (1-2), 263-271 https://doi.org/10.1016/j.physbeh.2007.05.021.

Minokoshi, Y., Shiuchi, T., Lee, S., Suzuki, A. & Okamoto, S. (2008). Role of hypothalamic AMP-kinase in food intake regulation. *Nutrition,* 24(9), 786-90. https://doi.org/10.1016/j.nut.2008.06.002.

Morris, C. J., Yang, J. N. & Scheer, F. A. J. L. (2012). The impact of the circadian timing system on cardiovascular and metabolic function. In A. Kalsbeek, M. Merrow, T. Roenneberg & R. G. Foster (Eds.), *The Neurobiology of Circadian Timing* (pp. 337-58). Progress in Brain Research. https://doi.org/10.1016/B978-0-444-59427-3.00019-8.

Morris, C. J., Yang, J. N., Garcia, J. I., Myers, S., Bozzi, I., Wang, W., Buxton, O. M., Shea, S. A. & Scheer, F. A. J. L. (2015). Endogenous circadian system and circadian misalignment impact glucose tolerance via separate mechanisms in humans. *Pnas*, 112 (17), E2225-E2234. https://doi.org/10.1073/pnas.1418955112.

Nagoshi, E., Saini, C., Bauer, C., Laroche, T., Naef, F. & Schibler, U. (2004). Circadian gene expression in individual fibroblasts: cellautonomous and self-sustained oscillators pass time to daughter cells. *Cell,* 119(5), 693-705. https://doi.org/10.1016/j.cell.2004.11.015.

Nakao, T., Kohsaka, A., Otsuka, T., Thein, Z. L., Le, H. T., Waki, H., Gouraud, S. S., Ihara, H., Nakanishi, M., Sato, F., Muragaki, Y. & Maeda, M. (2018). Impact of heart-specific disruption of the circadian clock on systemic glucose metabolism in mice. *The Journal of Biological and Medical Rhythm Research (Chronobiology International),* 35(4), 499-510. (Published online: 2017). https://doi.org/10.1080/07420528.2017.1415922.

Natalucci, G., Riedl, S., Gleiss, A., Zidek, T. & Frisch, H. (2005). Spontaneous 24-h ghrelin secretion pattern in fasting subjects: maintenance of a meal-related pattern. *European Journal of Endocrinology,* 152(6), 845-850. https://doi.org/10.1530/eje.1.01919.

O'Byrne, N. A., Yuen, F., Butt, W. Z. & Liu, P. Y. (2021). Sleep and circadian regulation of cortisol: A short review. *Current Opinion in Endocrine and Metabolic Research,* 18, 178-186 https://doi.org/10.1016/j.coemr.2021.03.011.

Oike, H., Oishi, K. & Kobori, M. (2014). Nutrients, Clock Genes, and Chrononutrition. *Curr Nutr Rep,* 3(3), 204–212. https://doi.org/10.1007/s13668-014-0082-6.

Oosterman, J. E., Kalsbeek, A., Fleur, S. E. & Belsham, D. D. (2015). Impact of nutrients on circadian rhythmicity, *American Journal of Physiology,* 308(5), 337-350. https://doi.org/10.1152/ajpregu.00322.2014.

Oosterman, J. E., Wopereis, S. & Kalsbeek, A. (2020). The circadian clock, shift work, and tissue-specific insulin resistance. *Endocrinology*, 161(12), bqaa180. https://doi.org/10.1210/endocr/bqaa180.

Orihara, K., Haraguchi, A. & Shibata, S. (2020). Crosstalk Among Circadian Rhythm, Obesity and Allergy. *Int. J. Mol. Sci.*, 21(5), 1884. https://doi.org/10.3390/ijms21051884.

Owens, N. D., Blitz, I. L., Lane, M. A., Patrushev, I., Overton, J. D., Gilchrist, M. J., Cho, K. W. & Khokha, M. K. (2016). Measuring absolute RNA copy numbers at high temporal resolution reveals transcriptome kinetics in development. *Cell Reports*, 14(3), 632–647. https://doi.org/10.1016/j.celrep.2015.12.050.

Pagano, E. S., Spinedi, E. & Gagliardino, J.J. (2017). White adipose tissue and circadian rhythm dysfunctions in obesity: pathogenesis and available therapies. *Neuroendocrinology,* 104 (4), 347–363. https://doi.org/10.1159/000453317.

Parameswaran, G. & Ray, D. W. (2022). Sleep, circadian rhythms, and type 2 diabetes mellitus. *Clinical endocrinology*, 96(1), 12-20. https://doi.org/10.1111/cen.14607.

Patterson, R. E., Laughlin, G. A., LaCroix, A. Z., Hartman, S. J., Natarajan, L., Senger, C. M., Martínez, M. E., Villaseñor, A., Sears, D. D., Marinac, C. R. & Gallo, L. C. (2015). Intermittent fasting and human metabolic health. *Journal of the Academy of Nutrition and Dietetics*, 115(8), 1203-1212. https://doi.org/10.1016/j.jand.2015.02.018.

Philippe, J. & Dibner, C. (2015). Thyroid circadian timing: roles in physiology and thyroid malignancies. *Journal of biological rhythms*, 30(2), 76-83. https://doi.org/10.1177/0748730414557634.

Poggiogalle, E., Jamshed, H. & Peterson, C. M. (2018). Circadian regulation of glucose, lipid, and energy metabolism in humans. *Metabolism*, 84, 11-27. https://doi.org/10.1016/j.metabol.2017.11.017.

Pogue-Geile, K. L., Lyons-Weiler, J. & Whitcomb, D. C. (2006). Molecular overlap of fly circadian rhythms and human pancreatic cancer. *Cancer letters*, 243(1), 55-57. https://doi.org/10.1016/j.canlet.2005.11.049.

Pot, G. K. (2018). Sleep and dietary habits in the urban environment: the role of chrononutrition. *Proceedings of the Nutrition Society,* 77(3), 189-198. https://doi.org/10.1017/S0029665117003974.

Qaid, M. M. & Abdelrahman, M. M. (2016). Role of insulin and other related hormones in energy metabolism—A review. *Cogent Food & Agriculture*, 2 (1), 1267691. http://dx.doi.org/10.1080/23311932.2016.1267691.

Reaven, G., Abbasi, F. & McLaughlin, T. (2004). Obesity, insulin resistance and cardiovascular disease. *Recent Prog Horm Res*, 59, 207-223. https://doi.org/10.1210/rp.59.1.207.

Reinke, H. & Asher, G. (2016). Circadian Clock Control of Liver Metabolic Functions. *Gastroenterology,* 150 (3), 574-580. https://doi.org/10.1053/j.gastro.2015.11.043.

Reppert, S. M. & Weaver, D. R. (2002). Coordination of circadian timing in mammals. *Nature,* 418, 935–941. https://doi.org/10.1038/nature00965.

Reutrakul, S., Hood, M. M., Crowley, S.J., Morgan, M. K., Teodori, M., Knutson, K. L. & Van Cauter, E. (2013). Chronotype is independently associated with glycemic control in type 2 diabetes. *Diabetes care*, 36(9), 2523-2529. https://doi.org/10.2337/dc12-2697.

Romon, M., Edme, J. L., Boulenguez, C., Lescroart, J. L. & Frimat, P. (1993). Circadian variation of diet-induced thermogenesis. *The American journal of clinical nutrition*, *57*(4), 476-480. https://doi.org/10.1093/ajcn/57.4.476.

Sadowski, S. M., Pusztaszeri, M., Brulhart-Meynet, M.C., Petrenko, V., De Vito, C., Sobel, J., Delucinge-Vivier, C., Kebebew, E., Regazzi, R., Philippe, J., Triponez, F. & Dibner, C. (2018). Identification of Differential Transcriptional Patterns in Primary and Secondary Hyperparathyroidism. *J Clin Endocrinol Metab,* 103 (6), 2189-98. https://doi.org/10.1210/jc.2017-02506.

Saha, S. & Sassone-Corsi, P. (2007). Circadian Clock and Breast Cancer: A Molecular Link. *Cell Cycle*, 6 (11), 1329-1331. https://doi.org/10.4161/cc.6.11.4295.

Saini, C., Liani, A., Curie, T., Gos, P., Kreppel, F., Emmenegger, Y., Bonacina, L., Wolf, J. P., Poget, Y. A., Franken, P. & Schibler, U. (2013). Real-time recording of circadian liver gene expression in freely moving mice reveals the phase-setting behavior of hepatocyte clocks. *Genes Dev,* 27, 1526-1536. https://doi.org/10.1101/gad.221374.113.

Sancar, G. & Brunner, M. (2014). Circadian clocks and energy metabolism. *Cellular and molecular life sciences*, 71, 2667-2680. https://doi.org/10.1007/s00018-014-1574-7.

Sato, T., Ida, T. & Kojima, M. (2017). Role of biological rhythms in the performance of physical activity. *J Phys Fitness Sports Med*, 6 (3), 125-134. https://doi.org/10.7600/jpfsm.6.125.

Sato, F., Kohsaka, A., Bhawal, U. K. & Muragaki, Y. (2018). Potential Roles of *Dec* and *Bmal1* Genes in Interconnecting Circadian Clock and Energy Metabolism. *Int. J. Mol. Sci*, 19 (3), 781. https://doi.org/10.3390/ijms19030781.

Serin, Y. & Tek, N. A. (2019). Effect of circadian rhythm on metabolic processes and the regulation of energy balance. *Annals of Nutrition and Metabolism*, 74(4), 322-330. https://doi.org/10.1159/000500071.

Shamseddeen, H., Getty, J. Z., Hamdallah, I. N. & Ali, M. R. (2011). Epidemiology and economic impact of obesity and type 2 diabetes. *Surg Clin North Am*, 91(6), 1163-1172. https://doi.org/10.1016/j.suc.2011.08.001.

Shi, S. Q., Ansari, T. S., McGuinness, O. P., Wasserman, D. H. & Johnson, C. H. (2013). Circadian Disruption Leads to Insulin Resistance and Obesity. *Current Biology*, 23(5), 372–381. http://doi.org/10.1016/j.cub.2013.01.048.

Shostak, A. (2017). Circadian Clock, Cell Division, and Cancer: From Molecules to Organism. *Int. J. Mol. Sci*, 18(4), 873. https://doi.org/10.3390/ijms18040873.

Sinturel, F., Makhlouf, A. M., Meyer, P., Tran, C., Pataky, Z., Golay, A., Rey, G., Howald, C., Dermitzakis, E. T., Pichard, C., Philippe, J., Brown, S. A. & Dibner, C. (2019). Cellular circadian period length inversely correlates with HbA1c levels in individuals with type 2 diabetes. *Diabetologia,* 62, 1453- 1462. https://doi.org/10.1007/s00125-019-4907-0.

Sinturel, F., Petrenko, V. & Dibner, C. (2020). Circadian clocks make metabolism run. *Journal of molecular biology*, *432*(12), 3680-3699. https://doi.org/10.1016/j.jmb.2020.01.018.

So, A. Y. L., Bernal, T. U., Pillsbury, M. L., Yamamoto, K. R. & Feldman, B. J. (2009). Glucocorticoid regulation of the circadian clock modulates glucose homeostasis. *Proceedings of the National Academy of Sciences,* 106 (41), 17582-17587. https://doi.org/10.1073/pnas.0909733106.

Sookoian, S., Gemma, C., Gianotti, T. F., Burgueño, A., Castaño, G. & Pirola, C. J. (2008). Genetic variants of clock transcription factor are associated with individual susceptibility to obesity. *American Journal of Clinical Nutrition*, 87 (6), 1606-1615. https://doi.org/10.1093/ajcn/87.6.1606.

Stenvers, D. J., Scheer, F. A. J. L., Schrauwen, P., la Fleur, S. E. & Kalsbeek, A. (2019). Circadian clocks and insulin resistance. *Nature Reviews Endocrinology,* 15(2), 75-89. https://doi.org/10.1038/s41574-018-0122-1.

Taheri, S., Lin, L., Austin, D., Young, T. & Mignot, E. (2004). Short sleep duration is associated with reduced leptin, elevated ghrelin, and increased body mass index. *PLoS Med*, 1(3), 210–7. https://doi.org/10.1371/journal.pmed.0010062.

Tang, Q., Cheng, B., Xie, M., Chen, Y., Zhao, J., Zhou, X. & Chen, L. (2017). Circadian clock gene Bmal1 inhibits tumorigenesis and increases paclitaxel sensitivity in tongue squamous cell carcinoma. *Cancer research*, 77(2), 532-544. https://doi.org/10.1158/0008-5472.CAN-16-1322.

Tsang, A. H., Barclay, J. L. & Oster, H. (2014). Interactions between endocrine and circadian systems. *J Mol Endocrinol*, 52(1), R1-16. https://doi.org/10.1530/JME-13-0118.

Walisser, J. A. & Bradfield, C. A. (2006). A time to divide: does the circadian clock control cell cycle? *Dev Cell*, 10(5), 539-40. https://doi.org/10.1016/j.devcel.2006.04.014.

Wang, X. S., Armstrong, M. E. G., Cairns, B. J., Key, T. J. & Travis, R. C. (2011). Shift work and chronic disease: the epidemiological evidence. *Occup. Med. (Lond.)*, 61(2), 78-89. https://doi.org/10.1093/occmed/kqr001.

Wefers, J., van Moorsel, D., Hansen, J., Connell, N. J., Havekes, B., Hoeks, J., Lichtenbelt, W. D. V. M., Duez, H., Phielix, E., Kalsbeek, A., Boekschoten, M. V., Hooiveld, G. J., Hesselink, M. K. C., Kersten, S., Staels, B., Scheer, F. A. J. L. & Schrauwen, P. (2018). Circadian misalignment induces fatty acid metabolism gene profiles and compromises insulin sensitivity in human skeletal muscle. *Proc Natl Acad Sci U S A*, 115(30), 7789-94. https://doi.org/10.1073/pnas.1722295115.

Vakili, H., Jin, Y. & Cattini, P. A. (2016). Evidence for a Circadian Effect on the Reduction of Human Growth Hormone Gene Expression in Response to Excess Caloric Intake. *J Biol Chem*, 291(26), 13823–13833. https://doi.org/10.1074/jbc.M116.722744.

Varela, L. & Horvath, T. L. (2012). Leptin and insulin pathways in POMC and AgRP neurons that modulate energy balance and glucose homeostasis. *EMBO Reports*, 13, 1079-1086. https://doi.org/10.1038/embor.2012.174.

Xie, Y., Tang, Q., Chen, G., Xie, M., Yu, S., Zhao, J. & Chen, L. (2019). New insights into the circadian rhythm and its related diseases. *Frontiers in Physiology*, 10, 682. https://doi.org/10.3389/fphys.2019.00682.

Yamazaki, S., Numano, R., Abe, M., Hida, A., Takahashi, R., Ueda, M., Block, G. D., Sakaki, Y., Menaker, M. & Tei, H. (2000). Resetting central and peripheral circadian oscillators in transgenic rats. *Science*, 288 (5466), 682–685. https://doi.org/10.1126/science.288.5466.682.

Ye, X., Li, M., Hou, T., Gao, T., Zhu, W. G. & Yang, Y. (2017). Sirtuins in glucose and lipid metabolism. *Oncotarget*, 8(1), 1845–1859. https://doi.org/10.18632/oncotarget.12157.

Yoo, S. H., Yamazaki, S., Lowrey, P. L., Shimomura, K., Ko, C. H., Buhr, E. D., Siepka, S. M., Hong, H. K., Oh, W. J., Yoo, O. J., Menaker, M. & Takahashi, J. S. (2004). PERIOD2:LUCIFERASE real-time reporting of circadian dynamics reveals persistent circadian oscillations in mouse peripheral tissues. *Proc. Natl. Acad. Sci. USA*, 101(15), 5339–5346. https://doi.org/10.1073/pnas.0308709101.

Zakhari, S. (2013). Alcohol Metabolism and Epigenetics Changes. *Alcohol Res.*, 35(1), 6–16.

Zhang, S., Dai, M., Wang, X., Jiang, S. H., Hu, L. P., Zhang, X. L. & Zhang, Z. G. (2020). Signalling entrains the peripheral circadian clock. *Cellular Signalling*, 69, 109433. https://doi.org/10.1016/j.cellsig.2019.109433.

Zimmermann-Belsing, T., Brabant, G., Holst, J. J. & Feldt-Rasmussen, U. (2003). Circulating leptin and thyroid dysfunction. *European Journal of Endocrinology*, 149 (4), 257–271. https://doi.org/10.1530/eje.0.1490257.

Chapter 7

The Circadian Immune System: Circadian Regulation of Innate Immunity and Adaptive Immunity

Mehmet Akif Gun*, **MD, PhD**
Department of Medical Microbiology, 19 May State Hospital, Samsun, Turkiye

Abstract

The immune system is a complex structure consisting of innate and adaptive immunity, which helps wound healing while protecting the body against pathogens and cancer cells. Innate immunity is the body's first line of defense, responding to pathogens with low specificity and in a short time frame. In contrast, adaptive immunity includes T and B cells and cells capable of presenting antigens to T cells. Internal clocks control the differentiation, development, and migration of immune cells. The circadian system creates a central clock located in the suprachiasmatic nucleus (SCN) of the hypothalamus and a set of peripheral clocks found in the gastrointestinal tract, liver, pancreas, skeletal muscle, fat, and other tissues. The circadian clock produces rhythms and the sleep-wake cycle; it also controls hormone levels, blood pressure, body temperature, cardiovascular and digestive systems, and the immune system. The circadian-regulated immune system has evolutionary benefits, such as activating the threat of pathogens at their height, the appropriate inflammatory response, and coordinating the metabolic processes and signals necessary for immune cell activation. Disruption in the circadian clock may cause metabolic and cardiovascular diseases and adversely affect the immune system. This section presents the relationship between

* Corresponding Author's Email: mehmetakif.gun@saglik.gov.tr.

In: Human Health is a Matter of Timing
Editors: Sumeyya Deniz Aybek, Gonca Gulbay and Mucahit Secme
ISBN: 979-8-89113-467-6

the circadian clock and the immune system. As the mechanisms between the clock and immunity are better understood, new approaches to treating diseases are hoped.

Keywords: circadian clock, immune system, innate immunity, adaptive immunity

Introduction

The immune system is a complex structure that helps wound healing while protecting the body against pathogens (such as viruses, bacteria, parasites), cancer cells, and innate and adaptive immunity are the two components of this system (Hunter et al., 2022; Nobis et al., 2018). Innate immunity is the body's first line of defense, responding to pathogens with low specificity and in a short time frame. Adaptive immunity includes T and B cells and cells that can present antigens to T cells (Cermakian et al., 2022; Nobis et al., 2018). The differentiation, development, and migration of immune cells are controlled by internal clocks (Mann et al., 2016; Scheiermann et al., 2018).

The circadian system creates a central clock located in the suprachiasmatic nucleus (SCN) of the hypothalamus and a set of peripheral clocks found in the gastrointestinal tract, liver, pancreas, skeletal muscle, fat, and other tissues (Poggiogalle et al., 2018; Buijs and Kalsbeek, 2001; Barclay et al., 2012). The signals of the clock regulate metabolism with factors such as nutrition, sleep, light, and the autonomous rhythms of peripheral tissues. The central clock regulates metabolism through cortisol, melatonin, and synaptic connections (Mohawk, 2012; Poggiogalle et al., 2018; Buijs and Kalsbeek, 2001; Barclay et al., 2012).

The circadian clock adapts to the earth's rotation and continues to produce rhythms of about 24 hours, even without daily environmental signals (zeitgebers) (Roenneberg and Merrow, 2016). In addition to the circadian clock sleep-wake cycle, it controls hormone levels, blood pressure, body temperature, cardiovascular and digestive systems, and the immune system (Ishida et al., 1999; Zhang et al., 2021; Panda et al., 2002; Carter et al., 2016; Reppert and Weaver, 2002). Daily variations are seen in immune system functions (Shimba and Ikuta, 2020). The immune system response to bacterial, viral, and parasitic infections varies within 24 hours (Jerigova et al., 2022; Jacobi et al., 2015). The circadian clock, which controls immune functions, ensures an optimum immune response when needed. While the circadian clock increases the immune system cell activity when the risk of infection is highest, it also contributes to avoiding unwanted conditions such as autoimmune diseases and allergic reactions by keeping the immune system cell activity limited at other times (Labrecque and Cermakian, 2015). The circadian clock is involved in antigen presentation and lymphocyte proliferation, as well as in cytokine production and the toll-like receptor (TLR) function (Scheiermann et al., 2013; Geiger et al., 2015). Pathogen interaction with the host, leukocyte movement, and activation of innate and adaptive immunity are immune functions under circadian control (Man et al., 2016; Curtis et al., 2014; Scheiermann et al., 2013; Labrecque and Cermakian, 2015). Circadian rhythm of the immune system; nerve signals are controlled by clock genes, especially glucocorticoid hormones (Shimba and Ikuta, 2020).

It has been shown that molecular clock proteins such as CLOCK, BMAL1, and REV-ERBa regulate the transcription of immune components. In contrast, the circadian transcription of immune genes can be controlled by clock-controlled transcription factors or regulatory RNAs (Silver et al., 2012; Gibbs et al., 2012; Spengler et al., 2012; Nguyen et al., 2013).

The circadian-regulated immune system has evolutionary benefits, such as activating the threat of pathogens at their height, the appropriate inflammatory response, and coordinating the metabolic processes and signals necessary for immune cell activation (Hunter et al., 2022; Yuan et al., 2020; Early and Curtis, 2016). However, disruption of the circadian clock may cause metabolic and cardiovascular diseases and adversely affect the immune system (Dumbell et al., 2016). This section presents the relationship between the circadian clock and the immune system.

Relationship between the Circadian Clock and Innate Immunity

The circadian clock attempts to keep the immune system in check, but infection and inflammation wreak havoc on circadian regulation (Abele et al., 2019). Innate immunity is the host's first line of defense, including the respiratory and gastrointestinal tract, the skin and mucosal surfaces, and the cellular components (Hunter et al., 2022; McDonald and Levy, 2019).

The white blood cells of the innate immunity system, hematopoietic stem progenitor cells (HSPCs), pass from the bone marrow to the circulation, and this transition is under circadian clock control. A correlation was found with HSPC activity, which peaks twice in the day-night cycle, with increased secretion of bone marrow norepinephrine and tumor necrosis factor (Baxter and Ray, 2020; Golan et al., 2018). The daytime tumor necrosis factor stimulates HSPC differentiation and causes increased vascular permeability. Nocturnal melatonin secretion is associated with the regeneration of HSPCs, the expression of surface c-Kit and CD150, and the potentiation of stem cells (Golan et al., 2018). The differentiation of HPSCs into mature innate immune cells is also under circadian clock control (Baxter and Ray, 2020; Keller et al., 2009; Silver et al., 2012; Wang et al., 2011; Ella et al., 2016).

The circadian clock acts on innate immune cells, including neutrophils, eosinophils, mast cells, monocytes, macrophages, natural killer (NK) cells, dendritic cells (DCs), microglia, and innate lymphoid cells (Scheiermann et al., 2018; Ella et al., 2016; Baumann et al., 2013; Wang et al., 2011; Nguyen et al., 2013; Keller et al., 2009; Silver et al., 2012; Arjona and Sarkar, 2005; Fonken et al., 2015; Teng et al., 2019). This clock mechanism is involved in mast cells' histamine release, allergic reactions, phagocytic activity of macrophages, and cytokine release of macrophages (Hunter et al., 2022; Baumann et al., 2013; Nakamura et al., 2017; Nakamura et al., 2014; Oliva-Ramírez et al., 2014; Keller et al., 2009; Gibbs et al., 2012). Antimicrobial activities of neutrophils are higher at 01:00 at night compared to 13:00 during the day, and superoxide production and Staphylococcus aureus phagocytosis are very high in this period (Abele et al., 2019; Ella et al., 2016). Additionally, it was observed that IgE-mediated mast cell responses vary over time through the IgE receptor FcεRI (Nakamura et al., 2014). The circadian clock plays a role in the regulation of plasma histamine levels through the organic cation transporter 3 (Oct 3), which is involved in the cellular transport of histamine (Nakamura et al., 2017). Disruption of the synchronization between the day-night cycle and the circadian clock causes a loss of rhythm, leading to the deterioration of the variability of plasma histamine levels at certain time intervals during the day (Abele et al., 2019; Nakamura et al., 2017).

Rev-ErbA is a nuclear hormone receptor and a core cellular clock protein, and it negatively affects immunity by disrupting the active inflammation structure (Gibbs et al., 2012). Loss of circadian clock structure can cause colitis, hepatosteatosis, dyslipidemia, and obesity (Baxter and Ray, 2020; Wang et al., 2018; Zhang et al., 2015).

NFIL3 (nuclear factor interleukin-3 regulated), called E4BP4, is a transcription suppressor exhaled from some human tissues. It is involved in circadian regulation and plays a role in nerve regeneration, energy metabolism, and immune cell differentiation. Its abnormal expression is associated with inflammation and metabolic diseases (Zeng et al., 2023; Kashiwada et al., 2010; Wang et al., 2017; Zhao et al., 2021).

NFIL3 is required to develop NK cells and innate lymphoid cells (ILCs) (Kostrzewski et al., 2018; Geiger et al., 2014; Seillet et al., 2014; Male et al., 2014; Kamizono et al., 2009). It is also thought to play a role in the development of regulatory T (Treg) cells and DCs (Male et al., 2012). NFIL3 is required to develop ILC1 and NK cells from a common ILC progenitor (Waggoner, 2020; Geiger et al., 2014; Seillet et al., 2014).

Disruption of circadian timing may adversely affect innate immunity, impairing the host's ability to fight pathogens. As a result, this may also lead to immunosuppression or chronic inflammatory diseases (Jerigova et al., 2022).

Relationship between the Circadian Clock and Adaptive Immunity

Data Either a previous infection or vaccination induces adaptive immunity. Adaptive immunity is also responsible for the recognition of 'non-self' antigens, forming pathogen-specific immune responses, and forming memory cells that enable rapid immune response when the infectious agent is reencountered (Hunter et al., 2022; Bonilla and Oettgen 2010). Innate immunity also interacts with adaptive immunity, including pattern recognition receptor (PRR)-mediated regulation of components required for antigen presentation and recognition (Downton et al., 2020; Hoebe et al., 2004).

The circadian clock controls adaptive immune system cells such as T and B lymphocytes and DCs, antigen-presenting cells (APCs) that lie between innate and adaptive immunity (Scheiermann et al., 2018; Druzd et al., 2017; Hemmers et al., 2015; Bollinger et al., 2011; Silver et al., 2012; Dimitrov et al., 2007). However, uncertainty about the effects of adaptive immune functions on daily rhythmicity continues (Bollinger et al., 2011; Hemmers and Rudensky, 2015).

Toll-like receptors (TLRs), located on the cell surface or in endosomal compartments, are responsible for immune recognition. Recognition of TLRs and subsequent binding to pathogen-associated molecular patterns (PAMPs) activate innate and adaptive immune responses (Kawai and Akira, 2010). One study demonstrated the rhythmic expression of TLR in splenic macrophages and a subset of splenocytes consisting of B cells, DCs, and macrophages (Abele et al., 2019; Silver et al., 2015).

T and B cells are in a circadian state of circulation between the blood, lymph, and lymphoid organs. In mammals, lymphocyte counts vary over 24 hours (Deprés-Brummer et al., 1997; Cermakian et al., 2022). In human peripheral blood, naive CD4 and CD8 T cells and total lymphocyte counts are highest at night and lowest during the day (Cermakian et al., 2022; Born et al., 1997; Dimitrov et al., 2009; Kirsch et al., 2012). The cortisol hormone is secreted by the adrenal glands and controls the circadian system. With the effect of cortisol, the number of T lymphocytes in humans' blood changes day and night (Dimitrov et al., 2009; Cermakian et al., 2022).

In a study examining subsets of CD4 and CD8 T lymphocytes in humans in which the effect of glucocorticoids was observed; Except for effector CD4 T lymphocytes, 24-hour changes in naive (CD45RA+CD62L+), central memory (CD45RA−CD62L+), and effector memory (CD45RA−CD62L−) blood cell counts were evaluated (Dimitrov et al., 2009). As a result of the evaluation, while the number of cells was at its peak at night, it was found to be the lowest in the afternoon. When exogenous cortisol is administered to the subjects in the evening hours when the T lymphocyte count is ordinarily high and endogenous cortisol is low, the T lymphocyte count decreases dramatically. When epinephrine was administered to subjects, a short-term increase in effector CD8 T was shown (Cermakian et al., 2022; Dimitrov et al., 2009). While glucocorticoids upregulate the expression of CXCR4 in naive memory and central memory CD4 and CD8 T lymphocytes, the glucocorticoid receptor antagonist mifepristone causes a decrease in the number of T lymphocytes (Dimitrov et al., 2009; Besedovsky et al., 2014).

Moreover, the glucocorticoid receptor activates the expression of the interleukin 7 receptor (IL7R), which stimulates the chemokine receptor CXCR4 and accelerates T lymphocyte migration by increasing the chemokine ligand CXCL12 in the spleen at night (Shimba et al., 2018). The loss of NFIL3 in T lymphocytes resulted in increased frequencies of T helper 17 (Th17) lymphocytes (Waggoner, 2020; Yu et al., 2013). The circadian clock also effectively differentiates CD4 T cells into Th17 and Tregs (Cermakian et al., 2022).

It is supposed that attention is drawn to the critical role of Th17 lymphocytes in intestinal health and immunity. In that case, the role of clock genes in Th17 homeostasis is to regulate the delicate balance required for optimal immune protection against pathogens with minimal tissue damage (Waggoner, 2020). The intrinsic clocks of lymphocytes and lymphocyte levels are controlled with autonomic neuronal innervation, glucocorticoids, chemokine receptors, and chemokine ligands (Cermakian et al., 2022).

Studies show that circadian clock components also control B lymphocytes, although relatively more limited than T lymphocytes (Cermakian et al., 2022). NFIL3 was involved in the development of ILCs, whereas BMAL1 is responsible for a similar effect in the development of B lymphocytes (Waggoner, 2020; Sun et al., 2006). Bmal1 (Brain and muscle arnt-like) is an essential factor in the transcription/translation feedback of the biological clock (Zheng et al., 2023). Significant reductions in immunoglobulin levels and peripheral B lymphocyte counts were observed in BMAL1 -/- mice (Waggoner, 2020; Sun et al., 2006).

The circadian clock controls the immune system, and disruption of circadian rhythms affects the immune response. Clock gene mutations or deletions (PER1-3 and BMAL1) cause disruption of circadian rhythms and altered macrophage function, resulting in increased inflammatory status (Abele et al., 2019; Wang et al., 2016). The deletion of PER1 in liver macrophages and Kupffer cells increased macrophage recruitment. It has been shown that this leads to an increase in lipopolysaccharide (LPS) and a higher incidence of death after the increase in proinflammatory cytokine release (Wang et al., 2016). This was attributed to the interaction between PER1, which inhibits the expression of C-C chemokine receptor 2, and the receptor gamma activated by the peroxisome proliferator (Wang et al., 2016).

In a study in mice, animals vaccinated using the TLR9 ligand as an adjuvant showed an effective adaptive immune response weeks later than those vaccinated 12 hours earlier (Silver et al., 2012). The influenza vaccine has been shown to have a better antibody response when administered in the morning than in the afternoon (Long et al., 2016).

Conclusion

Over time, our habits change, such as nutrition, reading, sleeping, sports, traveling, and etc. Our lifestyle has direct effects on the circadian clock and the immune system. Poor synchronization between these systems; increases the incidence of diabetes, hyperlipidemia, and obesity in the population. The digestive system, cardiovascular system diseases, cancer, and autoimmune diseases are also becoming more common in the human population. As the mechanisms between the clock and immunity are better understood, it will be easier to know what we do wrong and what we need to do better. Positive changes will emerge in our drug and immunotherapy approaches.

References

Abele, S. H., Meadows, K. E., Medeiros, D., & Silver, A. C. (2019). Time is on the Immune System's Side, Yes it is. *The Yale journal of biology and medicine*, *92*(2), 225–231.

Arjona, A., & Sarkar, D. K. (2005). Circadian oscillations of clock genes, cytolytic factors, and cytokines in rat NK cells. *Journal of immunology (Baltimore, Md. : 1950)*, *174*(12), 7618–7624. https://doi.org/10.4049/jimmunol.174.12.7618.

Barclay, J. L., Tsang, A. H., & Oster, H. (2012). Interaction of central and peripheral clocks in physiological regulation. *Progress in brain research*, *199*, 163–181. https://doi.org/10.1016/B978-0-444-59427-3.00030-7.

Baumann, A., Gönnenwein, S., Bischoff, S. C., Sherman, H., Chapnik, N., Froy, O., & Lorentz, A. (2013). The circadian clock is functional in eosinophils and mast cells. *Immunology*, *140*(4), 465–474. https://doi.org/10.1111/imm.12157.

Baxter, M., & Ray, D. W. (2020). Circadian rhythms in innate immunity and stress responses. *Immunology*, *161*(4), 261–267. https://doi.org/10.1111/imm.13166.

Besedovsky, L., Born, J., & Lange, T. (2014). Endogenous glucocorticoid receptor signaling drives rhythmic changes in human T-cell subset numbers and the expression of the chemokine receptor CXCR4. *FASEB journal : official publication of the Federation of American Societies for Experimental Biology*, *28*(1), 67–75. https://doi.org/10.1096/fj.13-237958.

Bollinger, T., Leutz, A., Leliavski, A., Skrum, L., Kovac, J., Bonacina, L., Benedict, C., Lange, T., Westermann, J., Oster, H., & Solbach, W. (2011). Circadian clocks in mouse and human CD^{4+} T cells. *PloS one*, *6*(12), e29801. https://doi.org/10.1371/journal.pone.0029801.

Bonilla, F. A., & Oettgen, H. C. (2010). Adaptive immunity. *The Journal of allergy and clinical immunology*, *125*(2 Suppl 2), S33–S40. https://doi.org/10.1016/j.jaci.2009.09.017.

Born, J., Lange, T., Hansen, K., Mölle, M., & Fehm, H. L. (1997). Effects of sleep and circadian rhythm on human circulating immune cells. *Journal of immunology (Baltimore, Md. : 1950)*, *158*(9), 4454–4464.10. 20. Cuesta M, Boudreau P, Dubeau-Laramee G, Cermakian N, Boivin DB (2016) Simulated night shift disrupts circadian rhythms of immune functions in humans. J Immunol 196:2466– 2475. https://doi.org/10.4049/jimmunol.1502422.

Buijs, R. M., & Kalsbeek, A. (2001). Hypothalamic integration of central and peripheral clocks. *Nature reviews. Neuroscience*, *2*(7), 521–526. https://doi.org/10.1038/35081582.

Carter, S. J., Durrington, H. J., Gibbs, J. E., Blaikley, J., Loudon, A. S., Ray, D. W., & Sabroe, I. (2016). A matter of time: study of circadian clocks and their role in inflammation. *Journal of leukocyte biology*, *99*(4), 549–560. https://doi.org/10.1189/jlb.3RU1015-451R.

Cermakian, N., Stegeman, S. K., Tekade, K., & Labrecque, N. (2022). Circadian rhythms in adaptive immunity and vaccination. *Seminars in immunopathology*, *44*(2), 193–207. https://doi.org/10.1007/s00281-021-00903-7.

Chloé C Nobis, Nathalie Labrecque, Nicolas Cermakian, From immune homeostasis to inflammation, a question of rhythms, Current Opinion in Physiology, Volume 5, 2018, Pages 90-98, ISSN 2468-8673, https://doi.org/10.1016/j.cophys.2018.09.001.

Curtis, A. M., Bellet, M. M., Sassone-Corsi, P., & O'Neill, L. A. (2014). Circadian clock proteins and immunity. *Immunity*, *40*(2), 178–186. https://doi.org/10.1016/j.immuni.2014.02.002.

Deprés-Brummer, P., Bourin, P., Pages, N., Metzger, G., & Lévi, F. (1997). Persistent T lymphocyte rhythms despite suppressed circadian clock outputs in rats. *The American journal of physiology*, *273*(6), R1891–R1899. https://doi.org/10.1152/ajpregu.1997.273.6.R1891.

Dimitrov, S., Benedict, C., Heutling, D., Westermann, J., Born, J., & Lange, T. (2009). Cortisol and epinephrine control opposing circadian rhythms in T cell subsets. *Blood*, *113*(21), 5134–5143. https://doi.org/10.1182/blood-2008-11-190769.

Dimitrov, S., Lange, T., Nohroudi, K., & Born, J. (2007). Number and function of circulating human antigen presenting cells regulated by sleep. *Sleep*, *30*(4), 401–411. https://doi.org/10.1093/sleep/30.4.401.

Downton, P., Early, J. O., & Gibbs, J. E. (2020). Circadian rhythms in adaptive immunity. *Immunology*, *161*(4), 268–277. https://doi.org/10.1111/imm.13167.

Druzd, D., Matveeva, O., Ince, L., Harrison, U., He, W., Schmal, C., Herzel, H., Tsang, A. H., Kawakami, N., Leliavski, A., Uhl, O., Yao, L., Sander, L. E., Chen, C. S., Kraus, K., de Juan, A., Hergenhan, S. M., Ehlers, M., Koletzko, B., Haas, R., Scheiermann, C. (2017). Lymphocyte Circadian Clocks Control Lymph Node Trafficking and Adaptive Immune Responses. *Immunity*, *46*(1), 120–132. https://doi.org/10.1016/j.immuni.2016.12.011.

Dumbell, R., Matveeva, O., & Oster, H. (2016). Circadian Clocks, Stress, and Immunity. *Frontiers in endocrinology*, *7*, 37. https://doi.org/10.3389/fendo.2016.00037.

Early, J. O., & Curtis, A. M. (2016). Immunometabolism: Is it under the eye of the clock?. *Seminars in immunology*, *28*(5), 478–490. https://doi.org/10.1016/j.smim.2016.10.006.

Ella, K., Csépányi-Kömi, R., & Káldi, K. (2016). Circadian regulation of human peripheral neutrophils. *Brain, behavior, and immunity*, *57*, 209–221. https://doi.org/10.1016/j.bbi.2016.04.016.

Fonken, L. K., Frank, M. G., Kitt, M. M., Barrientos, R. M., Watkins, L. R., & Maier, S. F. (2015). Microglia inflammatory responses are controlled by an intrinsic circadian clock. *Brain, behavior, and immunity*, *45*, 171–179. https://doi.org/10.1016/j.bbi.2014.11.009.

Geiger, S. S., Fagundes, C. T., & Siegel, R. M. (2015). Chrono-immunology: progress and challenges in understanding links between the circadian and immune systems. *Immunology*, *146*(3), 349–358. https://doi.org/10.1111/imm.12525.

Geiger, T. L., Abt, M. C., Gasteiger, G., Firth, M. A., O'Connor, M. H., Geary, C. D., O'Sullivan, T. E., van den Brink, M. R., Pamer, E. G., Hanash, A. M., & Sun, J. C. (2014). Nfil3 is crucial for development of innate lymphoid cells and host protection against intestinal pathogens. *The Journal of experimental medicine*, *211*(9), 1723–1731. https://doi.org/10.1084/jem.20140212.

Gibbs, J. E., Blaikley, J., Beesley, S., Matthews, L., Simpson, K. D., Boyce, S. H., Farrow, S. N., Else, K. J., Singh, D., Ray, D. W., & Loudon, A. S. (2012). The nuclear receptor REV-ERBα mediates circadian regulation of innate immunity through selective regulation of inflammatory cytokines. *Proceedings of the National Academy of Sciences of the United States of America*, *109*(2), 582–587. https://doi.org/10.1073/pnas.1106750109.

Golan, K., Kumari, A., Kollet, O., Khatib-Massalha, E., Subramaniam, M. D., Ferreira, Z. S., Avemaria, F., Rzeszotek, S., García-García, A., Xie, S., Flores-Figueroa, E., Gur-Cohen, S., Itkin, T., Ludin-Tal, A., Massalha, H., Bernshtein, B., Ciechanowicz, A. K., Brandis, A., Mehlman, T., Bhattacharya, S., … Lapidot, T. (2018). Daily Onset of Light and Darkness Differentially Controls Hematopoietic Stem Cell Differentiation and Maintenance. *Cell stem cell*, *23*(4), 572–585.e7. https://doi.org/10.1016/j.stem.2018.08.002.

Hemmers, S., & Rudensky, A. Y. (2015). The Cell-Intrinsic Circadian Clock Is Dispensable for Lymphocyte Differentiation and Function. *Cell reports*, *11*(9), 1339–1349. https://doi.org/10.1016/j.celrep.2015.04.058.

Hoebe, K., Janssen, E., & Beutler, B. (2004). The interface between innate and adaptive immunity. *Nature immunology*, *5*(10), 971–974. https://doi.org/10.1038/ni1004-971.

Hunter, F. K., Butler, T. D., & Gibbs, J. E. (2022). Circadian rhythms in immunity and host-parasite interactions. *Parasite immunology*, *44*(3), e12904. https://doi.org/10.1111/pim.12904.

Ishida, N., Kaneko, M., & Allada, R. (1999). Biological clocks. *Proceedings of the National Academy of Sciences of the United States of America*, *96*(16), 8819–8820. https://doi.org/10.1073/pnas.96.16.8819.

Jacobi, D., Liu, S., Burkewitz, K., Kory, N., Knudsen, N. H., Alexander, R. K., Unluturk, U., Li, X., Kong, X., Hyde, A. L., Gangl, M. R., Mair, W. B., & Lee, C. H. (2015). Hepatic Bmal1 Regulates Rhythmic Mitochondrial Dynamics and Promotes Metabolic Fitness. *Cell metabolism*, *22*(4), 709–720. https://doi.org/10.1016/j.cmet.2015.08.006.

Jerigova, V., Zeman, M., & Okuliarova, M. (2022). Circadian Disruption and Consequences on Innate Immunity and Inflammatory Response. *International journal of molecular sciences*, *23*(22), 13722. https://doi.org/10.3390/ijms232213722.

Kamizono, S., Duncan, G. S., Seidel, M. G., Morimoto, A., Hamada, K., Grosveld, G., Akashi, K., Lind, E. F., Haight, J. P., Ohashi, P. S., Look, A. T., & Mak, T. W. (2009). Nfil3/E4bp4 is required for the development and maturation of NK cells in vivo. *The Journal of experimental medicine*, *206*(13), 2977–2986. https://doi.org/10.1084/jem.20092176.

Kashiwada, M., Levy, D. M., McKeag, L., Murray, K., Schröder, A. J., Canfield, S. M., Traver, G., & Rothman, P. B. (2010). IL-4-induced transcription factor NFIL3/E4BP4 controls IgE class switching. *Proceedings of the National Academy of Sciences of the United States of America*, *107*(2), 821–826. https://doi.org/10.1073/pnas.0909235107.

Kawai, T., & Akira, S. (2010). The role of pattern-recognition receptors in innate immunity: update on Toll-like receptors. *Nature immunology*, *11*(5), 373–384. https://doi.org/10.1038/ni.1863.

Keller, M., Mazuch, J., Abraham, U., Eom, G. D., Herzog, E. D., Volk, H. D., Kramer, A., & Maier, B. (2009). A circadian clock in macrophages controls inflammatory immune responses. *Proceedings of the National Academy of Sciences of the United States of America*, *106*(50), 21407–21412. https://doi.org/10.1073/pnas.0906361106.

Kirsch, S., Thijssen, S., Alarcon Salvador, S., Heine, G. H., van Bentum, K., Fliser, D., Sester, M., & Sester, U. (2012). T-cell numbers and antigen-specific T-cell function follow different circadian rhythms. *Journal of clinical immunology*, *32*(6), 1381–1389. https://doi.org/10.1007/s10875-012-9730-z.

Kostrzewski, T., Borg, A. J., Meng, Y., Filipovic, I., Male, V., Wack, A., DiMaggio, P. A., & Brady, H. J. M. (2018). Multiple Levels of Control Determine How E4bp4/Nfil3 Regulates NK Cell Development. *Journal of immunology (Baltimore, Md. : 1950)*, *200*(4), 1370–1381. https://doi.org/10.4049/jimmunol.1700981.

Labrecque, N., & Cermakian, N. (2015). Circadian Clocks in the Immune System. *Journal of biological rhythms*, *30*(4), 277–290. https://doi.org/10.1177/0748730415577723.

Long, J. E., Drayson, M. T., Taylor, A. E., Toellner, K. M., Lord, J. M., & Phillips, A. C. (2016). Morning vaccination enhances antibody response over afternoon vaccination: A cluster-randomised trial. *Vaccine*, *34*(24), 2679–2685. https://doi.org/10.1016/j.vaccine.2016.04.032.

Male, V., Nisoli, I., Gascoyne, D. M., & Brady, H. J. (2012). E4BP4: an unexpected player in the immune response. *Trends in immunology*, *33*(2), 98–102. https://doi.org/10.1016/j.it.2011.10.002.

Male, V., Nisoli, I., Kostrzewski, T., Allan, D. S., Carlyle, J. R., Lord, G. M., Wack, A., & Brady, H. J. (2014). The transcription factor E4bp4/Nfil3 controls commitment to the NK lineage and directly regulates Eomes and Id2 expression. *The Journal of experimental medicine*, *211*(4), 635–642. https://doi.org/10.1084/jem.20132398.

Man, K., Loudon, A., & Chawla, A. (2016). Immunity around the clock. *Science (New York, N.Y.)*, *354*(6315), 999–1003. https://doi.org/10.1126/science.aah4966.

McDonald D. R., Levy O. 3 - Innate Immunity. In: Rich RR, Fleisher TA, Shearer WT, Schroeder HW, Frew AJ, Weyand CM, eds. Clinical Immunology, 5th ed. Elsevier; 2019:39–53.e1. https://doi.org/10.1016/B978-0-7020-6896-6.00003-X.

Mohawk, J. A., Green, C. B., & Takahashi, J. S. (2012). Central and peripheral circadian clocks in mammals. *Annual review of neuroscience*, *35*, 445–462. https://doi.org/10.1146/annurev-neuro-060909-153128.

Nakamura, Y., Ishimaru, K., Shibata, S., & Nakao, A. (2017). Regulation of plasma histamine levels by the mast cell clock and its modulation by stress. *Scientific reports*, *7*, 39934. https://doi.org/10.1038/srep39934.

Nakamura, Y., Nakano, N., Ishimaru, K., Hara, M., Ikegami, T., Tahara, Y., Katoh, R., Ogawa, H., Okumura, K., Shibata, S., Nishiyama, C., & Nakao, A. (2014). Circadian regulation of allergic reactions by the mast cell clock in mice. *The Journal of allergy and clinical immunology*, *133*(2), 568–575. https://doi.org/10.1016/j.jaci.2013.07.040.

Nguyen, K. D., Fentress, S. J., Qiu, Y., Yun, K., Cox, J. S., & Chawla, A. (2013). Circadian gene Bmal1 regulates diurnal oscillations of Ly6C(hi) inflammatory monocytes. *Science (New York, N.Y.)*, *341*(6153), 1483–1488. https://doi.org/10.1126/science.1240636.

Oliva-Ramírez, J., Moreno-Altamirano, M. M., Pineda-Olvera, B., Cauich-Sánchez, P., & Sánchez-García, F. J. (2014). Crosstalk between circadian rhythmicity, mitochondrial dynamics and macrophage bactericidal activity. *Immunology*, *143*(3), 490–497. https://doi.org/10.1111/imm.12329.

Panda, S., Antoch, M. P., Miller, B. H., Su, A. I., Schook, A. B., Straume, M., Schultz, P. G., Kay, S. A., Takahashi, J. S., & Hogenesch, J. B. (2002). Coordinated transcription of key pathways in the mouse by the circadian clock. *Cell*, *109*(3), 307–320. https://doi.org/10.1016/s0092-8674(02)00722-5.

Poggiogalle, E., Jamshed, H., & Peterson, C. M. (2018). Circadian regulation of glucose, lipid, and energy metabolism in humans. *Metabolism: clinical and experimental*, *84*, 11–27. https://doi.org/10.1016/j.metabol.2017.11.017.

Reppert, S. M., & Weaver, D. R. (2002). Coordination of circadian timing in mammals. *Nature*, *418*(6901), 935–941. https://doi.org/10.1038/nature00965.

Roenneberg, T., & Merrow, M. (2016). The Circadian Clock and Human Health. *Current biology : CB*, *26*(10), R432–R443. https://doi.org/10.1016/j.cub.2016.04.011.

Scheiermann, C., Gibbs, J., Ince, L., & Loudon, A. (2018). Clocking in to immunity. *Nature reviews. Immunology*, *18*(7), 423–437. https://doi.org/10.1038/s41577-018-0008-4.

Scheiermann, C., Kunisaki, Y., & Frenette, P. S. (2013). Circadian control of the immune system. *Nature reviews. Immunology*, *13*(3), 190–198. https://doi.org/10.1038/nri3386.

Seillet, C., Rankin, L. C., Groom, J. R., Mielke, L. A., Tellier, J., Chopin, M., Huntington, N. D., Belz, G. T., & Carotta, S. (2014). Nfil3 is required for the development of all innate lymphoid cell subsets. *The Journal of experimental medicine*, *211*(9), 1733–1740. https://doi.org/10.1084/jem.20140145.

Shimba, A., & Ikuta, K. (2020). Glucocorticoids Regulate Circadian Rhythm of Innate and Adaptive Immunity. *Frontiers in immunology*, *11*, 2143. https://doi.org/10.3389/fimmu.2020.02143.

Shimba, A., Cui, G., Tani-Ichi, S., Ogawa, M., Abe, S., Okazaki, F., Kitano, S., Miyachi, H., Yamada, H., Hara, T., Yoshikai, Y., Nagasawa, T., Schütz, G., & Ikuta, K. (2018). Glucocorticoids Drive Diurnal Oscillations in T Cell Distribution and Responses by Inducing Interleukin-7 Receptor and CXCR4. *Immunity*, *48*(2), 286–298.e6. https://doi.org/10.1016/j.immuni.2018.01.004.

Silver, A. C., Arjona, A., Hughes, M. E., Nitabach, M. N., & Fikrig, E. (2012). Circadian expression of clock genes in mouse macrophages, dendritic cells, and B cells. *Brain, behavior, and immunity*, *26*(3), 407–413. https://doi.org/10.1016/j.bbi.2011.10.001.

Silver, A. C., Arjona, A., Walker, W. E., & Fikrig, E. (2012). The circadian clock controls toll-like receptor 9-mediated innate and adaptive immunity. *Immunity*, *36*(2), 251–261. https://doi.org/10.1016/j.immuni.2011.12.017.

Silver, A. C., Buckley, S. M., Hughes, M. E., Hastings, A. K., Nitabach, M. N., & Fikrig, E. (2018). Daily oscillations in expression and responsiveness of Toll-like receptors in splenic immune cells. *Heliyon*, *4*(3), e00579. https://doi.org/10.1016/j.heliyon.2018.e00579.

Spengler, M. L., Kuropatwinski, K. K., Comas, M., Gasparian, A. V., Fedtsova, N., Gleiberman, A. S., Gitlin, I. I., Artemicheva, N. M., Deluca, K. A., Gudkov, A. V., & Antoch, M. P. (2012). Core circadian protein CLOCK is a positive regulator of NF-κB-mediated transcription. *Proceedings of the National Academy of Sciences of the United States of America*, *109*(37), E2457–E2465. https://doi.org/10.1073/pnas.1206274109.

Sun, Y., Yang, Z., Niu, Z., Peng, J., Li, Q., Xiong, W., Langnas, A. N., Ma, M. Y., & Zhao, Y. (2006). MOP3, a component of the molecular clock, regulates the development of B cells. *Immunology*, *119*(4), 451–460. https://doi.org/10.1111/j.1365-2567.2006.02456.x.

Teng, F., Goc, J., Zhou, L., Chu, C., Shah, M. A., Eberl, G., & Sonnenberg, G. F. (2019). A circadian clock is essential for homeostasis of group 3 innate lymphoid cells in the gut. *Science immunology*, *4*(40), eaax1215. https://doi.org/10.1126/sciimmunol.aax1215.

Waggoner S. N. (2020). Circadian Rhythms in Immunity. *Current allergy and asthma reports*, *20*(1), 2. https://doi.org/10.1007/s11882-020-0896-9.

Wang, S., Lin, Y., Yuan, X., Li, F., Guo, L., & Wu, B. (2018). REV-ERBα integrates colon clock with experimental colitis through regulation of NF-κB/NLRP3 axis. *Nature communications*, *9*(1), 4246. https://doi.org/10.1038/s41467-018-06568-5.

Wang, T., Wang, Z., Yang, P., Xia, L., Zhou, M., Wang, S., Du, J., & Zhang, J. (2016). PER1 prevents excessive innate immune response during endotoxin induced liver injury through regulation of macrophage recruitment in mice. *Cell death & disease*, *7*(4), e2176. https://doi.org/10.1038/cddis.2016.9.

Wang, X., Reece, S. P., Van Scott, M. R., & Brown, J. M. (2011). A circadian clock in murine bone marrow-derived mast cells modulates IgE-dependent activation in vitro. *Brain, behavior, and immunity*, *25*(1), 127–134. https://doi.org/10.1016/j.bbi.2010.09.007.

Wang, Y., Kuang, Z., Yu, X., Ruhn, K. A., Kubo, M., & Hooper, L. V. (2017). The intestinal microbiota regulates body composition through NFIL**3** and the circadian clock. *Science (New York, N.Y.)*, *357*(6354), 912–916. https://doi.org/10.1126/science.aan0677.

Wang, Y., Pati, P., Xu, Y., Chen, F., Stepp, D. W., Huo, Y., Rudic, R. D., & Fulton, D. J. (2016). Endotoxin Disrupts Circadian Rhythms in Macrophages via Reactive Oxygen Species. *PloS one*, *11*(5), e0155075. https://doi.org/10.1371/journal.pone.0155075.

Yu, X., Rollins, D., Ruhn, K. A., Stubblefield, J. J., Green, C. B., Kashiwada, M., Rothman, P. B., Takahashi, J. S., & Hooper, L. V. (2013). TH17 cell differentiation is regulated by the circadian clock. *Science (New York, N.Y.)*, *342*(6159), 727–730. https://doi.org/10.1126/science.1243884.

Yuan, Y., Wu, S., Li, W., & He, W. (2020). A Tissue-Specific Rhythmic Recruitment Pattern of Leukocyte Subsets. *Frontiers in immunology*, *11*, 102. https://doi.org/10.3389/fimmu.2020.00102.

Zeng, L., Chen, D., Xue, Y., Zhang, M., Wu, Y., & Yang, W. (2023). A new border for circadian rhythm gene NFIL3 in diverse fields of cancer. *Clinical & translational oncology : official publication of the Federation of Spanish Oncology Societies and of the National Cancer Institute of Mexico*, 10.1007/s12094-023-03098-5. Advance online publication. https://doi.org/10.1007/s12094-023-03098-5.

Zhang, Y., Fang, B., Emmett, M. J., Damle, M., Sun, Z., Feng, D., Armour, S. M., Remsberg, J. R., Jager, J., Soccio, R. E., Steger, D. J., & Lazar, M. A. (2015). GENE

REGULATION. Discrete functions of nuclear receptor Rev-erbα couple metabolism to the clock. *Science (New York, N.Y.)*, *348*(6242), 1488–1492. https://doi.org/10.1126/science.aab3021.

Zhang, Z., Zeng, P., Gao, W., Zhou, Q., Feng, T., & Tian, X. (2021). Circadian clock: a regulator of the immunity in cancer. *Cell communication and signaling : CCS*, *19*(1), 37. https://doi.org/10.1186/s12964-021-00721-2.

Zhao, Z., Yin, L., Wu, F., & Tong, X. (2021). Hepatic metabolic regulation by nuclear factor E4BP4. *Journal of molecular endocrinology*, *66*(1), R15–R21. https://doi.org/10.1530/JME-20-0239.

Zheng, Y., Pan, L., Wang, F., Yan, J., Wang, T., Xia, Y., Yao, L., Deng, K., Zheng, Y., Xia, X., Su, Z., Chen, H., Lin, J., Ding, Z., Zhang, K., Zhang, M., & Chen, Y. (2023). Neural function of Bmal1: an overview. *Cell & bioscience*, *13*(1), 1. https://doi.org/10.1186/s13578-022-00947-8.

Chapter 8

The Aging Clock

Dilek Arslan Ateşşahin[1,*], PhD
and Yusuf Muhammed Durna[2], MD
[1]Department of Plant and Animal Production, Baskil Vocational School, Firat University, Elazığ, Turkiye
[2]Department of Otolaryngology and Head and Neck Surgery, Private Practice, Istanbul, Turkiye

Abstract

The diurnal alternation between light and darkness, constituting a roughly 24-hour cycle, exerts a significant influence on the temporal orchestration of biological processes within living organisms. These cyclic modulations, encompassing physiological, biochemical, and behavioral manifestations, are collectively recognized as circadian rhythms. Extensive empirical investigations have consistently demonstrated a progressive decline in circadian rhythms throughout the lifespan of organisms. This attenuation is intrinsically associated with genetic modifications within circadian genes and perturbations within the molecular chronometer, thus correlating these alterations with the aging phenomenon. Aging, a complex and multifaceted phenomenon, is characterized by a myriad of biological, biochemical, and physiological transformations. Several intracellular pathways have direct influence over cellular and epigenetic mechanisms that govern the aging process. It has been ascertained that certain pathways implicated in nutrient sensing concurrently participate in the regulatory processes governing aging and the molecular chronometer. Furthermore, aging is intricately intertwined with perturbations in circadian rhythms and the modulation

[*] Corresponding Author's Email: datessahin@firat.edu.tr.

In: Human Health is a Matter of Timing
Editors: Sumeyya Deniz Aybek, Gonca Gulbay and Mucahit Secme
ISBN: 979-8-89113-467-6

of energy homeostasis, consequently affecting a plethora of metabolic pathways. Hence, therapeutic strategies aimed at the manipulation of circadian regulation, aging, maintenance of metabolic energy equilibrium, and nutrient sensing pathways hold substantial promise in enhancing the efficiency of interventions. In this chapter, the intricate interplay between the aging process and the circadian clock is meticulously examined and evaluated.

Keywords: aging, circadian clock, gene, metabolic pathway, energy balance

Introduction

Circadian rhythms represent intrinsic self-sustaining oscillatory patterns with a characteristic periodicity of approximately 24 hours. These rhythms are subject to entrainment by external environmental signals, a critical mechanism that allows organisms to adjust their physiological and behavioral patterns in anticipation of impending alterations in their surroundings (Bhadra et al., 2017; Blacher et al., 2022). The temporal organization of daily activities in all organisms is orchestrated through the interplay of solar and biological cycles. Solar cycles, stemming from the Earth's rotation, result in the periodic exposure and obscuration of its surface to sunlight. Concurrently, daily biological rhythms arise from the intrinsic circadian clock present across organisms spanning various taxonomic phyla. The oscillation between illumination and obscurity generates a diverse array of environmental cues, encompassing factors such as light, temperature, and resource availability, which possess the capacity to synchronize the inherent temporal regulatory systems within these organisms. The advent of mechanical timekeeping devices has introduced a third temporal dimension known as "social time," which exerts a significant impact on the daily routines of human beings. Despite the implementation of time zones to account for the constantly shifting solar timings, these divisions remain approximations. Consequently, the occurrence of sunrise and sunset occurs at varying social times within each designated time zone, as documented by Roenneberg et al., in 2007. Within mammals, a central timekeeping center, commonly referred to as the "pacemaker," is localized in the suprachiasmatic nucleus (SCN), situated above the point where the optic nerves intersect. This circadian pacemaker orchestrates physiological processes at various levels, from regulation of gene expression to the orchestration of intricate behaviors, such as sleep patterns and performance levels. In the absence of external influences from solar and societal temporal cues, a phenomenon known as "constant conditions," the endogenous biological rhytme operates with an intrinsic period that approximates 24 hours. In the context of real-world conditions, circadian clocks are typically synchronized to the 24-hour day by external time cues, commonly referred to as zeitgebers, as discussed by Roenneberg et al., in their work from 2003 and 2007. Among the various zeitgebers, light (and its absence, darkness) stands out as the most pivotal, as it also serves as the master regulator of the rhythmicity of all other environmental effects. In mammals, light is exclusively detected through ocular mechanisms, involving a combination of photoreceptor cells encompassing rods and cones. Furthermore, melanopsin has been identified, and it is distributed within the ganglion cell layer of the retina, as extensively detailed in works by Freedman et al., (1999), Hofman (2000), Panda et al., (2002), and Roenneberg et al., (2003).

The circadian clock assumes a prominent role within neuronal systems not only during the developmental stages but also as a pivotal factor throughout the aging process. It is conceivable that interventions, whether of a pharmacological or behavioral nature, aimed at enhancing the functionality of the circadian clock according to the intrinsic signals, may hold the key to mitigating the cognitive decline associated with aging and could potentially pave the way for future chronotherapeutic approaches to address age-related maladies. As posited by Van Drunen and Eckel-Mahan in 2023, this concept is increasingly gaining recognition. Additionally, the theory of DOHaD "Developmental Origin of Health and Disease," underpinned by mounting empirical support, underscores the notion that diseases linked to lifestyle are, in fact, shaped during the formative phases of an organism, commencing with fertilization and extending throughout the embryonic and neonatal stages. This paradigm is in line with the work of Heindel and Vandenberg in 2015. While established factors contributing to disease susceptibility encompass nutrition, stress, and exposure to environmental chemicals, emerging data propose the inclusion of circadian disruption in this roster. Over the course of the last decade, research has unveiled that the circadian system initiates its development prenatally, a process initiated through entrainment from the maternal environment. Notably, in humans, the suprachiasmatic nucleus (SCN) exhibits the expression of melatonin receptors as early as eighteen weeks of gestation, followed by the subsequent regulation of the expression of dopamine receptors at 22 weeks of gestational age, as indicated in the work of Reppert et al., (1988). Maternal hormones have been observed to traverse both the placenta and the fetal BB barrier, thereby stimulating the developing fetus, as demonstrated in the study by Okatani et al., (1998). Compelling data indicate the pivotal role of maternal rhythms in shaping the build of circadian rhythms in offspring (Van Drunen and Eckel-Mahan, 2023). Early perturbations of these rhythmic processes can result in cognitive and behavioral deficits in later developmental stages. Moreover, the aging process appears to exacerbate cognitive decline by compromising the functionality of the circadian clock. Consequently, the preservation of a robust internal circadian clock emerges as a central mechanism for retarding age-associated cognitive deterioration. Recent investigations have explored numerous pharmacological and behavioral interventions, primarily employing preclinical models, to assess whether fortifying the circadian clock's function can enhance circadian resilience across the aging trajectory and prevent cognitive decline, as documented by He et al., (2016), Kim et al., (2021), and Wirianto et al., (2022).

Age and Chronotype

The chronotype, the temporal preference in individuals, is known to be influenced by various factors, encompassing genetic determinants (Vink et al., 2001), environmental variables (Roenneberg et al., 2003a), and the factor of age (Roenneberg et al., 2003a; Park et al., 2002; Duffy and Czeisler, 2002; Dijk et al., 2000). Additionally, a noteworthy pattern emerges regarding the maturation of the chronotype, where females generally exhibit an earlier chronotype compared to males. Women typically reach their peak lateness earlier than men, displaying a later chronotype throughout most of their adulthood. Intriguingly, this sex-based discrepancy, which should be distinguished from gender, diminishes around the age of fifty, as elucidated in studies by Hollander et al. (2001) and Roenneberg et al. (2007). It is noteworthy that individuals over sixty years of age, transition to even earlier chronotypes than they exhibited during childhood. The intricate interplay between age and sex, in conjunction with an understanding of how social schedules, particularly those experienced, can influence sleep-wake behavior, not only enables the accurate estimation of chronotype but also permits the standardization of an individual's chronotype, rendering it independent of age and sex. These crucial adjustments serve as a foundational requirement for genetic and epidemiological investigations, as highlighted in the work by Roenneberg et al. (2007).

Molecular Relationships between Aging and the Circadian Clock

Aging is a multifaceted process characterized by the progressive deterioration of organismal functions, directed by a combination of environmental and genetic factors. Numerous regulatory systems are implicated in the modulation of aging, with most of these systems susceptible to the effects of aging itself. Awareness that the functionality of the circadian rhythm can be affected by the aging process has been well-established. Moreover, changes in wake-sleep patterns and oscillations in physiological parameters in aging individuals. It is only in recent years, however, that the hypothesis suggesting the reciprocal influence of the biological clock on the aging process has gained traction, primarily rooted in observations conducted in model organisms, as expounded by Kondratov in 2007. The accumulating body of evidence underscores the intricate and multifaceted influences between the circadian rhythm and the aging mechanism, further underscoring that the impact of the circadian mechanisms on aging is contingent on the interplay and equilibrium of various circadian proteins, as elucidated in works by Khapre et al., (2010) and Welz and Benitah (2020).

In mammals, the orchestration of circadian rhythms is achieved through the synchronization of biological processes by the light-entrained basic pacemaker situated in the SCN within the hypothalamus. In the neurons of the suprachiasmatic nucleus, the intricate regulation of circadian rhythms is facilitated by transcription-translation feedback, which involves the core clock stimulator protein BMAL1/CLOCK and the repressor proteins PER/CRY, culminating in the generation of circadian molecular elements. Subsequently, these transcription factors translocate to the nucleus, where they engage in binding to consensus enhancer box (E-box) Deoxyribonucleic acid (DNA) patterns that regulate related genes with the circadian rhythm. Peripheral cells within the organism also possess their own autonomous circadian clocks, which are regulated by an identical transcription factor feedback loop, as expounded in works by Herzog and Tosini (2001), Albrecht and Eicheley (2003), and Blacher et al., (2022). When examining related to genes with circadian across various organs, the data reveal that nearly half of all protein-coding genes have the capacity to undergo diurnal regulation in distinct tissues, as corroborated by studies conducted by Zhang et al., in 2014 and Blacher et al., in 2022. This tissue-specific modulation of circadian gene expression plays a pivotal role in the regulation of crucial cellular processes for the preservation and dynamic adaptation of individual organ functions throughout the circadian cycle. In the context of the diurnal rhythmicity of immune responses spans a broad spectrum, encompassing processes such as leukocyte processing, immunosurveillance, the specific acting of pathogens, and the activation of the defensive immune process, as outlined by the work of Blacher et al., (2022). In the context of the innate immune system, critical constituents of myeloid responses, including the phagocytic steps, produce of cytokines and chemokines, cellular mechanisms, and the expression of Toll-like receptors, exhibit a tightly regulated diurnal rhythm with distinct circadian phases. This regulation has been substantiated by multiple studies, including those conducted by Hayashi et al., (2007), Leone et al., (2012), Oliva-Ramírez et al., (2014), Geiger et al., (2019), and Blacher et al., (2022). The temporal coordination of the first immune cell basis serves to uphold homeostasis by orchestrating a well-ordered sequence of immune defense responses against pathogens, as expounded upon in the work of Blacher et al., (2022). The process of aging is notably marked by an elevated susceptibility to a variety of diseases, among them cancer, cardiovascular disease, metabolic syndrome, and neurodegeneration. These common diseases exhibit a strong correlation with age-related alterations in immune function, influencing both their onset and progression. The aging process is further characterized by a significant dysregulation of immune functionality, including a shift towards myeloid cell differentiation over lymphoid cells, as documented in the work by Rossi et al., (2008). Additionally, aging is associated with disturbances in mitochondrial respiration and energy metabolism, rendering individuals more vulnerable to viral and bacterial infections. Furthermore, a state of persistent low-grade inflammation becomes a hallmark of the aging immune system, as illuminated by research conducted by Hofman (2000) and Blacher et al., (2022).

The amygdala, a crucial brain region, is responsible for regulating social behaviors and anxiety. Among its various nuclei, the lateral amygdaloid nucleus (LAN), the basal amygdaloid nucleus (BAN), and the medial amygdaloid nucleus (MAN) are particularly significant components of the amygdaloid complex. Emotional responses, such as anxiety, exhibit temporal variations over the course of a day, a phenomenon termed circadian (where "circa" denotes "about" and "diem" signifies "day"). Moreover, age-related changes in emotional responses indicate a regulatory role of the amygdala's function by the biological clock, which, in turn, is influenced by the aging process. To explore the interaction between circadian influences and age-related changes in the amygdala, a study examined circadian variances between the early light phase and early dark phase of the day, alongside the age-related changes in the expression of the neuronal nuclear protein (NeuN) and the neural plasticity marker phosphorylated mitogen-activated protein kinase 1/2 (p42/44-MAPK) within the LAN, BAN, and MAN subregions of the amygdala in both young and middle-aged mice. The findings revealed heightened levels of NeuN and p42/44-MAPK during the light phase, signifying a robust correlation between neuronal activity in the amygdala and the circadian system. In contrast, the group of middle-aged mice demonstrated decreased expression levels of these neuronal proteins in the amygdala, suggesting a substantial interaction between the circadian system and aging in modulating the functional state of neurons within the amygdala, as elucidated in the work by Ali and Nasr in 2023.

In addition to the influence of endogenous factors, circadian events are also activated by external stimuli, including dietary input, hormones, and other environmental cues. At the genetic level, the circadian clock comprises an intricate network of interlocked central dogma feedback loops. The central molecular components of this machinery consist of the transcription factors of CLOCK and Brain and Muscle ARNT-Like 1 (BMAL1), which build heterodimers and show affinity for E-box promoters. This interaction leads to the activation of a substantial number of clock-controlled genes (CCGs). It is emphasized that circadian events regulate the cyclic expression of approximately 10-20% of genes in any given cell, as reported by Aguilar-Arnal and Sassone-Corsi in 2013. However, emerging research suggests that a more extensive array of genes may undergo circadian regulation, contingent upon nutritional and metabolic factors, as indicated by findings by Eckel-Mahan et al., in 2013. Crucially, epigenetic mechanisms emerge as key contributors to the precise orchestration of circadian transcription. Researchers have demonstrated the importance of epigenetic control in maintaining the harmonious functioning of circadian rhythms, as evident in studies conducted by Asher et al., in 2008, Nakahata et al., in 2008, and Aguilar-Arnal et al., in 2013. The circadian rhythmicity plays a fundamental role in homeostatic control, exerting influence over a myriad of physiological steps in cellular processes. As such, disruptions in circadian rhythmicity have been linked to a range of pathologies, encompassing conditions such as obesity, diabetes, eating-sleeping disorders, neurological and psychiatric disorders.

It is worth noting that many of these diseases are not only associated with aging but are disorders that manifest in tandem with the aging process. Daily fluctuations in hormone levels, which encompass melatonin and cortisol, alongside alterations in body temperature and the sleep-wakefulness cycle, undergo modification as individuals age. These age-related changes result in disturbances within these daily cycles, characterized by decreases in their amplitude and shifts in their phase, as evidenced by the research conducted by Hofman and Swaab in 2006 and Orozco-Solis, and Sassone-Corsi in 2014. This experiment provides additional support for the concept that the circadian clock may influence the pace of aging. Early studies in rodents have also contributed to this notion, demonstrating that grafting fetal suprachiasmatic nuclei (SCN) into aged hamsters, particularly in a model known as taus/+, not only restores behavioral rhythmicity but also extends their lifespan, as documented by Hurd and Ralph in 1998. This observation aligns with findings showing that the transplantation of the pineal gland from young to older mice is capable of prolonging lifespan. In this context, the hormone melatonin serves as a potent synchronizer. The synthesis and release of melatonin exhibit fluctuations in response to the day-night cycles under sympathetic control (Haus, 2007; Perreau-Lenz et al., 2005). Furthermore, beyond its well-documented chronobiological functions, melatonin also exerts immunomodulatory, neuroendocrine, and antioxidant effects, all of which collectively develop into its anti-aging qualities, as indicated by research conducted by Poeggeler in 2005. Notably, the amplitude of melatonin amount displays gradual decreases with aging, as substantiated by various studies, including those by Kondratov et al., in 2006, Bellet et al., in 2011, Khapre et al., in 2014, and Orozco-Solis and Sassone-Corsi in 2014.

The circadian regulation and the response to genotoxic stress can indeed contribute to the clock-based regulation of the aging process. However, it is important to recognize that the circadian clock extends its control to various organism systems that are related to be intricately associated with aging. These systems include the regulation of metabolism, as underscored by Green et al., in 2008, as well as the management of oxidative stress responses, as elucidated in the works by Hardeland et al., in 2003 and Kondratov in 2007. Aging is often characterized by an increase in free radicals and reactive oxygen species (ROS) in cells. Elevated ROS levels can lead to oxidative stress, causing damage to proteins, lipids, and DNA. The progressive accumulation of such damage has been proposed as a potential cause or significant contributor to the development of various age-related diseases, as documented by Droge in 2002, and, potentially, to the aging process itself, as indicated in studies by Khapre et al., in 2010 and Welz and Benitah in 2020.

Conclusion

Circadian research represents an interdisciplinary field that integrates genetics, medicine, molecular biology, physiology, biochemistry, and psychiatry to unravel the underlying mechanisms of the biological clock present in all the phylum of organisms. These circadian clocks, when isolated from external temporal cues, maintain their own distinct periodicity, which may not precisely align with a 24-hour cycle. They achieve synchronization with the Earth's daily rotation through a process known as entrainment. Circadian clocks exert control and influence over a wide spectrum of functions, spanning from gene expression and physiological processes to behavior and cognitive functions. Furthermore, recent evidence has shed light on the mechanisms that show the relationships of aging and pathologies associated with circadian rhythmicity. Notably, cellular energy and nutrient sensing mechanisms have emerged as pivotal players in both the circadian period and the aging events. Recent research has elucidated a definite relationship between the circadian event and nutrient intake. Additionally, nutrient habits are ultimately effective and related to the anti-aging and homeostatic potential of organisms. Consequently, the prospect of targeting circadian clocks through dietary interventions or pharmacological approaches opens up a promising avenue in the realm of anti-aging therapy, emphasizing the significance of circadian rhythms and longevity. As a result, therapeutic strategies focused on the circadian regulation of metabolism and physiology warrant serious consideration in the quest for novel anti-aging interventions.

References

Aguilar-Arnal, L., & Sassone-Corsi, P. (2013). The circadian epigenome: How metabolism talks to chromatin remodeling. *Current Opinion in Cell Biology, 25*(2), 170-176.

Aguilar-Arnal, L., Hakim, O., Patel, V. R., Baldi, P., Hager, G. L., & Sassone-Corsi, P. (2013). Cycles in spatial and temporal chromosomal organization driven by the circadian clock. *Nature Structural & Molecular Biology, 20*(10), 1206-1213.

Albrecht, U., & Eichele, G. (2003). The mammalian circadian clock. *Current Opinion in Genetics & Development, 13*(3), 271–277. doi: 10.1016/S0959-437X(03)00055-8.

Ali, A. A. H., & Nasr, A. N. A. (2023). Circadian and Age-Related Changes in the Expression of NeuN and p42/44-MAPK in Mouse Amygdaloid Complex. *Egyptian Academic Journal of Biological Science, 15*(1), 63-77.

Asher, G., Gatfield, D., Stratmann, M., Reinke, H., Dibner, C., Kreppel, F., Mostoslavsky, R., Alt, F. W., & Schibler, U. (2008). SIRT1 regulates circadian clock gene expression through PER2 deacetylation. *Cell, 134*, 317-328.

Bellet, M. M., Orozco-Solis, R., Sahar, S., Eckel-Mahan, K., & Sassone-Corsi, P. (2011). The time of metabolism: NAD+, SIRT1, and the circadian clock. *Cold Spring Harbor Symposia on Quantitative Biology, 76*, 31-38.

Bhadra, U., Takkar, N., Das, P., & Pal Bhadra, M. (2017). Evolution of circadian rhythms: From bacteria to humans. *Sleep Medicine, 35*, 49–61.

Blacher, E., Tsai, C., Litichevskiy, L., Shipony, Z., Iweka, C. A., Schneider, K. M., Chuluun, B., Heller, H. C., Menon, V., Thaiss, C. A., & Andreasson, K. I. (2022). Aging disrupts circadian gene regulation and function in macrophages. *Nature Immunology, 23*, 229-236.

Dijk, D. J., Duffy, J. F., & Czeisler, C. A. (2000). Contribution of circadian physiology and sleep homeostasis to age-related changes in human sleep.

Dröge, W. (2002). Free radicals in the physiological control of cell function. *Physiological Reviews, 82*, 47-95.

Duffy, J. F., & Czeisler, C. A. (2002). Age-related change in the relationship between circadian period, circadian phase, and diurnal preference in humans. *Neuroscience Letters, 318*(3), 117–120.

Eckel-Mahan, K. L., Patel, V. R., de Mateo, S., Orozco-Solis, R., Ceglia, N. J., Sahar, S., Dilag-Penilla, S. A., Dyar, K. A., Baldi, P., & Sassone-Corsi, P. (2013). Reprogramming of the circadian clock by nutritional challenge. *Cell, 155*, 1464-1478.

Freedman, M. S., Lucas, R. J., Soni, B., Von Schantz, M., Muñoz, M., David-Gray, Z., & Foster, R. (1999). Regulation of mammalian circadian behavior by non-rod, non-cone, ocular photoreceptors. *Science, 284*(5413), 502-504.

Geiger, S. S., Curtis, A. M., O'Neill, L. A. J., Siegel, R. M. (2019). Daily variation in macrophage phagocytosis is clock-independent and dispensable for cytokine production. *Immunology, 157*, 122–136.

Green, C. B., Takahashi, J. S., & Bass, J. (2008). The meter of metabolism. *Cell, 134*, 728–742.

Hardeland, R., Coto-Montes, A., Poeggeler, B. (2003). Circadian rhythms, oxidative stress, and antioxidative defense mechanisms. *Chronobiology International, 20*, 921–962.

Haus, E. (2007). Chronobiology in the endocrine system. *Advances in Drug Delivery Reviews, 59*, 985-1014.

Hayashi, M., Shimba, S., Tezuka, M. (2007). Characterization of the molecular clock in mouse peritoneal macrophages. *Biological and Pharmaceutical Bulletin, 30*, 621–626.

He He, B., Nohara, K., Park, N., Park, Y. S., Guillory, B., Zhao, Z., Garcia, J. M., Koike, N., Lee, C. C., Takahashi, J. S., Yoo, S. H., & Chen, Z. (2016). The small molecule nobiletin targets the molecular oscillator to enhance circadian rhythms and protect against metabolic syndrome. *Cell metabolism, 23*(4), 610-621. doi: 10.1016/j.cmet. 2016.03.007.

Heindel, J. J., & Vandenberg, L. N. (2015). Developmental origins of health and disease: A paradigm for understanding disease cause and prevention. *Current Opinion in Pediatrics, 27*, 248–253. doi: 10.1097/MOP.0000000000000191.

Herzog, E. D., & Tosini, G. (2001). The mammalian circadian clock shop. *Seminars in Cell and Developmental Biology, 12*, 295–303.

Hofman, M. A. (2000). The human circadian clock and aging. *Chronobiology International, 17*(3), 245-259. doi: 10.1081/CBI-10010104.

Hofman, M. A., & Swaab, D. F. (2006). Living by the clock: The circadian pacemaker in older people. *Ageing Research Reviews, 5*, 33-51.

Hollander, L. E., Freeman, E. W., Sammel, M. D., Berlin, J. A., Grisso, J. A., Battistini, M. (2001). Sleep quality, estradiol levels, and behavioral factors in late reproductive age women. *Obstetrics & Gynecology, 98*(3), 391–397.

Hurd, M. W., & Ralph, M. R. (1998). The significance of circadian organization for longevity in the golden hamster. *Journal of Biological Rhythms, 13*, 430-436.

Kang, T. H., Reardon, J. T., Kemp, M., Sancar, A. (2009). Circadian oscillation of nucleotide excision repair in mammalian brain. *Proceedings of the National Academy of Sciences of the United States of America, 106*, 2864–2867.

Khapre, R. V., Kondratova, A. A., Patel, S., Dubrovsky, Y., Wrobel, M., Antoch, M. P., Kondratov R. V. (2014). BMAL1-dependent regulation of the mTOR signaling pathway delays aging. *Aging (Albany, NY), 6*, 48-57.

Khapre, R. V., Samsa, W. E., Kondratov, R. V. (2010). Circadian regulation of cell cycle: Molecular connections between aging and the circadian clock. *Annals of Medicine, 42*(6), 404-415. doi: 10.3109/07853890.2010.499134.

Kim, E., Nohara, K., Wirianto, M., Escobedo Jr, G., Lim, J. Y., Morales, R., Yoo, S. H., & Chen, Z. (2021). Effects of the clock modulator nobiletin on circadian rhythms and pathophysiology in female mice of an Alzheimer's disease model. *Biomolecules, 11*(7), 1004. doi: 10.3390/biom11071004.

Kondratov, R. V., Kondratova, A. A., Gorbacheva, V. Y., Vykhovanets, O. V., Antoch, M. P. (2006). Early aging and age-related pathologies in mice deficient in BMAL1, the core component of the circadian clock. *Genes & Development, 20*, 1868-1873.

Kondratov, R. V. (2007). A role of the circadian system and circadian proteins in aging. *Ageing Research Reviews, 6*, 12-27.

Leone, M. J., Marpegan, L., Duhart, J. M., Golombek, D. A. (2012). Role of proinflammatory cytokines on lipopolysaccharide-induced phase shifts in locomotor activity circadian rhythm. *Chronobiology International, 29*, 715-723.

Nakahata, Y., Kaluzova, M., Grimaldi, B., Sahar, S., Hirayama, J., Chen, D., Guarente, L. P., Sassone-Corsi, P. (2008). The NAD+-dependent deacetylase SIRT1 modulates CLOCK-mediated chromatin remodeling and circadian control. *Cell, 134*, 329-340.

Okatani, Y., Okamoto, K., Hayashi, K., Wakatsuki, A., Tamura, S., Sagara, Y. (1998). Maternal-fetal transfer of melatonin in pregnant women near term. *Journal of Pineal Research, 25*, 129–134.

Oliva-Ramírez, J., Moreno-Altamirano, M. M. B., Pineda-Olvera, B., Cauich-Sánchez, P., Javier Sánchez-García, F. (2014). Crosstalk between circadian rhythmicity, mitochondrial dynamics, and macrophage bactericidal activity. *Immunology, 143*, 490–497.

Orozco-Solis, R., & Sassone-Corsi, P. (2014). Circadian clock: Linking epigenetics to aging. *Current Opinion in Genetics & Development, 26*, 66–72. http://dx.doi.org/10.1016/j.gde.2014.0.

Panda, S., Sato, T. K., Castrucci, A. M., Rollag, M. D., DeGrip, W. J., Hogenesch, J. B., Provencio, I., & Kay, S. A. (2002). Melanopsin (Opn4) requirement for normal light-induced circadian phase shifting. *Science*, *298*(5601), 2213-2216.

Park, Y. M., Matsumoto, K., Seo, Y. J., Kang, M. J., Nagashima, H. (2002). Changes of sleep or waking habits by age and sex in Japanese. *Perceptual and Motor Skills, 94*, 1199–1213.

Perreau-Lenz, S., Kalsbeek, A., Van Der Vliet, J., Pe´vet, P., Buijs, R. M. (2005). In vivo evidence for a controlled offset of melatonin synthesis at dawn by the suprachiasmatic nucleus in the rat. *Neuroscience, 130*, 797-803.

Poeggeler, B. (2005). Melatonin, aging, and age-related diseases: Perspectives for prevention, intervention, and therapy. *Endocrine, 27*, 201-212.

Reppert, S. M., Weaver, D. R., Rivkees, S. A., & Stopa, E. G. (1988). Putative melatonin receptors in a human biological clock. *Science, 242*, 78–81. doi: 10.1126/ science.2845576.

Roenneberg, T., Daan, S., Merrow, M. (2003). The art of entrainment. *Journal of Biological Rhythms, 18*(3), 183–194.

Roenneberg, T., Wirz-Justice, A., Merrow, M. (2003). Life between clocks—daily temporal patterns of human chronotypes. *Journal of Biological Rhythms, 18*(1), 80–90.

Roenneberg, T., Kuehnle, T., Juda, M., Kantermann, T., Allebrandt, K., Gordijn, M., Merrow, M. (2007). Epidemiology of the human circadian clock. *Sleep Medicine Reviews, 11*, 429-438.

Rossi, D. J., Jamieson, C. H., Weissman, I. L. (2008). Stems cells and the pathways to aging and cancer. *Cell, 132*, 681-696.

Van Drunen, R., Eckel-Mahan, K. (2023). Circadian rhythms as modulators of brain health during development and throughout aging. *Frontiers in Neural Circuits, 16*. https://doi.org/10.3389/fncir.2022.1059229.

Vink, J. M., Groot, A. S., Kerkhof, G. A., Boomsma, D. I. (2001). Genetic analysis of morningness and eveningness. *Chronobiology International, 18*(5), 809–822.

Welz, P. S., Benitah, S. A. (2020). Molecular Connections Between Circadian Clocks and Aging. *Journal of Molecular Biology, 432*, 3661-3679. https://doi.org/10.1016/j.jmb. 2019.12.036.

Wirianto, M., Wang, C. Y., Kim, E., Koike, N., Gomez-Gutierrez, R., Nohara, K., Escobedo G. Jr, Choi J. M., Han C., Yagita K., Jung S. Y., Soto C, Lee H. K., Morales R, Yoo S. H., & Chen, Z. (2022). The clock modulator Nobiletin mitigates astrogliosis-associated neuroinflammation and disease hallmarks in an Alzheimer's disease model. *The FASEB Journal*, *36*(3). doi: 10.1096/fj.202101633R.

Zhang, R., Lahens, N. F., Ballance, H. I., Hughes, M. E., Hogenesch, J. B. (2014). A circadian gene expression atlas in mammals: Implications for biology and medicine. *Proceedings of the National Academy of Sciences of the United States of America, 111*, 16219–16224.

Chapter 9

The Circadian Rhythm and Light Influence on Skin Health and Disorders

Seyfullah Yücel*, MD

Department of Internal Medicine, Kahramanmaras Necip Fazıl City Hospital, Kahramanmaras, Turkiye

Abstract

Organisms have an internal rhythm that helps them anticipate and adapt to daily changes in the environment. The timing of the circadian clock, which is synchronized with the light-dark cycle over a period of about 24 hours, is adjusted by light-triggering signals sent from the retina to the suprachiasmatic nucleus. Food intake, exercise, temperature, and other inputs affect the clocks of peripheral tissues, including the skin. Disruption of the circadian rhythm has been linked to a wide range of dermatological problems. Studies have shown that earlier exposure to ultraviolet light can continue to damage the skin even in the dark, and this has shown that skin cell repair peaks at night. In this book chapter, we discuss the complex interaction between the core clock network and key physiological processes in the skin, such as homeostasis, regeneration, and immune and stress responses. Afterward, we discuss studies involving the circadian clock and skin diseases, including skin cancer, sunburn, hair loss, aging, infections, inflammation, skin diseases, and wound healing. A better understanding of the role that circadian rhythm plays in overall skin health will help doctors provide optimal treatment to patients, including the use of topical medications at the most effective times during a 24-hour cycle and appropriate recommendations regarding skin care.

* Corresponding Author's Email: seyfullahyucel016@gmail.com.

In: Human Health is a Matter of Timing
Editors: Sumeyya Deniz Aybek, Gonca Gulbay and Mucahit Secme
ISBN: 979-8-89113-467-6

Keywords: aging, cancer, circadian clock, skin diseases

Introduction

The skin, which makes up the bulk of the body, plays an important role in defense mechanisms against the environment, including toxins, microorganisms, and radiation (Wong et al., 2016; Zouboulis, 2009). However, the skin is an important part of organism homeostasis, with fat storage and hormone production, including vitamin D.

The circadian clock, an internal autonomous clock that controls different functions of the body day and night, affects skin stem cell metabolism and proliferation, DNA repair, stimulus response, and the expression of multiple genes that mediate immunity. Circadian clock research has elucidated the key regulatory mechanisms that contribute to skin cancer, aging, inflammatory, and other skin diseases. Existing clinical trials have begun to use these findings to develop treatments based on the principles of circadian medicine. Although circadian dermatology is a new field, research on the circadian clock continues to unravel the complex regulation system of the skin.

Understanding the role of the circadian clock in skin may provide new insights into the pathogenesis and treatment of skin diseases. To this end, we will review the role of the circadian clock in the skin, highlight the latest findings in the field, and discuss the role of circadian clock disruption in skin diseases.

Circadian Rhythm

Although sunlight is an important regulator of circadian rhythms, there is not enough information about the effects of UV radiation on circadian rhythms (Kawara et al., 2002). Although it is known that 10% of genes in the body have circadian oscillations, circadian rhythms affect many physiological functions. The group of genes under circadian control includes genes involved in cell proliferation, DNA damage repair response, cell cycle and cell cycle arrest, and apoptosis (Sancar et al., 2010). Light plays an important role in the regulation of circadian rhythms in the body. Circadian rhythms are entrained by a central pacemaker in the SCN region of the brain when light is perceived by the retina (Reppert et al., 2002). Thus, it can adjust its body clock according to the light/dark cycles in the environment. Because light has a significant impact on circadian rhythm patterns, disturbances in natural light patterns, such as the increased use of artificial light at night, can cause irregularities in circadian rhythms. Disrupted circadian rhythms can cause a variety of negative health problems. Obesity, diabetes, and cardiovascular disease can be affected by circadian rhythm disturbances. Changes in eating habits and sleep patterns lead to decreased leptin levels and a reversal of cortisol release patterns, as well as insulin, postprandial glucose, and mean arterial pressure (Scheer et al., 2009). However, epidemiological studies show an increased risk of metabolic disease for alternate shift and night shift workers compared to day workers (De Bacquer et al., 2009; Pietroiusti et al., 2010).

A study on the effects of UV light on keratinocytes has shown that UVB can suppress most of the genes involved in circadian rhythm regulation for up to 24 hours (Kawara et al., 2002). A recent study has shown that circadian rhythms can have a protective effect on skin against UVB damage (Gaddameedhi et al., 2011). The Xeroderma pigmentosum group A (XPA) protein has a very important place in the DNA damage repair in the body as it is one of the proteins that perform DNA excision repair. Gaddameedhi et al. (2011) showed that XPA is released through circadian rhythmicity in the skin, reaching its lowest level in the early morning and peaking in mice in the early evening. Mice exposed to UVB light in the early morning showed a frequency five times higher and a faster skin cancer growth rate than mice exposed to the same UVB light in the early evening. This suggests that the normal circadian rhythm is important in the body's natural defenses against UV-induced skin cancer and should be taken into account when examining UV light exposure and cancer. With this study, the authors suggested that the circadian rhythm could be used to reduce the incidence of skin cancer in humans. Because the core circadian clock and its outputs showed contrasting stages in mice (being nocturnal species) versus humans (being diurnal species), the authors of this study predicted that humans would be less prone to the carcinogenic effect of UV radiation early in the day and would have a higher repair rate in the morning.

Circadian Rhythm and Skin

Acting as a protective barrier against external stressors and toxins, the skin is a multi-layered organ that houses various cell types to prevent hormone synthesis and perform many tasks, such as dehydration (Wong et al., 2016; Zouboulis, 2009). In humans and mice, the skin consists of three main layers:

the epidermis, dermis, and hypodermis; Each layer has its own unique active circadian clocks.

Light plays an important role in circadian rhythm regulation due to its effect on the central pacemaker in the SCN. Furthermore, light can play a secondary role in the regulation of circadian rhythms through the regulation of the pineal hormone melatonin. In recent studies, melatonin has been established to be a pleiotropic bioregulator with a multitude of functions (Pandi-Perumal et al., 2006; Hardeland and Pandi-Perumal, 2005; Hardeland, 2005). Defensive responses have been shown to be involved in the modulation of anti-jet delay and tumor growth inhibitor effects, as well as acting as a potent antioxidant, chemotoxicity-reducing agent, and putative anti-aging agent (Carrillo-Vico et al., 2004; Guerrero et al., 2002; Jung et al., 2006; Herxheimer et al., 2002; Poeggeler et al., 1993; Tan et al., 2002; Karasek et al., 2002; Reiter et al., 1999; Reiter et al., 2002). These pleiotropic properties are of particular interest to researchers about this endogenous factor. The effects of melatonin on cellular and organism health have led to research on the mechanical effects of melatonin against various stresses, including the oxidative stress produced by UV exposure. Melatonin levels vary with the circadian rhythm and are typically low during the day and high at night (Schernhammer et al., 2001). Exposure to light leads to a rapid drop in melatonin levels and a decrease in melatonin production due to negative feedback (Gupta et al., 2013). Melatonin has been associated with the suppression of ultraviolet (UV) damage in skin cells, hair growth, antitumor, and wound healing effects (Kleszczyński et al., 2011; Gupta et al., 2013, Ozler et al., 2010). Oral melatonin supplements are widely used to improve sleep quality and sleep comfortably, and studies have shown that taking melatonin externally stimulates the secretion of nocturnal melatonin (Lewy et al., 1992 and Deacon et al., 1995). Circadian rhythm is thought to have many different effects on skin, from transepidermal water loss to keratinocyte proliferation, and is associated with the risk of cancer and other diseases (Matsunaga et al., 2014). It has also been shown that the repair of DNA-damaged skin cells peaks at night as a result of UV exposure (Yosipovitch et al., 1998). Furthermore, DNA damage may continue on the skin in the dark even with previous exposure to UV light (Premi et al., 2015).

In addition to the SCN, the circadian system is also made up of peripheral circadian oscillators in many cells, including the skin. The skin contains circadian clock genes that are involved in regulating the circadian rhythm (Zanello et al., 2000). As a result of circadian rhythm changes in the stratum corneum, skin permeability is higher in the evening (Yosipovitch et al., 1998).

Aquaporin 3 (AQP3) is produced in the epidermis and is regulated by molecular clocks that aid in transepidermal water loss (Matsunaga et al., 2014). Since transepidermal water loss is associated with increased pruritus in cases of atopic dermatitis, increased itching is observed at night in patients with atopic dermatitis (Patel et al., 2007). The effect of topical medications on the skin is also associated with the circadian rhythm. Skin penetration of hydrophilic and lipophilic topical drugs is at its maximum around 4:00 a.m. with slowing absorption during daylight hours (Reinberg et al., 1995).

Another component that can affect the absorption and effectiveness of topical medications is the blood flow to the skin. Skin blood flow rate has also been shown to be influenced by the circadian rhythm and increases in the late afternoon and at night (Smolander et al., 1993). Circadian rhythm blood flow rates have been shown to be maintained even during treatment with topical corticosteroids (Yosipovitch et al., 1998). Vasodilation and increased skin blood flow have been shown to accelerate diffusion and drug passage from tissues into the systemic circulation (Lemmer et al., 1994).

The proliferation of keratinocytes has also been found to alter with the circadian rhythm, with peak proliferation occurring around midnight (Frentz et al., 1991). Cortisol levels also vary throughout the day, with a natural drop in cortisol levels in the evening, which may be a factor that increases complaints in patients with inflammatory skin conditions that increase itching at night (Gupta et al., 2013). Most patients with inflammatory dermatosis, including psoriasis and atopic dermatitis, have increased nocturnal itching (Ozler et al., 2010). The circadian rhythm also controls skin temperature and core body temperature (Yosipovitch et al., 1998).

Circadian Rhythm and Skin Diseases

Since the circadian rhythm affects many skin processes, including immunity, metabolism, cell proliferation, and DNA damage repair, it comes to mind that circadian dysregulation may contribute to the occurrence and progression of skin diseases. The link between circadian dysfunction and skin diseases is being studied in both laboratory and clinical settings. In the lab, chronic jet lag, prolonged light exposure, and flashlight treatment at night caused circadian disruption in mice. Human studies mostly focus on epidemiological data collected from shift workers and aim to determine the relationship between circadian disturbances due to shift work and diseases. In this regard, we focus on the effect of the circadian clock on various skin diseases such as skin cancer, sunburn, aging, hair loss, inflammatory diseases, and wound healing.

Skin Cancer

Skin cancers are classified into two main headings: carcinoma and melanoma. Carcinomas, such as squamous cell and basal cell carcinomas, are caused by keratinocytes. Melanomas are derived from melanocytes (Simoes et al., 2015). Carcinomas are more common, and melanomas are more deadly, and metastasize through the blood (Lubov et al., 2021). UV radiation is a potent mutagen that is considered the main cause of human skin cancers (Leffell et al., 2007). Exposure to both the sun and indoor UV rays contributes to the carcinogenesis of the skin. The cellular effects of UV radiation are induced primarily through a chain of events that cause the induction of DNA lesions. The chemical nature and effectiveness of the formation of DNA lesions largely depend on the type and wavelength of UV radiation and the base composition of the DNA at the lesion site (Runger, 2007; Yagura et al., 2011). Different wavelengths of UV radiation indicate different levels of skin penetration, which causes different effects (Agar et al., 2004). UV radiation from the sun can be divided into three types according to its wavelength: UVA, UVB, and UVC. UVC is the most harmful of all, and most of it is absorbed by the ozone layer. At the same time, most of the UVA and a small percentage of UVB still reach the Earth. These two wavelengths are absorbed by the skin and cause DNA mutations with different modes of action. While UVB accounts for only a small fraction of the UV radiation that reaches the Earth's surface, it is thought to be most responsible for skin cancers. UVB has been shown to have less penetration power than UVA and mainly affects the epidermal basal layer of the skin.

Solar UV radiation is the primary source for the occurrence of skin cancers, which more often affect the Caucasian population. The estimated incidence rate for these cancers is ~1 million new cases diagnosed each year in the United States alone (Jemal et al., 2010). Non-melanoma skin cancers, consisting of squamous cell carcinomas (SCCs) and basal cell carcinomas (BCCs), which account for ~96% of all skin cancers, are melanoma (Bowden et al., 2004; Cemal et al., 2010). Most skin cancers develop in areas of the skin that come into contact with the sun. While non-melanoma skin cancers are more benign, melanoma, the least common form of skin cancer, usually has a high mortality rate. Skin cancer caused by UV radiation involves three distinct stages defined as initiation, progression, and ascension, mediated by changes in cellular, biochemical, and molecular mechanisms. Initiation is the beginning of the process of photocarcinogenesis, which involves genetic changes in which DNA translational changes occur. When these mutations occur, they are thought to be irreversible. These DNA mutations cause changes in signal transduction that cause clonal expansion of initiated cells, but clonal expansion is still thought to be reversible. If the initiated cells undergo clonal expansion and the processes of carcinogenesis cannot be stopped, tumor progression begins with the malignant transformation of papillomas into carcinomas (Ananthaswamy et al., 1990; Melnikova et al., 2005).

Epidemiological studies linking occupational working hours and circadian disruption to cancer risk have highlighted the effect of the circadian clock in several types of cancer, including melanoma (Sandu et al., 2015).

The skin is protected from UV radiation by melanin (Sarkar and Gaddameedhi, 2020). The core clock component, BMAL1, is involved in the production of melanin, along with the microphthalmia-associated transcription factor (MITF), which is the main regulator of melanogenesis. MITF indicates the levels of rhythmic expression related to BMAL1. By overexpressing BMAL1, melanin from the melanogenesis pathway was correspondingly higher, providing greater protection for skin cells against damage from UV radiation (Sarkar et al., 2021).

In addition to controlling susceptibility to UV-induced DNA damage and cancer onset, the watch plays a role in the progression of skin cancer in at least two ways. On the one hand, cancerous cells abnormally have clock genes, which leads to impaired clock function (Masri et al., 2015). On the other hand, mutations in core clock genes are associated with melanoma progression (Gutierrez and Arbesman, 2016). Recent studies have targeted components of the circadian clock to normalize tumor cell circadian rhythms in cancer treatment (Masri et al., 2015).

A comparison of gene expression data from human melanoma and healthy skin samples shows a downregulation of clock genes in melanoma (De Assis et al., 2018). Increased regulation of oncogenes, such as RAS, lengthens the duration of the clock by indicating mechanisms that disrupt the circadian mechanism in the progression of cancer (Relogio et al., 2014). In oncogenic keratinocytes, the circadian mechanism is disrupted; Ablation of the tumor suppressor gene PTEN increases BMAL1 in hair follicle stem cells, revealing the regulatory effect of tumor suppressors on the components of the core clock (Zagni et al., 2017).

In addition to impaired circadian clock function in melanoma cells, circadian clock irregularities also act on other oncogenic mechanisms. Myeloid-specific BMAL1 knockout causes metabolic dysregulation in macrophages, thereby facilitating immune suppression and melanoma tumor burden (Alexander et al., 2020). Given that circadian clock dysfunction increases tumor proliferation, aiming to improve the function of the clock may facilitate the management of the fight against cancer. Stimulation of circadian rhythmicity by dexamethasone in tumor cells slows melanoma growth in vivo in mice (Kiessling et al., 2017). This response is clock-related since disabling BMAL 1 in tumors prevents the growth-inhibiting effect of dexamethasone. Pharmacological studies have also targeted components of the circadian clock, the nuclear hormone receptors NR1D1 and NR1D2, to stimulate apoptosis in cancer cells (Sulli et al., 2018). By administering agonists of these receptors, senescent cells, such as those of melanocytic nevi, undergo cell death, indicating that treatments targeting core clock machines impair melanoma proliferation. Current cancer treatments can target circadian clock machines but use the clock by modulating time to administer treatment. Looking at the mechanism of action of chemotherapeutic cisplatin, its toxicity to melanoma cells varies throughout the day, indicating that melanoma treatment is more beneficial for patients in the morning (Dakup et al., 2018).

In summary, the circadian clock plays a role in the onset and progression of skin cancer. The rhythmicity of the clock regulates the repair of DNA damage, thereby regulating the susceptibility to UV-induced DNA damage and cancer onset. Carcinomas and melanomas often promote cell cycle transitions and cell proliferation by reducing clock function. Therapeutically targeting of core clock genes to restore clock function may be a promising approach to cancer treatment.

Sunburn

Short-term exposure to excessive UV radiation causes sunburn. DNA damage due to UV radiation leads to the onset of an inflammatory process characterized by pain, redness, and swelling of the skin (De Assis et al., 2021). On human skin, radiation in the evening (between 7 p.m. and 9 p.m.) causes more severe redness than between 7 a.m. and 9 p.m., indicating that human skin is more sensitive to radiation in the evening hours (Nikkola et al., 2018). UV-induced DNA damage is related to acute inflammatory processes, but the effect of UV radiation on the skin depends on the time of day due to DNA damage repair and the recording of the cell cycle (De Assis et al., 2021; Nikkola et al., 2018).

Hair Loss

Hair loss, also known as alopecia, is one of the most common skin problems. Although it usually occurs on the scalp, hair loss can affect any hair-bearing part of the body. The most common form of alopecia is androgenetic alopecia, which affects both women and men, despite a different pattern of hair loss. There is also an aging-related hair loss that is not associated with androgenetic alopecia (Geyfman et al., 2015). Alopecia areata is an autoimmune disease characterized by hair loss. Another type of alopecia is scar alopecia, which are inflammatory condition that leads to the permanent loss of hair follicles and the destruction of bulging stem cells of the hair follicle (Vary, 2015). Given the regulatory role of the circadian clock in hair follicles, it is thought that clock disturbances may contribute to hair loss and aging-related hair loss. However, evidence of this has not been adequately demonstrated in epidemiological studies. The clearest evidence of the circadian clock's role in hair loss comes from mouse studies showing that the clock stops cell division in growing hair follicles. Therefore, when γ radiation is applied to anagen hair follicles in the morning, when mitosis peaks, it causes more hair loss than in the evening when mitosis levels decrease (Plikus et al., 2013). Based on this finding in mice, it is estimated that evening radiation will cause more hair loss than morning radiation in humans. Therefore, it may be better to arrange radiotherapy treatment in the morning to minimize hair follicle damage during treatment.

Aging

At the organism level, aging is linked to circadian rhythm, as indicated by features such as improved sleep patterns, flattened body temperature fluctuation, and decreased activity levels during wakefulness (Hood and Amir, 2017). Characteristics of aging on the skin include lines and wrinkles, hair loss, dryness, a thin epidermis, slow wound healing, and easy breakage, as well as skin fragility. Endogenous aging, which is one of the causes of skin aging, is strongly correlated with chronological age. Intrinsic aging mechanisms include oxidative damage to DNA and proteins produced by metabolism, stem cell dysfunction, accumulation of genetic mutations, and changes in hormones. Other causes of aging include UV radiation, mainly in external skin aging mechanisms, but also other factors such as pollution and smoking (Bonte et al., 2019). Because circadian rhythms in the skin can protect cells from UV-induced DNA damage by regulating cell proliferation, circadian reprogramming and cell cycle shifts caused by internal aging may contribute to external skin aging (Geyfman et al., 2012). Additionally, clock-related hormone dysfunction caused by internal aging, although it does not affect skin function, can facilitate external skin aging. The hormone melatonin is one of the hormones that regulate peripheral clocks, and its receptor is found in the skin (Slominski AT et al., 2018). The melatonin receptor MT1 has an important role in DNA repair, as it activates the P53-dependent DNA damage response (Santoro et al., 2013). On human skin, MT1 levels decrease as we age, resulting in increased sensitivity to UV radiation (Dong K et al., 2020).

Skin Infections

The circadian clock regulates daily rhythms in innate immunity (Plikus et al., 2015; Scheiermann et al., 2013). The circadian clock regulates immune responses to infections in the digestive tract, respiratory system, liver, and other body parts (Sundar et al., 2015; Sengupta et al., 2019; Chen et al., 2020; Bellet et al., 2013). For example, the severity of parasitic infections on the skin varies daily. In vitro experiments confirm that the binding of the parasite to mouse macrophages occurs through a circadian rhythm and depends on the circadian mechanism, which also regulates the time-dependent release of cytokines and chemokines (Kiessling et al., 2015). Although there are few studies on circadian regulation of the skin's defenses against viral infections, studies in other organs show that the circadian clock plays a role in regulating this activity. Skin has the task of defending against many viruses, which are biological entities that can only develop and multiply in a living cell. Mice infected with influenza or herpes viruses intranasally during the day have a higher burden of infection and death than mice infected at night (Edgar et al., 2016).

Inflammatory skin diseases

Inflammatory responses are related to circadian rhythms (Greenberg et al., 2020). Disruption of the circadian rhythm can lead to inflammatory diseases. For example, in mice, chronic jet lag causes ulcerative dermatitis (Kettner et al., 2016). Atopic dermatitis and psoriasis are two of the most common autoimmune skin diseases. Both diseases are related to circadian rhythms. In humans, disruption of the circadian clock during the night shift is associated with psoriasis (Lu et al., 2019; Li et al., 2013). Psoriasis symptoms have a diurnal rhythm, with more than 70% of patients reporting itching that increases in severity in the evening or at night (Ferguson et al., 2021). Itching that occurs at night disrupts sleep patterns, which increases the severity of the disease and disrupts circadian rhythms. This circadian disruption also contributes to the development of metabolic diseases such as obesity, which may be causally linked to psoriasis (Rodrigues et al., 2021).

Conclusion

Light, melatonin, and circadian rhythms are all intertwined in a complex system. The balance required for proper maintenance of this system depends on exposure to the proper amount of light. The disruption of our light-dark cycles caused by the overuse of artificial lights disrupts the balance of circadian rhythms.

Circadian medicine is an important component of preventive medicine and patient care and is receiving more and more attention. Studies in model animals and cultured human cells show how disruption of circadian rhythms through clock gene manipulations can contribute to the development and progression of various skin diseases, including cancer, radiation-induced hair loss, sunburns, aging, inflammatory diseases, infections, and wounds. Additionally shift work, social jet lag, sleep disturbances, and excessive exposure to light at night have all been common causes of circadian rhythm disturbance in modern society. Shift workers are more prone to skin diseases such as psoriasis, itching, dandruff/seborrheic dermatitis, dry skin, acne, and melanoma.

Therefore, maintaining normal sleep patterns and avoiding shift work will be beneficial to minimize the risk and severity of skin diseases. While it makes sense that a healthy lifestyle aimed at maintaining normal circadian rhythms can improve skin health, a better understanding of circadian regulation is needed to develop new strategies to address circadian-related conditions and diseases.

References

Agar, N. S., G. M. Halliday, R. S. Barnetson, H. N. Ananthaswamy, M. Wheeler, and A. M. Jones (2004) The basal layer in human squamous tumors harbors more UVA than UVB fingerprint mutations: The role of UVA in human skin carcinogenesis. *Proc. Natl Acad. Sci. USA*101, 4954–4959.

Alexander R. K., Liou Y. H., Knudsen N. H., Starost K. A., Xu C., Hyde A. L, Liu S., Jacobi D., Liao N. S. ve Lee C. H. (2020) Bmal1 mitokondriyal entegre eder.

Ananthaswamy, H. N. and W. E. Pierceall (1990) Molecular mechanisms of ultraviolet radiation carcinogenesis. *Photochemistry. Photobiol*. 52, 1119–1136.

Bellet, M. M., Deriu, E., Liu, J. Z., Grimaldi, B., Blaschitz, C., Zeller, M., Edwards, R. A., Sahar, S., Dandekar, S., Baldi, P., George, M. D., Raffatellu, M., and Sassone-Corsi, P. (2013) The circadian clock regulates host response to salmonella. *Proc Natl Acad Sci USA* 110, 9897–9902.

Bonte F., Girard D., Archambault J. C. and Desmouliere A. (2019) Skin changes during aging. *Subcellular biochemistry*, pp. 249–280, Springer Singapore.

Bruguerolle, B., Giaufre, E., & Prat, M. (1991). Temporal changes in transcutaneous passage of drugs: the case of lidocaine in children and rats. *Chronobiology international*, *8*(4), 277-282. https://doi.org/10.3109/07420529109063932.

Carrillo-Vico, A., J. R. Calvo, P. Abreu, P. J. Lardone, S. Garcia-Maurino, R. J. Reiter, and J. M. Guerrero (2004) Evidence and physiological significance of melatonin synthesis by human lymphocytes: Possible role as an intracrine, autocrine, and/or paracrine substance. *FASEB J*. 18, 537–539.

Chen L., Li S., Nie J., Zhao J., Yu S., Li Y. and Peng J. (2020) Bmal1 regulates clotting factor biosynthesis in mouse liver in streptococcal oralis infection. *Pre-cell infected microbiome* 10, 530190.

Dakup P. P., Porter K. I., Little A. A., Gajula R. P., Zhang H., Skornyakov E., Kemp M. G., Van Dongen H. P. A., and Gaddameedhi S. (2018) The circadian clock regulates cisplatin-induced toxicity and tumor regression in melanoma mice and human models. *Oncodestination* 9, 14524–14538.

de Assis L. V. M., Kinker G. S., Moraes M. N., Markus R. P., Fernandes P. A. and de Castrucci (2018) Expression of the circadian clock gene BMAL1 is positively associated with antitumor immunity and patient survival in metastatic melanoma. *Front Oncol* 8, 185.

de Assis L. V. M., Tonolli P. N., Moraes M. N., Baptista M. S. and Lauro Castrucci (2021) How does the skin perceive sunlight? An integrative view of light-sensing molecules. *J Photochem Photobiol,* C 47, 100403.

De Bacquer, D., M. Van Risseghem, E. Clays, F. Kittel, G. De Backer, and L. Braeckman (2009) Rotational shift work and metabolic syndrome: A prospective study. *Int. J. Epidemiol.* 38, 848–854.

Deacon, S., & Arendt, J. (1995). Melatonin-induced temperature suppression and acute phase shift effects are associated in humans in a dose-dependent manner. *Brain research*, *688*(1-2), 77-85. https://doi.org/10.1016/0006-8993(95)96872-i.

Edgar R. S., Stangherlin A., Nagy A. D., Nicoll M. P., Efstathiou S., O'Neill J. S. and Reddy A. B. (2016) Cell autonomic regulation of herpes and influenza virus infection by circadian clock. *Proc Natl Acad Sci* 113, 10085.

Frentz, G., Møller, U., Hölmich, P., & Christensen, I. J. (1991). On circadian rhythms in human epidermis cell proliferation. *Acta dermato-venereologica*, *71*(1), 85-87. doi: 10.12688/f1000research.11770.1.

Gaddameedhi, S., C. P. Selby, W. K. Kaufmann, R. C. Smart and A. Sancar (2011) Control of skin cancer by circadian rhythm. *Proc. Natl Acad. Sci. USA* 108, 18790–18795.

Geyfman M., Kumar V., Liu Q., Ruiz R., Gordon W., Espitia F., Cam E., Millar S. E., Smyth P., Ihler A. et al. (2012) Brain and muscle arnt-like protein-1 (BMAL1) controls circadian cell proliferation and susceptibility to UVB-induced DNA damage in the epidermis. *Proc Natl Acad Sci* 109, 11758–11763.

Geyfman M., Plikus M. V., Treffeisen E., Andersen B. and Paus R. (2015) Resting From Now: Redefining Telogen as the maintenance phase of the hair growth cycle. *Biol Rev Camb Philos Soc* 90, 1179 1196.

Greenberg E. N., Marshall M. E., Jin S., Venkatesh S., Dragan M., Tsoi L. C., Gudjonsson J. E., Nie Q., Takahashi J. S. and Andersen B. (2020) Circadian control of interferon-sensitive gene expression in murine skin. *Proc Natl Aca Sci USA* 117, 5761–5771.

Guerrero, J. M. and R. J. Reiter (2002) Melatonin-immune system relationships. Curly. Top of the page. *Med. Chemistry* 2, 167-179.

Gupta, M. A. and Gupta, A. K. (2013). Sleep-wake disorders and dermatology. *Dermatology Clinics*, *31*(1), 118-126. https://doi.org/10.1016/j.clindermatol. 2011.11.016.

Gutierrez D. and Arbesman J. (2016) Link with circadian dysrhythmias, physiological abnormalities, and skin cancer. *Int J Mol Sci* 17, 621.

Hardeland, R. (2005) Antioxidative protection by melatonin – Numerous mechanisms ranging from radical detoxification to radical avoidance. *Endocrine* 27, 119–130.

Hardeland, R. and S. R. Pandi-Perumal (2005) Melatonin, a potent agent in antioxidative defense: acts as a natural food ingredient, gastrointestinal factor, drug and prodidrug. *Nutr. Metab.* (London). 2, 22.

Herxheimer, A. and K. J. Petrie (2002) Melatonin for the prevention and treatment of jet lag. *Cochrane Database System Rev.* CD001520. https://doi.org/10.1002/14651858. CD001520.

Hood S. and Amir S. (2017) The aging clock: Circadian rhythms and later life. *Journal of Clinical Investigations* 127, 437–446.

Jacob H., Curtis, and Kearney C. J. (2020) Clock therapeutics: Circadian medicine in the treatment of chronic inflammatory diseases. *Biochem Pharmacol* 182, 114254.

Jemal, A., R. Siegel, J. Q. Xu, and E. Ward (2010) *Cancer statistics*, 2010. CA-Cancer J. Clin. 60, 277–300.

Jung, B. and N. Ahmad (2006) Melatonin in cancer management: Progress and promise. *Cancer Res.* 66, 9789–9793.

Karasek, M. and R. J. Reiter (2002) Melatonin and aging. *Neuroendocrinole. Lett.* 23, 14–16.

Kawara, S., R. Mydlarski, A. J. Mamelak, I. Freed, B. Wang, H. Watanabe, G. Shivji, S. K. Tavadia, H. Suzuki, G. A. Bjarnason, R. K. Jordanand D. N. Sauder (2002) Low-dose ultraviolet B rays alter mRNA expression of circadian clock genes in cultured human keratinocytes. *J. Investment. Dermatol. 119*, 1220–1223.

Kettner N. M., Voicu H., Finegold M. J., Coarfa C., Sreekumar A., Putluri N., Katchy C. A., Lee C., Moore D. D. and Fu L. (2016) suppress hepatocarcinogenesis of circadian homeostasis of liver metabolism. *Cancer Cell* 30, 909–924.

Kiessling S., Beaulieu-Laroche L., Blum I. D., Landgraf D., Welsh D. K., Storch K. F., Labrecque N, and Cermakian N (2017) Increased circadian clock function in cancer cells inhibits tumor growth. *BMC Biol* 15, 13.

Kiessling S., Dubeau-Laramee G., Ohm H., Labrecque N., Olivier M. and Cermakian N. (2017) The circadian clock in immune cells controls the magnitude of leishmania parasitic infection. *Science Representative* 7, 10892.

Kleszczyński, K., Hardkop, L. H., and Fischer, T. W. (2011). Different effects of melatonin as a dermato-endocrine regulator that prevents UV damage in a wide range. *Dermato-endocrinology,3*(1), 27-31.doi:/10.3390/ijms17060801.

Leffell, D. J. and D. E. Brash (1996) Sunlight and skin cancer. *Science.* 275, 52-53.

Lemmer, B., & Bruguerolle, B. (1994). Chronopharmacokinetics: is it clinically significant? *Clinical pharmacokinetics*, *26*(6), 419-427. https://doi.org/10.2165/00003088-199426060-00001.

Lewy, A. J., Ahmed, S., Jackson, J. M. L., & Sack, R. L. (1992). Melatonin alters human orcadian rhythms according to a phase-response curve. *Chronobiology international*, *9*(5), 380-392. https://doi.org/10.3109/07420529209064550.

Li W. Q, Qureshi A. A., Schernhammer E. S., and Han J. (2013) Alternating night shift work and psoriasis risk in U.S. women. *J Invest in Dermatol* 133, 565–567.

Lu F., Suggs A., Ezaldein H. H., Ya J., Fu P., Jamora J., Verallo-Rowel V., and Baron E. D. (2019) Impact of shift work and inadequate sleep on self-reported skin conditions: A survey of call center agents in the Philippines. *Hours and Sleep* 1, 273–279.

Lubov J., Cvammen W. and Kemp M. (2021) Effect of circadian clock on skin physiology and cancer development. *International J Mol Sci* 22, 6112.

Masri S., Kinouchi K. and Sassone-Corsi P. (2015) Circadian clocks, epigenetics and cancer. *Curr opin Oncol* 27, 50–56.

Matsunaga, N., Itcho, K., Hamamura, K., Ikeda, E., Ikeyama, H., Furuichi, Y., & Ohdo, S. (2014). The 24-hour rhythm of Aquaporin-3 function in the epidermis is regulated by molecular clocks. *Journal of Investigative Dermatology*, 134(6), 1636-1644. https://doi.org/10.1038/jid.2014.13.

Melnikova, V. O. and H. N. Ananthaswamy (2005) Cellular and molecular events leading to the development of skin cancer. Usual. Res.-Fundam. *Mol. Mech. Mutagen*. 571, 91–106.

Nikkola V., Gro€nroos M., Huotari-Orava R., Kautiainen H., Ylianttila L., Karppinen T., Partonen T. and Snellman E. (2018) Circadian time effects on NB-UVB-induced erythema in vivo in human skin. *Invest in Dermatol* 138, 464-467.

Özler, M., Şimşek, K., Özkan, C. Akgul, E. O., Topal, T., Oter, S., and Korkmaz, A. Comparison of the effect of topical and systemic melatonin administration on delayed wound healing in rats undergoing pinealectomy. *Scand J Clinical Laboratory Investment.* In 2010; 70(6):447–452. https://doi.org/10.3109/00365513.2010.506926.

Pandi-Perumal, S. R., V. Srinivasan, G. J. M. Maestroni, D. P. Cardinali, B. Poeggeler and R. Hardeland (2006) Melatonin - Nature's most versatile biological signal? *Feb. J.* 273, 2813–2838.

Patel, T., Ishiuji, Y., & Yosipovitch, G. (2007). Night itching: why do we itch at night? *Acta dermato-venereologica, 87*(4), 295-298. https://doi.org/10.2340/00015555-0280.

Pietroiusti, A., A. Neri, G. Somma, L. Coppeta, I. Iavicoli, A. Bergamaschi and A. Magrini (2010) Incidence of metabolic syndrome among healthcare workers on the night shift. *Occupation. Environ. Med.* 67, 54-57.

Plikus M. V., Van Spyk E. N., Pham K., Geyfman M., Kumar V., Takahashi J. S. and Andersen B. (2015) Circadian clock in the skin: Implications of adult stem cells for tissue regeneration, cancer, aging and immunity. *J Biol Rhythms* 30, 163–182.

Plikus M. V., Vollmers C., de la Cruz D., Chaix A., Ramos R., Panda S., and Chuong C. M. (2013) The local circadian clock enables cell cycle progression of transient ascending cells during the regenerative hair cycle. *Proc Natl Acad Sci* 110, E2106–E2115.

Poeggeler, B., R. J. Reiter, D. X. Tan, L. D. Chen and L. C. Manchester (1993) Melatonin, hydroxyl radical mediated oxidative damage and aging: a hypothesis. *J. Epiphysis Fig.* 14, 151–168.

Premi, S., Wallisch, S., Mano, C. M., Weiner, A. B., Bacchiocchi, A., Wakamatsu, K., ... & Brash, D. E. (2015). Chemical stimulation of melanin derivatives induces DNA photoproducts long after exposure to UV rays. *Science, 347*(6224), 842-847. https://doi.org/10.1126/science.1256022.

Reinberg, A. E., Soudant, E., Koulbanis, C., Bazin, R., Nicolai, A., Mechkouri, M., & Touitou, Y. (1995). Dependence on circadian dosing time on forearm skin penetration of methyl and hexyl nicotinate. *Life sciences, 57*(16), 1507-1513. https://doi.org/10.1016/0024-3205(95)02123-z.

Reiter, R. J., D. X. Tan, L. C. Manchester and M. R. El-Sawi (2002) Melatonin reduces oxidant damage and promotes mitochondrial respiration. Ann. NY Acad. Sci. 959, 238–250.

Reiter, R. J., D. X. Tan, S. J. Kim, L. C. Manchester, W. B. Qi, J. J. Garcia, J. C. Cabrera, G. El-Sokkary, and V. Rouvier-Garay (1999) Increased oxidative damage indices in lifelong melatonin-deficient rats. *Mechanical Aging Giant.* 110, 157–173.

Relogio A., Thomas P., Medina-Perez P., Reischl S., Bervoets S., Gloc E., Riemer P., Mang-Fatehi S., Maier B., Sch€afer R. et al. (2014) Ras-mediated deregulation of the circadian clock in cancer. *PLoS Genet* 10, e1004338.

Reppert, S. M. and D. R. Weaver (2002) Coordination of circadian timing in mammals. *Nature* 418, 935–941.

Rodrigues G. D., Fiorelli E. M., Furlan L., Montano N. and Tobaldini E. (2021) Obesity and sleep disorders: the question of "chicken or egg." *Eur J Intern Med* 10, 16.

Runger, T. M. (2007) How different wavelengths of the ultraviolet spectrum contribute to skin carcinogenesis: the role of cellular damage responses. *J. Investment. Dermatol.* 127, 2103–2105.

Sancar, A., L. A. Lindsey-Boltz, T. H. Kang, J. T. Reardon, J. H. Lee and N. Öztürk (2010) Circadian clock control of cellular response to DNA damage. *Feb. Lett.* 584, 2618–2625.

Sandu C., Liu T., Malan A., Challet E., Pevet P., and Felder-Schmittbuhl M. P. (2015) Circadian clocks in rat skin and dermal fibroblasts: Different effects of aging, temperature, and melatonin. *Cell Mole Life Sci* 72, 2237–2248.

Santoro R., Mori F., Marani M., Grasso G., Cambria M. A., Blandino G., Muti P. and Strano S. (2013) Blockage of melatonin receptors impairs p53-mediated prevention of DNA damage accumulation. *Carcinogenesis* 34, 1051–1061.

Sarkar S. and Gaddameedhi S. (2020) Solar ultraviolet-induced DNA damage response: A history of melanocytes in transformation to peripheral melanomagenesis. *Near Mol Mutagen* 61, 736–751.

Sarkar S., Porter K. I., Daqup P. P., Gajula R. P., Koritala B. S. C,. Hylton R., Kemp M. G., Wakamatsu K. and Gaddameedhi S. (2021) The circadian clock protein BMAL1 regulates melanogenesis in melanoma cells. *Pigment Cell Mel Res* 34, 955.

Scheer, F. A. J. L., M. F. Hilton, C. S. Mantzoros, and S. A. Shea (2009) Adverse metabolic and cardiovascular consequences of circadian misalignment. *Proc. Natl Acad. Sci. USA* 106, 4453–4458.

Scheiermann C., Kunisaki Y. and Frenette P. S. (2013) Circadian control of the immune system. *Nat Rev Immuno* 13, 190-198.

Schernhammer E. S., Laden F., Speizer F. E. and others. Alternating night shifts and the risk of breast cancer at 17. Women involved in nurses' health work. *J Natl Cancer Lecturer* 2001; 93(20):1563–1568. https://doi.org/10.1093/jnci/93.20.1563.

Sengupta S., Tang S. Y., Devine J. C., Anderson S. T., Nayak S., Zhang S. L., Valenzuela A., Fisher D. G., Grant G. R., Lopez C. B. et al. (2019) Circadian control of lung inflammation in influenza infection. *Nat Commune* 10, 4107.

Simoes M. C. F., Sousa J. J. S. and Pais A. A. C. C. (2015) Skin cancer and new treatment perspectives: a review. *Cancer Lett* 357, 8–42.

Slominski A. T., Hardeland R., Zmijewski M. A., Slominski R. M., Reiter R. J. and Paus R. (2018) Melatonin: A skin perspective on production, metabolism and functions. *Journal of Investigative Dermatology* 138, 490–499.

Smolander, J., Härmä, M., Lindgvist, A., Kolari, P., & Laitinen, L. A. (1993). Circadian change in peripheral blood flow depending on core temperature at rest. *European journal of applied physiology and occupational physiology*, *67*, 192-196. https://doi.org/10.1007/BF00376666.

Sulli G., Rommel A., Wang X., Kolar M. J., Puca F., Saghatelian A., Plikus M. V., Verma I. M. and Panda S. (2018) Pharmacological activation of REV-ERBs is lethal in cancer and oncogene-induced aging. *Nature* 553, 351–355.

Sundar I. K., Yao H., Sellix M. T. and Rahman I. (2015) Circadian molecular clock in lung pathophysiology. *J Physiol Lung Cell Mole Physyol* 309, L1056–L1075.

Tan, D. X., R. J. Reiter, L. C. Manchester, M. T. Yan, M. El-Sawi, R. M. Sainz, J. C. Mayo, R. Kohen, M. Allegra, and R. Hardeland (2002) Chemical and physical properties and potential mechanisms: Melatonin as a broad-spectrum antioxidant and free radical scavenger. *Curly. Top of the page. Med. Chemistry* 2, 181–197.

Vary J. C. (2015) Selected disorders of skin appendages are acne, alopecia, hyperhidrosis. *Med Clin North* 99, 1195–1211.

Wong R., Geyer S., Weninger W., Guimberteau J. C. and Wong J. K. (2016) Dynamic anatomy and pattern of the skin. *Exp Dermatol* 25, 92–98.

Yagura, T., K. Makita, H. Yamamoto, C. F. M. Menck and A. P. Schuch (2011) Biological sensors for solar ultraviolet radiation. *Sensors* 11, 4277–4294.

Yosipovitch, G., Xiong, G. L., Haus, E., Sackett-Lundeen, L., Ashkenazi, I., & Maibach, H. I. (1998). Time-dependent variations of skin barrier function in humans: transepidermal water loss, stratum corneum hydration, skin surface pH, and skin temperature. *Journal of investigative dermatology*, *110*(1), 20-23. https://doi.org/10.1046/j.1523-1747.1998.00069.x.

Zagni C, Almeida L. O., Balan T., Martins M. T., Rosselli-Murai L. K., Papagerakis P, Castilho RM and Squarize CH (2017) PTEN mediates the activation of the core clock protein BMAL1 and the accumulation of epidermal stem cells. *Stem Cell Representative* 9, 304–314.

Zanello, S. B., Jackson, D. M., and Holick, M. F. (2000). Expression of circadian clock genes, clock and period1 in human skin. *Journal of investigative dermatology*, 115(4), 757-760. https://doi.org/10.1046/j.1523-1747.2000.00121.x.

Zouboulis C. C. (2009) Skin as an endocrine organ. *Dermato-Endocrinole* 1, 250–252.

Chapter 10

The Circadian Control of the Cardiovascular System and Cardiovascular Diseases

Yasemin Doğan*, **MD**
Department of Cardiology, Kayseri City Hospital, Kayseri, Turkiye

Abstract

There is a close relationship between intrinsic circadian clocks and cardiovascular functions, according to the growing evidence. Some well-known circadian rhythms are diurnal changes in blood pressure and heart rate. Circadian changes are also observed in platelet aggregation, endothelial function, and thrombus formation. The onset of several cardiovascular diseases (CVDs) and events such as arrhythmia, myocardial infarction, sudden cardiac death, and stroke also reveal temporal trends. Moreover, epidemiological studies and strong evidence found in animal models reveal that disrupted circadian rhythms are risk factors for several cardiovascular diseases, which may have a time-dependent influence. This chapter presents current knowledge regarding the effects of circadian rhythms on cardiovascular functions and cardiovascular diseases. A better understanding of the mechanisms between circadian rhythms and cardiovascular diseases will lead to the emergence of new treatment options for these diseases.

Keywords: cardiology, circadianrhythm, peripheral clocks

---

* Corresponding Author's Email: klavuz35@hotmail.com.

In: Human Health is a Matter of Timing
Editors: Sumeyya Deniz Aybek, Gonca Gulbay and Mucahit Secme
ISBN: 979-8-89113-467-6

Introduction

Circadian rhythm refers to an endogenous biorhythm with a 24-hour cycle driven by a periodic and intrinsic molecular clock adapting individuals' physiological activities and behaviors to the changes in the external environment (Roenneberg & Merrow 2005; Harmer & Kay 2001).

Almost all cardiovascular (CV) variables such as blood pressure, heart rate, circulating catecholamines, coagulation factors, and vascular endothelial function differ according to the different times of the day in day/night patterns. For example, while typical morning behaviors lead to an increase in sympathetic tone, vasoconstriction, peripheral arterial pressure, heart rate, blood pressure, and thrombocyte aggregation, they cause a decline in parasympathetic tone and vascular endothelial function. Sudden increases in energy consumption necessary to make the activity of the metabolic and circulatory systems ready soon after awakening are provided with circulating cortisol and body temperature. Fluctuations affecting cardiovascular endogenous circadian rhythm arise from the negative feedback effect of daily environmental and behavioral changes. Organisms prepare for the cycles of fasting/feeding and resting/activity with circadian timing in order to ideally adapt to the predictable changes around. The master pacemaker present in the suprachiasmatic nucleus (SCN) of the hypothalamus in mammals controls peripheral clocks in other tissues in detail to synchronize all present clocks (Lowrey & Takahashi 2011; Dibner et al., 2010). Interactional transcription-translation auto-regulatory feedback loop with the core clock genes such as Clock (circadian locomotor output cycles kaput), *BMAL1* (brain and muscle aryl-hydrocarbon receptor nuclear translocator-like 1) and *CRY*1/2 (cryptochrome1/2) induces molecular circadian clock. The CLOCK and BMAL1 proteins bind to E-box elements in promoter regions of clock-controlled genes (CCGs) such as many significant genes regarding cardiovascular and renal function by collectively forming a heterodimer (Zhang & Pollock, 2020; Lutshumba et al., 2018). When the CRY and PER proteins accumulate and become completely superfluous in the cytoplasm, they both translocate to the nucleus where the transcription of the heterodimeric activator is shut down (Duong et al., 2011). Additionally, ROR (RAR-related orphan receptor), one of the nuclear receptors, is activated, and RORE (ROR element) is suppressed by REV-ERB (subfamily1 of nuclear receptor, group D) so that CLOCK and BMAL1 transcriptions are directly controlled (Guillaumond et al., 2005). Furthermore, PPAR*γ*, another nuclear receptor is integrated in this loop and targeted by BMAL1, as it directly binds to PPRE (PPAR response element) in its promoter (Wang et al., 2008). All PPAR isoforms that are dynamic but coordinated exhibited diurnal expression at different points of time in the tissues of mice.

Circadian Rhythms in Cardiovascular Function

The circadian system consists of a central clock located in the suprachiasmatic nucleus (SCN) of the hypothalamus and a range of peripheral clocks located in the other tissues of the body. Peripheral clocks in the cardiovascular systems are located in the endothelium, vascular smooth muscle cells, and aorta. The central clock regulates hormone release, body temperature, sleep/wake cycles, and various rhythmic cycles including blood pressure and heart rate by means of peripheral clocks (Aoyama & Shibata, 2017). The autonomic nervous system with parasympathetic and sympathetic effects plays a role in the relationship between the central clock and peripheral clocks. Glucocorticoids and mineralocorticoids are also within this signal transducing chain. Circadian clocks are described in all CV cellular types including cardiomyocytes. The local heart clock is located in the working myocardial cells and the cardiac conduction system. As a general concept, circadian clocks temporarily divide biological processes to let a cell/organ ideally respond to fluctuations throughout 24 hours and provide a selective advantage. The heart deals with two main behavioral cycles during the day: Sleep-wake and fed-fast cycles. These cycles are associated with demand for energy, neural stimulation, hormones, nutrients, oxygen level, body temperature, and significant fluctuations in shear stress. Consistent with the nature of transcription, circadian clocks generally direct cellular functions to provide modulation of genes that are not the components of the nucleus clock. All types of cells are connected with the molecular clock, so that the cardiovascular system can respond to peripheral diurnal variations in synchronization with heart rate-blood pressure. This ensures that the peripheral clocks and the central clock work in coordination. As in the other organs, approximately 5%-10% of genes expressed in the heart show a circadian release. The nucleus clock machine directly regulates the clock-controlled genes at the transcription level, which is provided directly with DNA binding, improvement in coregulators, and modification of histone tails and chromatin. Molecular rhythms are sensitively regulated with regulation after transcription, changes after transcription, reregulation of chromatin, intracellular localization, and clock proteins (Kim & Lazar, 2020).

Disruptions of normal day and night cycles such as jet-lag cause desynchronization between central and peripheral clocks and lead kinetics in clock genes and organs to change. Circadian clocks control a large number of tissue-specific clock-controlled genes (CCGs). Disruption of this mechanism will potentially start a series of biochemical and physiological chain reactions contributing to the incidence of cardiovascular disorders (CVDs). The circadian rhythm regulates the rhythmic release of cardiac genes and proteins, cardiac contractility, and metabolism (Martino et al., 2004). Eventually, we observe daily physiological and behavioral rhythms most of which are crucial for cardiovascular systems by means of outputs of this cellular mechanism (Martino & Young, 2015; Martino & Sole, 2009). For example, our pulse rate and blood pressure increase during the daytime and decrease at night. Normal cardiovascular rhythms help individuals prepare for the physiological demands of activity throughout the day through rest and renewing at night. Our endocrine hormones are released by the circulation, which is related to the cardiovascular system. For example, catecholamines peak during the daytime and decline at night in healthy individuals in parallel with our epinephrine and norepinephrine sympathetic and parasympathetic tendencies (Linsell et al., 1985; Scheer et al., 2011; Furlan et al., 1990; Richards et al., 1986).

Moreover, immune cells and cytokines, coagulation factors, and other classical biomarkers in the circulation reveal a daily routine similar to normal cardiovascular physiology (Martino et al., 2004; Martino et al., 2007). Increasing cortisol levels during the mornings and melatonin reaching peak levels at night are the signs of circadian rhythm and daily homeostasis (Mavroudis et al., 2012). These daily rhythms collectively help maintain normal cardiovascular function in healthy people.

Blood Pressure and Circadian Rhythm

The day/night pattern of blood pressure is clearly evident. It is generally lower during sleep than during wakefulness and has a characteristic fluctuation after awakening. It exhibits parallelism with adverse cardiac events. Fluctuation of systolic blood pressure to 10 mmHg within 2 hours just after awakening in elderly patients with hypertension is associated with a 22% higher risk of stroke independently of 24-hour mean blood pressure (Kario & Pickering, 2003). No decline in blood pressure at night is a sensitive sign of CV mortality. Each 10 mmHg increase in night systolic BP means a 21% higher risk of CV mortality, and each 5 mmHg increase in diastolic blood pressure means a 9% higher risk (Dolan et al., 2005).

These time-dependent effects are not only the results of the sleep/wake cycle or rhythms in neuroendocrine compounds but can also be attributed to fluctuations in cardiac-blood veins throughout the day. Regulators of blood pressure such as plasma epinephrine, norepinephrine, cortisol, cardiac vagal tone, and heart rate reveal circadian fluctuation as well (Burgess et al., 1997). The autonomic nervous system is associated with a 24-hour mean blood pressure. Plasma norepinephrine is higher during wake than during sleep and brings about increasing blood pressure. Dipper and non-dipper tension playing an important role in cardiovascular mortality are affected by autonomic nervous system dysfunction as well. In addition, decreased function of smooth muscle cells independent from the state of tension is independently associated with decreasing blood pressure at night. Clinical studies have associated Na transport in the kidney and abnormal circadian rhythms with salt sensitivity and non-dipper hypertension (Uzu et al., 1996; Kimura & Fukuda, 2010; Sinha & Agarwal, 2015). However, the exact role of the circadian system in non-dipper hypertension has not been enlightened yet. Blood vessels also reveal circadian rhythmicity. For example, approximately 5% of all genes in the aorta are rhythmic (Rudic et al., 2005). Vascular endothelium and vascular smooth muscle cells are crucial in the regulation of vascular resistance and blood pressure. The genes exhibiting circadian rhythms in animals are involved in the structural integrity of vascular smooth muscle cells (Chalmers et al., 2008).

Peripheral clocks in smooth muscles, perivascular adipose tissues, liver, adrenal gland, and kidney play a role in the regulation of blood pressure rhythm. A disrupted circadian rhythm of blood pressure is associated with adverse cardiorenal outcomes and an increased risk of cardiovascular mortality. BMAL1 deletion in mice disrupts circadian rhythm in vascular smooth muscle cells. Thus, it advances the circadian phases of systolic and diastolic blood pressure and removes the circadian variation of the pulse pressure (Xie et al., 2015). The kidney is necessary for long-term regulation of blood pressure and about 13% of protein-coding genes in the kidney are rhythmic. PER1 plays a crucial role in terms of BP and affects sodium retention by regulating aldosterone levels (Richards et al., 2013; Gumz et al., 2009; Stow et al., 2012). The shift work causing misalignment in circadian rhythm is associated with an increase in cancer and cardiovascular diseases. Studies have revealed that long-term shift work increases inflammatory markers (C-reactive protein (CRP), interleukin-6, resistin, and TNFα) and causes an increase in systolic and diastolic blood pressures (Morris et al.,

2016; Morris et al., 2017). It has been revealed that the increase in interleukin-6, resistin, and TNFα levels has a role in the progression of hypertension through activation of inflammation and endothelial dysfunction (Fang et al., 2013). The decrease in accompanying cardiac vagal modulation and the disruption of normal circadian rhythms cause an increase in the risk of CVD.

Atherosclerosis and Circadian Rhythm

The incidence of myocardial infarction associated with the autonomic nervous system has a 24-hour model (Muller et al., 1985). The risks triggering potential cardiovascular diseases such as sympathetic activity, shear stress, and an increase in blood pressure increase during mornings (Manfredini et al., 1996). Animal studies have revealed that the peripheral clock has a crucial role. Platelet aggregation and coagulation, ventricular repolarization abnormalities, and other several cardiovascular risk factors are regulated by peripheral circadian clocks, which explains that the incidence of cardiovascular events peaks during specific times of the day (Shea et al., 2011; Dashti et al., 2016; Scheer & Shea, 2014). The time of myocardial infarction is related to the outcomes. If myocardial infarction occurs during the early hours of the morning myocardial injury and dysfunction can be higher compared to the infarction occurring in the afternoon. However, not all studies claim the same data (Ammirati et al., 2013). Sleep disorders, jet lag, and shift work disrupt circadian rhythm and increase the risk of metabolic syndrome, myocardial infarction, ischemic stroke, and early death (Vyas et al., 2012; Esquirol et al., 2011). Patients are generally exposed to stimuli, loud noise, and frequent patient-personnel interactions, especially at night during hospitalization due to an acute disease. The circadian rhythm and sleep pattern are disrupted as a result the daily routine is affected in the intensive care unit. Systematic inflammatory responses and local events critical for the healing process occur following an acute myocardial infarction. Reviews on mice claim that disruptions in circadian rhythm and sleep pattern within the first few hours following myocardial infarction cause impairment in cellular recovery and deterioration in long-term outcomes. Cytokines are released rhythmically from inflammatory cells including neutrophils with a molecular clock, which provides adaptation to circadian rhythm in mammals (Aroca-Crevillén et al., 2020; Hidalgo et al., 2019).

Studies on ischemia in mice have revealed that the chemokine receptor CXCR2 increases neutrophil infiltration at night, which results in more heart injury caused by myocardial infarction (Schloss et al., 2016). Some circadian patterns have been detected in the release of hemostasis molecules playing a role in thrombosis, procoagulation factors such as the von Willebrand factor, factors VII, VIII, IX, and X, and anticoagulation factors such as antithrombin (AT), protein C, and protein S. It has been revealed that molecules involved in fibrinolysis (D-dimers and factor X) and the activity of plasminogen activator inhibitor-1 (PAI-1) peak in the mornings (Scheer & Shea, 2014). Platelet production and aggregation are regulated by the central clock through thrombopoietin (Pritchett & Reddy, 2015; Andrews et al., 1996) and peak in number in the mornings, while the activity of activation molecules such as platelet factor 4 (CXCL4) and B-thromboglobulin (B-TG) peaks in the afternoon (Jafri et al., 1992). The synthesis of nitric oxide (NO) decreases under physiological conditions during the daytime and a decrease in vasodilatation occurs as a result. It works at night with a mechanism in contrast with that (Kanabrocki et al., 2001). A decrease in NO synthesis and cardiovascular events such as stroke and atherosclerosis-induces acute myocardial infarction caused by endothelial dysfunction associated with increasing vasoconstriction and hypercoagulopathy occur more often in the morning hours. It has been revealed that there is the link between clock genes and proteins and thrombosis and fibrinolysis factors (Tsimakouridze et al., 2015). PAI-1 gene transcription is regulated by both CLOCK and BMAL, which can be given as an example. It may be related to high fibrinogen levels in BMAL1, vWF, and PAI-1 creating a prothrombotic state with an increased risk of thrombosis (Somanath et al., 2011). How circadian rhythm affects the pathophysiology of thrombosis can be clarified with the identification of circadian-clock genes regulating thrombosis.

Cardiovascular events occur more often in the early morning hours. The incidence of both AMI and cardiac death in the morning is higher. Circulating neutrophils associated with inflammation can migrate more rapidly to the myocardium in the mornings and thereby trigger a stronger proinflammatory response by increasing the expression of the C-X-C chemokine receptor type 2 (CXCR2). Some of these findings have not been confirmed in humans yet (Lecour et al., 2022).

Gene disruption of BMAL-CLOCK may be triggering the diurnal secretion of fatty acid oxidation of KLF15, which is a transcriptional activity clock protein. BMAL-CLOCK mice increase the size of the infarction in cardiomyocytes and cause sudden cardiac death while PER2 and REV-ERB α/β decrease the size of the infarction (Durgan et al., 2010; Nakashima et al., 2017; Schroder et al., 2015). PER2 decreases infarction size by decreasing fatty acid oxidation and glycolysis through the adenosine Adora2b receptor (Eckle et al., 2012). Similar findings have also been found in the genes in fibroblasts in remodeling after AMI. Fibroblasts and cardiomyocytes cause deletion in clock genes, a decrease in left ventricle ejection fraction, and an increase in the size of increased left ventricles (Bennardo et al., 2016). The sleep/wake cycle in mammals is regulated by melatonin which is a hormone secreted by the epiphysis at night. Melatonin has anti-inflammatory and antioxidant features, which are related to daily hormonal regulation. Melatonin levels provide cardiac protection and cause a decrease in the risk of AMI. Melatonin protects endothelial cells after ischemia-reperfusion injury by inhibiting autophagy (Chen et al., 2018).

Cardiac Arrhythmia and Circadian Rhythm

Heart rate, electrophysiological parameters in the ECG such as QRS and QTC, and heart rate variation change throughout a day in healthy individuals. The variation in electrophysiological parameters is regulated by both the (central) autonomic nervous system and peripheral circadian clocks. Peripheral circadian clocks regulate the expression and function of sodium, potassium, and calcium channels. Disruption of the molecular circadian clock, especially in cardiomyocytes in animal models, causes a decrease in the variation of pulse rate (Bray et al., 2008). The local cardiac circadian clock has been controlled by HCN4 protein (Hyperpolarization activated cyclic nucleotide-gated potassium channel 4) HCN4 mRNA and the funny current (I_f), which is the corresponding current according to a recent preliminary report. The higher heart rate can be clearly explained with the higher density of I_f in the wake time. According to two studies, cardiomyocyte-specific disruption in the local cardiac clock (cardiomyocyte-specific CLOCK or BMAL1 knockout) decreases circadian rhythm in heart rate but it does not abolish it. Therefore, it is possible to say that the local cardiac clock contributes to the circadian rhythm in the heart rate. On the contrary, the circadian rhythm in heart rate is driven by the central SCN clock. When mice are subjected to bilateral thermal ablation of the SCN, the circadian rhythm is lost in heart rate (Tong et al., 2013).

Mice that have deficient vasoactive intestinal peptide, which is an important molecule in SCN, experience the same. Moreover, circadian rhythm is lost or dampened in heart rate as a result of global knockout of CLOCK and BMAL1, the core circadian clock genes (both central SCN clock and local circadian clocks are disrupted). It is claimed that the circadian rhythm in heart rate is controlled by the SCN clock with circadian variation in the autonomic tone to the sinus node. SCN clock specifically uses an increase in vagal tone at night here. It also controls the release of other neurohumoral factors in a circadian manner; however, how it affects the circadian rhythm in heart rate has not been well clarified yet. Studies on day/night variations in HRV (heart rate variability) apparently support the role of autonomic tone. According to the experiment by Tong et al. on the role of the autonomic nervous system in the heart, the circadian rhythm was lost, which may not be related to the well-known actions of the autonomic nervous system on ionic conductance. In this respect, Tong et al. explained in their two studies that there was a loss of circadian rhythm in the expression of ion channels under the same conditions, which suggests that ion channel transcription is affected by the autonomic nervous system (Tong et al., 2013). Furthermore, it has been revealed that circadian gene expression and local cardiac clock are stimulated by adrenergic agonists. Circadian PER expression is induced by isoproterenol in ventricular explants of mice while BMAL1, PER, and REV-ERB circadian expression is induced by noradrenaline in cardiomyocytes of rats.

PR and QT intervals are extended during night rest, as well as QRS. Sinus pauses (<2 seconds), sinus bradycardia, first-degree ventricular block, and second-degree atrioventricular block (Wenckebach) were found as the most common electrocardiographic changes at night, which can be explained by changes in electrical features of cells present in atrioventricular (AV)node, the sinus node, ventricular muscle, and His-Purkinje system. Nocturnal bradyarrhythmia, the clinical relevance of which is difficult to determine, is quite prevalent in the general population (Gula et al., 2004). Patients with sinus node dysfunction have been reported with an early loss of circadian heart rate variability. The frequency of bradyarrhythmias that have clinical significance increases at night, which can be concluded that they have a circadian pattern. Paroxysmal atrioventricular block can be given as an example, since its incidence increases between 2:00 and 4:00 am (Saito et al., 2014).

The slowing conduction velocity of myocardial cells and lower firing of the intrinsic pacemaker of the sinus node are among the leading underlying mechanisms of nocturnal bradycardization. In the sinus node, the pacemaker current I_f is regulated and the local clock is established by Hyperpolarization Activated Cyclic Nucleotide gated potassium channel 4 (HCN4), which is one of the ionic channels. Changes in electrical properties in a healthy individual will result in a lower heart rate at night, while significant pauses or AV block may occur in individuals with an abnormal conduction system.

Except for atrial fibrillation, supraventricular tachycardia episodes occur more often during the daytime. While paroxysmal supraventricular tachycardia occurs more often in the afternoon (Burgess et al., 1997; Uzu et al., 1996) paroxysmal atrial fibrillation occurs more often during the night (Irwin et al., 1988, Watanabe et al., 2002; Gillis et al., 2001). The affected arrhythmogenic substrate can cause circadian variations to act as a trigger in autonomic tone. More frequent paroxysmal and persistent episodes of nocturnal atrial fibrillation can be explained by an increase in nocturnal vagal tone (Mitchell et al., 2003). Patients who have permanent atrial fibrillation can have circadian oscillation because their ventricular response daily varies like in the sinus rhythm. The average heart rate is higher in people with inappropriate sinus tachycardia than in those with normal sinus rhythm, but no changes have been observed in normal diurnal variation. It has been concluded that there may be an intrinsic sinus node abnormality in these individuals, which may cause a higher 24-hour mean heart rate. The risk of sudden cardiac death and ventricular arrhythmia is higher in the early morning. Increased repolarization dispersion and increased activity of the sympathetic nervous system promoting early afterdepolarization, reentry, and calcium overload may be stated among the several mechanisms explaining that morning peak (Gardner et al., 2016). L-type calcium channels are functioning and expressed in a circadian manner. Fatal arrhythmias may be triggered by early afterdepolarizations promoted in the case of circadian variance in L-type calcium conductance (Diekman & Wei, 2021). Individuals with severe ventricular systolic dysfunction may not have circadian variability of ventricular arrhythmias. The increased activity of the sympathetic nervous system disrupting the circadian pattern has explained this absence.

The morning peak in sudden cardiac death has been associated with episodes of myocardial ischemia in the general population. However, there may be some other factors affecting it such as the predominance and increase of sympathetic system activity in arrhythmic risk or cortisol release (Gamble et al., 2014). The circadian pattern of ventricular arrhythmias was not affected by a present coronary artery disease in individuals with structural heart disease. Ventricular arrhythmias associated with some channelopathies such as Brugada syndrome are likely to have a nocturnal distribution in which it peaks between midnight and early morning, which suggests that not all cardiac problems have the same circadian pattern. Genotype is the determinant of circadian variations in long QT syndrome. Ventricular arrhythmias occur more frequently during sleep or at rest in type 3, which means they are more frequent at night. Sympathetic stimulation (mostly in the mornings) is the time when arrhythmic events mostly occur in type 1 and type 2 (Takigawa et al., 2012). The data above conclude that ventricular arrhythmias are significantly predisposed or triggered by the activity of the sympathetic or parasympathetic nervous system; however, this predisposition or trigger may be stronger in different periods of time.

Conclusion

Circadian clocks have been found in all cell types in the heart and vasculature, and many important biological processes, such as heart rate, blood pressure, metabolism, and hormone levels, show daily fluctuations. Clinical studies show that circadian rhythms driven by the molecular clock play an important role in the pathophysiology of conditions such as atherosclerosis, blood pressure irregularities, and arrhythmias. Targeting circadian mechanisms and molecules, provides therapeutic benefit by interfering with pathological processes and reducing cardiovascular morbidity and mortality. More complicatedly, circadian disruption not only impairs cardiovascular functions, but has also been linked to diseases such as obesity, diabetes, immune disorders, and mental illness that may affect each other. Therefore, control or prevent circadian rhythm related diseases and becomes crucial for cardiovascular functions.

References

Ammirati, E., Maseri, A., & Cannistraci, C. V. (2013). Still need for compelling evidence to support the circadian dependence of infarct size after ST-elevation myocardial infarction. *Circulation research*, 113(4), e43–e44. https://doi.org/10.1161/CIRCRESAHA.113.301908.

Andrews, N. P., Gralnick, H. R., Merryman, P., Vail, M., & Quyyumi, A. A. (1996). Mechanisms underlying the morning increase in platelet aggregation: a flow cytometry study. *Journal of the American College of Cardiology,* 28(7), 1789–1795. https://doi.org/10.1016/S0735-1097(96)00398-1.

Aoyama, S., & Shibata, S. (2017). The Role of Circadian Rhythms in Muscular and Osseous Physiology and Their Regulation by Nutrition and Exercise. *Frontiers in neuroscience*, *11*, 63. https://doi.org/10.3389/fnins.2017.00063.

Aroca-Crevillén, A., Adrover, J. M., & Hidalgo, A. (2020). Circadian Features of Neutrophil Biology. *Frontiers in immunology*, 11, 576. https://doi.org/10.3389/fimmu.2020.00576.

Bennardo, M., Alibhai, F., Tsimakouridze, E., Chinnappareddy, N., Podobed, P., Reitz, C., Pyle, W. G., Simpson, J., & Martino, T. A. (2016). Day-night dependence of gene expression and inflammatory responses in the remodeling murine heart post-myocardial infarction. American journal of physiology. *Regulatory, integrative and comparative physiology,* 311(6), R1243–R1254. https://doi.org/10.1152/ajpregu.00200.2016.

Bray, M. S., Shaw, C. A., Moore, M. W., Garcia, R. A., Zanquetta, M. M., Durgan, D. J., Jeong, W. J., Tsai, J. Y., Bugger, H., Zhang, D., Rohrwasser, A., Rennison, J. H., Dyck, J. R., Litwin, S. E., Hardin, P. E., Chow, C. W., Chandler, M. P., Abel, E. D., & Young, M. E. (2008). Disruption of the circadian clock within the cardiomyocyte influences myocardial contractile function, metabolism, and gene expression. American journal of physiology. *Heart and circulatory physiology,* 294(2), H1036–H1047. https://doi.org/10.1152/ajpheart.01291.2007.

Burgess, H. J., Trinder, J., Kim, Y., & Luke, D. (1997). Sleep and circadian influences on cardiac autonomic nervous system activity. *The American journal of physiology,* 273(4), H1761–H1768. https://doi.org/10.1152/ajpheart.1997.273.4.H1761.

Chalmers, J. A., Martino, T. A., Tata, N., Ralph, M. R., Sole, M. J., & Belsham, D. D. (2008). Vascular circadian rhythms in a mouse vascular smooth muscle cell line (Movas-1). American journal of physiology. *Regulatory, integrative and comparative physiology*, 295(5), R1529–R1538. https://doi.org/10.1152/ajpregu.90572.2008.

Chen, W. R., Liu, H. B., Chen, Y. D., Sha, Y., Ma, Q., Zhu, P. J., & Mu, Y. (2018). Melatonin Attenuates Myocardial Ischemia/Reperfusion Injury by Inhibiting Autophagy Via an AMPK/mTOR Signaling Pathway. *Cellular physiology and biochemistry: international journal of experimental cellular physiology, biochemistry, and pharmacology*, 47(5), 2067–2076. https://doi.org/10.1159/000491474.

Dashti, H. S., Aslibekyan, S., Scheer, F. A., Smith, C. E., Lamon-Fava, S., Jacques, P., Lai, C. Q., Tucker, K. L., Arnett, D. K., & Ordovás, J. M. (2016). Clock Genes Explain a Large Proportion of Phenotypic Variance in Systolic Blood Pressure and This Control Is Not Modified by Environmental Temperature. *American journal of hypertension*, 29(1), 132–140. https://doi.org/10.1093/ajh/hpv082.

Dibner, C., Schibler, U., & Albrecht, U. (2010). The mammalian circadian timing system: organization and coordination of central and peripheral clocks. *Annual review of physiology*, 72, 517–549. https://doi.org/10.1146/annurev-physiol-021909-135821.

Diekman, C. O., & Wei, N. (2021). Circadian Rhythms of Early Afterdepolarizations and Ventricular Arrhythmias in a Cardiomyocyte Model. *Biophysical journal,* 120(2), 319–333. https://doi.org/10.1016/j.bpj.2020.11.2264.

Dolan, E., Stanton, A., Thijs, L., Hinedi, K., Atkins, N., McClory, S., Den Hond, E., McCormack, P., Staessen, J. A., & O'Brien, E. (2005). Superiority of ambulatory over clinic blood pressure measurement in predicting mortality: the Dublin outcome study. *Hypertension* (Dallas, Tex: 1979), 46(1), 156–161. https://doi.org/10.1161/01.HYP.0000170138.56903.7a.

Duong, H. A., Robles, M. S., Knutti, D., & Weitz, C. J. (2011). A molecular mechanism for circadian clock negative feedback. *Science* (New York, N.Y.), 332(6036), 1436–1439. https://doi.org/10.1126/science.1196766.

Durgan, D. J., Pulinilkunnil, T., Villegas-Montoya, C., Garvey, M. E., Frangogiannis, N. G., Michael, L. H., Chow, C. W., Dyck, J. R., & Young, M. E. (2010). Short communication: ischemia/reperfusion tolerance is time-of-day-dependent: mediation by the cardiomyocyte circadian clock. *Circulation research,* 106(3), 546–550. https://doi.org/10.1161/CIRCRESAHA.109.209346.

Eckle, T., Hartmann, K., Bonney, S., Reithel, S., Mittelbronn, M., Walker, L. A., Lowes, B. D., Han, J., Borchers, C. H., Buttrick, P. M., Kominsky, D. J., Colgan, S. P., & Eltzschig, H. K. (2012). Adora2b-elicited Per2 stabilization promotes a HIF-dependent metabolic switch crucial for myocardial adaptation to ischemia. *Nature medicine*, 18(5), 774–782. https://doi.org/10.1038/nm.2728.

Esquirol, Y., Perret, B., Ruidavets, J. B., Marquie, J. C., Dienne, E., Niezborala, M., & Ferrieres, J. (2011). Shift work and cardiovascular risk factors: new knowledge from the past decade. *Archives of cardiovascular diseases,* 104(12), 636–668. https://doi.org/10.1016/j.acvd.2011.09.004.

Fang, C., Lei, J., Zhou, S. X., Zhang, Y. L., Yuan, G. Y., & Wang, J. F. (2013). Association of higher resistin levels with inflammatory activation and endothelial dysfunction in patients with essential hypertension. *Chinese medical journal*, 126(4), 646–649.

Furlan, R., Guzzetti, S., Crivellaro, W., Dassi, S., Tinelli, M., Baselli, G., Cerutti, S., Lombardi, F., Pagani, M., & Malliani, A. (1990). Continuous 24-hour assessment of the neural regulation of systemic arterial pressure and RR variabilities in ambulant subjects. *Circulation,* 81(2), 537–547. https://doi.org/10.1161/01.cir.81.2.537.

Gamble, K. L., Berry, R., Frank, S. J., & Young, M. E. (2014). Circadian clock control of endocrine factors. Nature reviews. *Endocrinology*, 10(8), 466–475. https://doi.org/10.1038/nrendo.2014.78.

Gardner, R. T., Ripplinger, C. M., Myles, R. C., & Habecker, B. A. (2016). Molecular Mechanisms of Sympathetic Remodeling and Arrhythmias. Circulation. *Arrhythmia and electrophysiology,* 9(2), e001359. https://doi.org/10.1161/CIRCEP.115.001359.

Gillis, A. M., Connolly, S. J., Dubuc, M., Yee, R., Lacomb, P., Philippon, F., Kerr, C. R., Kimber, S., Gardner, M. J., Tang, A. S., Molin, F., Newman, D., Abdollah, H., & PA3. Atrial Pacing Peri-ablation for Prevention of Atrial Fibrillation Trial (2001). Circadian variation of paroxysmal atrial fibrillation. PA3 Investigators. Atrial Pacing Peri-ablation for Prevention of Atrial Fibrillation Trial. *The American journal of cardiology,* 87(6), 794–A8. https://doi.org/10.1016/s0002-9149(00)01509-5.

Guillaumond, F., Dardente, H., Giguère, V., & Cermakian, N. (2005). Differential control of Bmal1 circadian transcription by REV-ERB and ROR nuclear receptors. *Journal of biological rhythms, 20*(5), 391–403. https://doi.org/10.1177/0748730405277232.

Gula, L. J., Krahn, A. D., Skanes, A. C., Yee, R., & Klein, G. J. (2004). Clinical relevance of arrhythmias during sleep: guidance for clinicians. *Heart* (British Cardiac Society), 90(3), 347–352. https://doi.org/10.1136/hrt.2003.019323.

Gumz, M. L., Stow, L. R., Lynch, I. J., Greenlee, M. M., Rudin, A., Cain, B. D., Weaver, D. R., & Wingo, C. S. (2009). The circadian clock protein Period 1 regulates expression of the renal epithelial sodium channel in mice. *The Journal of clinical investigation*, 119(8), 2423–2434. https://doi.org/10.1172/JCI36908.

Harmer, S. L., Panda, S., & Kay, S. A. (2001). Molecular bases of circadian rhythms. *Annual review of cell and developmental biology,* 17, 215–253. https://doi.org/10.1146/annurev.cellbio.17.1.215.

Hidalgo, A., Chilvers, E. R., Summers, C., & Koenderman, L. (2019). The Neutrophil Life Cycle. *Trends in immunology,* 40(7), 584–597. https://doi.org/10.1016/j.it.2019.04.013.

Irwin, J. M., McCarthy, E. A., Wilkinson, W. E., & Pritchett, E. L. (1988). Circadian occurrence of symptomatic paroxysmal supraventricular tachycardia in untreated patients. *Circulation,* 77(2), 298–300. https://doi.org/10.1161/01.cir.77.2.298.

Jafri, S. M., VanRollins, M., Ozawa, T., Mammen, E. F., Goldberg, A. D., & Goldstein, S. (1992).Circadian variation in platelet function in healthy volunteers. *The American journal of cardiology*, 69(9), 951–954. https://doi.org/10.1016/0002-9149(92)90799-5.

Kanabrocki, E. L., George, M., Hermida, R. C., Messmore, H. L., Ryan, M. D., Ayala, D. E., Hoppensteadt, D. A., Fareed, J., Bremner, F. W., Third, J. L., Shirazi, P., & Nemchausky, B. A. (2001). Day-night variations in blood levels of nitric oxide, T-TFPI, and E-selectin. Clinical and applied thrombosis/hemostasis : *official journal of the International Academy of Clinical and Applied Thrombosis/Hemostasis,* 7(4), 339–345. https://doi.org/10.1177/107602960100700417.

Kario, K., Shimada, K., & Pickering, T. G. (2003). Clinical implication of morning blood pressure surge in hypertension. *Journal of cardiovascular pharmacology*, 42 Suppl 1, S87–S91. https://doi.org/10.1097/00005344-200312001-00019.

Kim, Y. H., & Lazar, M. A. (2020). Transcriptional Control of Circadian Rhythms and Metabolism: A Matter of Time and Space. *Endocrine reviews,* 41(5), 707–732. https://doi.org/10.1210/endrev/bnaa014.

Kimura, G., Dohi, Y., & Fukuda, M. (2010). Salt sensitivity and circadian rhythm of blood pressure: the keys to connect CKD with cardiovascular events. Hypertension research: *official journal of the Japanese Society of Hypertension*, 33(6), 515–520. https://doi.org/10.1038/hr.2010.47.

Lecour, S., Du Pré, B. C., Bøtker, H. E., Brundel, B. J. J. M., Daiber, A., Davidson, S. M., Ferdinandy, P., Girao, H., Gollmann-Tepeköylü, C., Gyöngyösi, M., Hausenloy, D. J., Madonna, R., Marber, M., Perrino, C., Pesce, M., Schulz, R., Sluijter, J. P. G., Steffens, S., Van Linthout, S., Young, M. E., Van Laake, L. W. (2022). Circadian rhythms in ischaemic heart disease: key aspects for preclinical and translational research: position paper of the ESC working group on cellular biology of the heart. Cardiovascular research, 118(12), 2566–2581. https://doi.org/10.1093/cvr/cvab293.

Linsell, C. R., Lightman, S. L., Mullen, P. E., Brown, M. J., & Causon, R. C. (1985). Circadian rhythms of epinephrine and norepinephrine in man. *The Journal of clinical endocrinology and metabolism,* 60(6), 1210–1215. https://doi.org/10.1210/jcem-60-6-1210.

Lowrey, P. L., & Takahashi, J. S. (2011). Genetics of circadian rhythms in Mammalian model organisms. *Advances in genetics,* 74, 175–230. https://doi.org/10.1016/B978-0-12-387690-4.00006-4.

Lutshumba, J., Liu, S., Zhong, Y., Hou, T., Daugherty, A., Lu, H., Guo, Z., & Gong, M. C. (2018). Deletion of BMAL1 in Smooth Muscle Cells Protects Mice From Abdominal Aortic Aneurysms. Arteriosclerosis, thrombosis, and vascular biology, 38(5), 1063–1075. https://doi.org/10.1161/ATVBAHA.117.310153.

Manfredini, R., Gallerani, M., Portaluppi, F., & Fersini, C. (1996). Relationships of the circadian rhythms of thrombotic, ischemic, hemorrhagic, and arrhythmic events to blood pressure rhythms. *Annals of the New York Academy of Sciences,* 783, 141–158. https://doi.org/10.1111/j.1749-6632.1996.tb26713.x.

Martino, T., Arab, S., Straume, M., Belsham, D. D., Tata, N., Cai, F., Liu, P., Trivieri, M., Ralph, M., & Sole, M. J. (2004). Day/night rhythms in gene expression of the normal murine heart. *Journal of molecular medicine (Berlin, Germany),* 82(4), 256–264. https://doi.org/10.1007/s00109-003-0520-1.

Martino, T. A., & Sole, M. J. (2009). Molecular time: an often overlooked dimension to cardiovascular disease. *Circulation research,* 105(11), 1047–1061. https://doi.org/10.1161/CIRCRESAHA.109.206201.

Martino, T. A., Tata, N., Belsham, D. D., Chalmers, J., Straume, M., Lee, P., Pribiag, H., Khaper, N., Liu, P. P., Dawood, F., Backx, P. H., Ralph, M. R., & Sole, M. J. (2007). Disturbed diurnal rhythm alters gene expression and exacerbates cardiovascular disease with rescue by resynchronization. *Hypertension* (Dallas, Tex.: 1979), 49(5), 1104–1113. https://doi.org/10.1161/HYPERTENSIONAHA.106.083568.

Martino, T. A., & Young, M. E. (2015). Influence of the cardiomyocyte circadian clock on cardiac physiology and pathophysiology. *Journal of biological rhythms,* 30(3), 183–205. https://doi.org/10.1177/0748730415575246.

Mavroudis, P. D., Scheff, J. D., Calvano, S. E., Lowry, S. F., & Androulakis, I. P. (2012). Entrainment of peripheral clock genes by cortisol. *Physiological genomics,* 44(11), 607–621. https://doi.org/10.1152/physiolgenomics.00001.2012.

Mitchell, A. R., Spurrell, P. A., & Sulke, N. (2003). Circadian variation of arrhythmia onset patterns in patients with persistent atrial fibrillation. *American heart journal,* 146(5), 902–907. https://doi.org/10.1016/S0002-8703(03)00405-8.

Morris, C. J., Purvis, T. E., Mistretta, J., Hu, K., & Scheer, F. A. J. L. (2017). Circadian Misalignment Increases C-Reactive Protein and Blood Pressure in Chronic Shift Workers. *Journal of biological rhythms*, 32(2), 154–164. https://doi.org/10.1177/0748730417697537.

Morris, C. J., Purvis, T. E., Hu, K., & Scheer, F. A. (2016). Circadian misalignment increases cardiovascular disease risk factors in humans. *Proceedings of the National Academy of Sciences of the United States of America,* 113(10), E1402–E1411. https://doi.org/10.1073/pnas.1516953113.

Muller, J. E., Stone, P. H., Turi, Z. G., Rutherford, J. D., Czeisler, C. A., Parker, C., Poole, W. K., Passamani, E., Roberts, R., & Robertson, T. (1985). Circadian variation in the frequency of onset of acute myocardial infarction. *The New England journal of medicine*, 313(21), 1315–1322. https://doi.org/10.1056/NEJM198511213132103.

Nakashima, H., Mashimo, Y., Kurobe, M., Muto, S., Furudono, S., & Maemura, K. (2017). Impact of Morning Onset on the Incidence of Recurrent Acute Coronary Syndrome and Progression of Coronary Atherosclerosis in Acute Myocardial Infarction.

Circulation journal : official journal of the Japanese Circulation Society, 81(3), 361–367. https://doi.org/10.1253/circj.CJ-16-0817.

Pritchett, D., & Reddy, A. B. (2015). Circadian Clocks in the Hematologic System. *Journal of biological rhythms,* 30(5), 374–388. https://doi.org/10.1177/0748730415592729.

Richards, A. M., Nicholls, M. G., Espiner, E. A., Ikram, H., Cullens, M., & Hinton, D. (1986). Diurnal patterns of blood pressure, heart rate and vasoactive hormones in normal man. Clinical and experimental hypertension. Part A, *Theory and practice,* 8(2), 153–166. https://doi.org/10.3109/10641968609074769.

Richards, J., Cheng, K. Y., All, S., Skopis, G., Jeffers, L., Lynch, I. J., Wingo, C. S., & Gumz, M. L. (2013). A role for the circadian clock protein Per1 in the regulation of aldosterone levels and renal Na+ retention. American journal of physiology. *Renal physiology,* 305(12), F1697–F1704. https://doi.org/10.1152/ajprenal.00472.2013.

Roenneberg, T., & Merrow, M. (2005). Circadian clocks - the fall and rise of physiology. Nature reviews. *Molecular cell biology,* 6(12), 965–971. https://doi.org/10.1038/nrm1766.

Rudic, R. D., McNamara, P., Reilly, D., Grosser, T., Curtis, A. M., Price, T. S., Panda, S., Hogenesch, J. B., & FitzGerald, G. A. (2005). Bioinformatic analysis of circadian gene oscillation in mouse aorta. *Circulation,* 112(17), 2716–2724. https://doi.org/10.1161/CIRCULATIONAHA.105.568626.

Saito, K., Takeda, S., Saito, Y., Kawamura, M., Yoshikawa, Y., Yano, H., & Sata, M. (2014). Electrocardiographic and chronobiological features of paroxysmal AV block recorded by ambulatory electrocardiography. *The journal of medical investigation : JMI,* 61(3-4), 380–387. https://doi.org/10.2152/jmi.61.380.

Scheer, F. A., Michelson, A. D., Frelinger, A. L., 3rd, Evoniuk, H., Kelly, E. E., McCarthy, M., Doamekpor, L. A., Barnard, M. R., & Shea, S. A. (2011). The human endogenous circadian system causes greatest platelet activation during the biological morning independent of behaviors. *PloS one,* 6(9), e24549. https://doi.org/10.1371/journal.pone.0024549.

Scheer, F. A., & Shea, S. A. (2014). Human circadian system causes a morning peak in prothrombotic plasminogen activator inhibitor-1 (PAI-1) independent of the sleep/wake cycle. *Blood*, 123(4), 590–593. https://doi.org/10.1182/blood-2013-07-517060.

Schloss, M. J., Horckmans, M., Nitz, K., Duchene, J., Drechsler, M., Bidzhekov, K., Scheiermann, C., Weber, C., Soehnlein, O., & Steffens, S. (2016). The time-of-day of myocardial infarction onset affects healing through oscillations in cardiac neutrophil recruitment. *EMBO molecular medicine,* 8(8), 937–948. https://doi.org/10.15252/emmm.201506083.

Schroder, E. A., Burgess, D. E., Zhang, X., Lefta, M., Smith, J. L., Patwardhan, A., Bartos, D. C., Elayi, C. S., Esser, K. A., & Delisle, B. P. (2015). The cardiomyocyte molecular clock regulates the circadian expression of Kcnh2 and contributes to ventricular repolarization. *Heart rhythm,* 12(6), 1306–1314. https://doi.org/10.1016/j.hrthm.2015.02.019.

Shea, S. A., Hilton, M. F., Hu, K., & Scheer, F. A. (2011). Existence of an endogenous circadian blood pressure rhythm in humans that peaks in the evening. *Circulation research,* 108(8), 980–984. https://doi.org/10.1161/CIRCRESAHA.110.233668.

Sinha, A. D., & Agarwal, R. (2015). The complex relationship between CKD and ambulatory blood pressure patterns. *Advances in chronic kidney disease,* 22(2), 102–107. https://doi.org/10.1053/j.ackd.2015.01.003.

Somanath, P. R., Podrez, E. A., Chen, J., Ma, Y., Marchant, K., Antoch, M., & Byzova, T. V. (2011). Deficiency in core circadian protein Bmal1 is associated with a prothrombotic and vascular phenotype. *Journal of cellular physiology*, 226(1), 132–140. https://doi.org/10.1002/jcp.22314.

Stow, L. R., Richards, J., Cheng, K. Y., Lynch, I. J., Jeffers, L. A., Greenlee, M. M., Cain, B. D., Wingo, C. S., & Gumz, M. L. (2012). The circadian protein period 1 contributes to blood pressure control and coordinately regulates renal sodium transport genes. *Hypertension* (Dallas, Tex.: 1979), 59(6), 1151–1156. https://doi.org/10.1161/HYPERTENSIONAHA.112.190892.

Takigawa, M., Kawamura, M., Noda, T., Yamada, Y., Miyamoto, K., Okamura, H., Satomi, K., Aiba, T., Kamakura, S., Sakaguchi, T., Mizusawa, Y., Itoh, H., Horie, M., & Shimizu, W. (2012). Seasonal and circadian distributions of cardiac events in genotyped patients with congenital long QT syndrome. *Circulation journal : official journal of the Japanese Circulation Society,* 76(9), 2112–2118. https://doi.org/10.1253/circj.cj-12-0213.

Tong, M., Watanabe, E., Yamamoto, N., Nagahata-Ishiguro, M., Maemura, K., Takeda, N., Nagai, R., & Ozaki, Y. (2013). Circadian expressions of cardiac ion channel genes in mouse might be associated with the central clock in the SCN but not the peripheral clock in the heart. *Biological rhythm research,* 44(4), 519–530. https://doi.org/10.1080/09291016.2012.704801.

Tsimakouridze, E. V., Alibhai, F. J., & Martino, T. A. (2015). Therapeutic applications of circadian rhythms for the cardiovascular system. *Frontiers in pharmacology*, 6, 77. https://doi.org/10.3389/fphar.2015.00077.

Uzu, T., Kazembe, F. S., Ishikawa, K., Nakamura, S., Inenaga, T., & Kimura, G. (1996). High sodium sensitivity implicates nocturnal hypertension in essential hypertension. *Hypertension* (Dallas, Tex.: 1979), 28(1), 139–142. https://doi.org/10.1161/01.hyp.28.1.139.

Vyas, M. V., Garg, A. X., Iansavichus, A. V., Costella, J., Donner, A., Laugsand, L. E., Janszky, I., Mrkobrada, M., Parraga, G., & Hackam, D. G. (2012). Shift work and vascular events: systematic review and meta-analysis. *BMJ* (Clinical research ed.), 345, e4800. https://doi.org/10.1136/bmj.e4800.

Wang, N., Yang, G., Jia, Z., Zhang, H., Aoyagi, T., Soodvilai, S., Symons, J. D., Schnermann, J. B., Gonzalez, F. J., Litwin, S. E., & Yang, T. (2008). Vascular PPARgamma controls circadian variation in blood pressure and heart rate through Bmal1. *Cell metabolism, 8*(6), 482–491. https://doi.org/10.1016/j.cmet.2008.10.009.

Watanabe, M., Nakagawa, M., Nobe, S., Ohie, T., Takahashi, N., Hara, M., Yonemochi, H., Ito, M., & Saikawa, T. (2002). Circadian variation of short-lasting asymptomatic paroxysmal supraventricular tachycardia. *Journal of electrocardiology*, 35(2), 135–138. https://doi.org/10.1054/jelc.2002.31820.

Xie, Z., Su, W., Liu, S., Zhao, G., Esser, K., Schroder, E. A., Lefta, M., Stauss, H. M., Guo, Z., & Gong, M. C. (2015). Smooth-muscle BMAL1 participates in blood pressure circadian rhythm regulation. *The Journal of clinical investigation*, 125(1), 324–336. https://doi.org/10.1172/JCI76881.

Zhang, D., & Pollock, D. M. (2020). Diurnal Regulation of Renal Electrolyte Excretion: The Role of Paracrine Factors. *Annual review of physiology*, *82*, 343–363. https://doi.org/10.1146/annurev-physiol-021119-034446.

Chapter 11

The Circadian Clock in Neuroinflammation and Neurogenetic Disorders

Zeynep Birsu Cincin[1,3], PhD and Soner Sahin[2,3,*], MD, PhD

[1]Department of Medical Biochemistry, Istanbul Nişantaşı University, Istanbul, Turkey
[2]Department of Neurosurgery, Istanbul Nişantaşı University, Istanbul, Turkey
[2]Department of Health Ecosystem, Istanbul Nişantaşı University, Istanbul, Turkey

Abstract

The circadian rhythm is responsible for regulating the biological events that take part in the functional coordination of the organism according to the environmental effects of the organism. Therefore, circadian rhythm disorder has been shown to be a risk factor in developing essential diseases, including cancer, mental and metabolic disorders, autoimmune diseases, cancer, and neurodegenerative and neurogenetic diseases. Neurogenetic disease commonly involves disorders impairing the nervous and muscle system function. Symptoms may develop as weakness, stiffness, loss of muscle control, twitching, spasms, and myalgic attack. Three different circadian rhythm changes have been defined in neurogenetic disorders as behavioural disorders, physiological changes, and irregularities in molecular systems. Additionally, it has been shown to manage cerebral vascular hemodynamics, which has been shown to be associated with circadian rhythm changes in neuroinflammatory molecules that can cause the progression of neurogenetic diseases. In this book chapter, neurogenetic diseases associated with circadian rhythm are defined, and the correlation between circadian rhythm irregularity and disease development is tried to explain.

---

[*] Corresponding Author's Email: sahin.soner@nisantasi.edu.tr.

In: Human Health is a Matter of Timing
Editors: Sumeyya Deniz Aybek, Gonca Gulbay and Mucahit Secme
ISBN: 979-8-89113-467-6

The increase in preclinical molecular studies to treat circadian rhythm-related neurogenetic diseases will lead to significant developments in the clinical field. In this way, therapeutic methods will be developed to improve neurogenetic diseases more effectively with new chronotherapy strategies.

Keywords: circadian system, neurogenetic, inflammation, brain health

Introduction

The circadian rhythm, deriving its name from the Latin words "circa" and "diem," implying "approximately a day," orchestrates biochemical, physiological, and behavioural processes in a 24-hour cycle (Muraro et al., 2013). Circadian rhythms are intrinsic biological oscillations for approximately 24 hours that regulate numerous physiological processes such as sleep-wake cycles, hormonal release, metabolism, and immune responses (Neves et al., 2022). This innate biological clock is maintained by a set of 'clock genes' (Cox et al., 2019). Through intricate transcription-translation feedback loops, these genes produce proteins that regulate circadian rhythms (Takahashi, 2017). Any disruption in these clock genes or proteins could impact the circadian rhythm, potentially leading to various health disorders (Roenneberg and Merrow, 2016). Recent scientific exploration has revealed a potential correlation between the circadian system and the occurrence of neuroinflammatory and neurogenetic disorders (Zielinski and Gibbons, 2022). Understanding this connection promises potential diagnostic and therapeutic implications. Emerging evidence suggests that various factors can disrupt these rhythms, including neuroinflammation and neurogenetic disorders (Srinivasan and Walker, 2022). In recent years, the intimate connection between the brain and the immune system has been brought to light, with neuroinflammation and neurogenetic disorders being recognized as significant influencers of the internal biological clock of the body, the circadian rhythm (Carter et al., 2021). This book chapter explores this complex relationship in a detailed and integrated view, underscoring its importance in human health and disease.

Understanding the Relationship of Neuroinflammation and Neurogenetic Diseases in the Circadian Clock

Neuroinflammation: Mechanisms, Implications, and Therapeutic Approaches

Neuroinflammation, while initially a protective response, can lead to a self-perpetuating cycle of neuronal damage and inflammation when dysregulated, therefore, it has an essential impact on the pathogenesis of numerous neurodegenerative and psychiatric disorders (Benallague et al., 2022). Although various mechanisms were related to neuroinflammation, much remains to be discovered. Future research focusing on developing novel anti-inflammatory and pro-resolution therapies could provide groundbreaking advancements in the treatment of neuroinflammation-associated disorders (Bersano et al., 2023). However, the challenge remains to selectively target harmful inflammation while preserving the beneficial aspects of the neuroinflammatory response (Federico et al., 2022).

Neuroinflammation, characterized by enabling immune cells to be active within the central nervous system (CNS), is a complex biological response to harmful stimuli such as pathogens, damaged neurons, or toxic metabolites (Amonollahi et al., 2023). This protective mechanism involves the release of inflammatory mediators to eliminate the cause of cell injury and initiate tissue repair (Huang et al., 2022). However, chronic or unresolved neuroinflammation may exacerbate neurological damage, contributing to various neurodegenerative diseases (Gorgi, 2022). This section will explore the intricate mechanisms of neuroinflammation, its role in neurological disorders, and potential therapeutic interventions.

The CNS comprises a unique immune environment that primarily involves microglia, the immune cells in the brain and spinal cord, and other immune components such as astrocytes and invading peripheral immune cells (Feldman, 2022). Neuroinflammation initiates when these cells detect tissue damage or infection, activating microglia and astrocytes (Kwon, 2022; Tran et al., 2022). Microglia, often termed the CNS's macrophages, exhibit a variety of receptors that can identify pathogen-associated molecular patterns (PAMPs) and danger-associated molecular patterns (DAMPs) (Kumar, 2019). Upon detection, they transform from a surveillant state to an active state, releasing various inflammatory mediators such as cytokines, chemokines, and reactive oxygen species (ROS) (Serna-Rodríguez et al., 2022). Concurrently, activated astrocytes amplify the inflammatory response by producing additional cytokines and chemokines, thereby attracting peripheral immune cells into the CNS (Lopez-Rodriguez et al., 2021). While acute neuroinflammation is a protective mechanism to restore CNS homeostasis, chronic or uncontrolled neuroinflammation can lead to detrimental effects (Brandl et al., 2023). Excessive release of pro-inflammatory mediators and ROS can cause neuronal damage, disrupt the blood-brain barrier (BBB), and induce apoptosis (Candelario et al., 2022). This prolonged inflammation is involved in the pathogenesis of various neurological disorders.

Neurodegenerative diseases such as Alzheimer's disease, Parkinson's disease, and multiple sclerosis are characterized by sustained neuroinflammation (Lempriere, 2023). In these conditions, the perpetual cycle of neuronal damage and the inflammatory response exacerbates disease progression (Leng and Edison, 2021). Moreover, neuroinflammation has been associated with psychiatric disorders such as depression, schizophrenia, and autism, suggesting a broader role of neuroinflammation beyond neurodegeneration (Monji and Mizoguchi,2022). Given the fundamental role of neuroinflammation in neurodegenerative and psychiatric disorders, therapeutic strategies aim to modulate this inflammatory response (Kölliker-Frers et al., 2021; Mishra et al., 2021). Nonsteroidal anti-inflammatory drugs (NSAIDs) and corticosteroids have been widely used to attenuate inflammation, but their long-term use can lead to significant side effects.

Targeting specific molecular pathways involved in neuroinflammation presents a promising strategy. For example, inhibitors of the NLRP3 inflammasome, a protein complex that regulates the release of pro-inflammatory cytokines, have shown potential in preclinical models of Alzheimer's disease and multiple sclerosis (Huang et al., 2021; Zhu et al., 2021). Another emerging approach involves biologics, such as monoclonal antibodies against specific inflammatory mediators. For instance, the monoclonal antibody aducanumab, targeting amyloid-beta, a protein that accumulates and induces inflammation in Alzheimer's disease, has shown promise in clinical trials (Athar et al.,2021). Moreover, therapies that aim to improve the inherent resolution pathways of the brain, which naturally terminate inflammation and restore homeostasis, represent another avenue of research, thus enhancing anti-inflammatory cytokines or promoting microglial apoptosis after their activation (Fyfe, 2022).

Neuroinflammation and Circadian Clock

Neuroinflammation refers to the inflammation of nervous tissue, which can be a response to infection, injury, toxic metabolites, or autoimmunity (Ingelfinger et al., 2022). Evidence from various studies suggests that disruption of circadian rhythm can trigger neuroinflammation (Zielinski and Gibbons, 2022).

The cyclical expression of clock genes in immune cells and the brain ensures a time-dependent regulation of immune response, with an optimum balance between pro-inflammatory and anti-inflammatory reactions (Villasana-Salazae and Vezzani, 2023; Herhengan et al., 2020). Neuroinflammation is the inflammation of nervous tissue, often as a reaction to injury, infection, or autoimmune disorders (Won et al., 2021). This inflammation can impact brain functions, including regulating circadian rhythms (Lie et al., 2022; Shimba and Ikuta, 2020). The immune system and circadian clock have a bidirectional relationship where the immune response is under circadian control, and conversely, immune signals can affect the circadian clock (Wang and Li, 2021). This dynamic interplay indicates that a dysregulated immune response, such as persistent inflammation, can disrupt the normal rhythm of the circadian clock (Lananna and Musiek, 2020). Disruption of the circadian rhythm can lead to a persistent pro-inflammatory state, contributing to chronic neuroinflammation (Lindahl and Bryceson, 2022). This dysregulated immune response can aggravate neurodegenerative diseases such as Alzheimer's, Parkinson's, and multiple sclerosis, characterized by chronic neuroinflammation (Dhapola et al., 2021). Experimental models have shown that pro-inflammatory cytokines such as IL-1β, TNFα, and IL-6 can alter the phase and amplitude of circadian rhythms, suggesting that inflammation-induced circadian disruption may contribute to the pathogenesis of several neurodegenerative and psychiatric diseases (Musiek and Holtzman,2016; Mogi et al., 2018; Griffin et al., 2019).

Circadian Clock and Neurogenetic Disorders

Neurogenetic disorders, including Huntington's disease, Fragile X syndrome, and Down syndrome, are characterized by genetic abnormalities affecting the nervous system's structure and function (Wilson et al., 2023). Research has shown a correlation between the severity of circadian disruption and the severity of neurologic symptoms in these disorders. These findings suggest that the circadian clock is not only a bystander affected by the neuropathological process but may play a central role in the pathogenesis and progression of these diseases. The underlying mechanism of this disruption may be related to the direct effects of genetic mutations on clock gene function or indirect effects on neuronal circuits that regulate the circadian clock. In many neurogenetic disorders, gene mutations linked to the circadian clock have been identified (Cedernaes et al., 2019). For instance, in Huntington's disease, mutations in the Huntingtin gene disrupt the functioning of proteins within the circadian clock machinery, leading to alterations in sleep-wake patterns, hormone secretion, and other circadian-controlled functions (Saade-Lemus and Videnovic, 2023). Similarly, in Down syndrome, abnormalities in the CLOCK gene have been associated with disturbed sleep and cognitive deficits (Lovos et al., 2021). Many of these disorders present with disruptions in the sleep-wake cycle or other circadian-related disturbances. In Fragile X syndrome, the mutation in the FMR1 gene has been found to affect the expression of several clock genes, thereby disrupting circadian rhythms and leading to sleep disorders commonly seen in these patients (Dueck et al., 2020). Collectively, these examples highlight the crucial role of the circadian clock in the manifestation and progression of neurogenetic disorders.

Therapeutic Implications

Given the intertwined relationship between circadian rhythm, neuroinflammation, and neurogenetic disorders, a potential therapeutic approach could involve manipulating the circadian clock (Mishra et al., 2021). Chronotherapy, a treatment that aligns with the circadian rhythms of the body, could be viable (Lee et al., 2021). It may involve adjusting the timing of medication or light therapy to synchronize with the patient's circadian rhythm, thereby reducing symptoms and enhancing the efficacy of treatments (Dong et al., 2020). Moreover, developing drugs that can modulate the activity of clock genes or their downstream targets could offer promising therapeutic avenues (Moradi and Dashti, 2022). These interventions could alleviate symptoms and slow disease progression in neuroinflammatory and neurogenetic disorders (Guo et al., 2021).

Understanding the complex relationship between neuroinflammation, neurogenetic disorders, and the circadian clock can open novel therapeutic avenues (Zhou et al., 2022). Strategies such as chronotherapy, which aligns treatment administration with the circadian rhythms of the body, can optimize treatment outcomes for various conditions (Yu et al., 2022). For neuroinflammatory and neurogenetic disorders, interventions that restore circadian homeostasis, such as light therapy, sleep hygiene, or pharmacological modulation of clock genes, may provide beneficial effects.

Conclusion

The interconnection between the circadian clock, neuroinflammation, and neurogenetic disorders sheds light on the complex nature of these disorders. Although much progress has been made in understanding the role of the circadian clock in these diseases, there still need to be significant knowledge gaps, particularly in the underlying molecular mechanisms. Future research is essential to deepen our understanding and leverage this knowledge to develop more effective diagnostics and therapeutic strategies. This approach may provide novel insights, revealing a new horizon in for the management and treatment of neuroinflammatory and neurogenetic disorders.

In conclusion, the circadian clock plays a pivotal role in maintaining the functional integrity of the nervous system. Disruptions caused by neuroinflammation and neurogenetic disorders can result in circadian dysregulation, which can contribute to disease pathogenesis. Although significant strides have been made in understanding this complex relationship, more research is warranted to unravel the mechanistic details fully. This knowledge could lead to the development of innovative therapeutic strategies to restore the integrity of the circadian rhythm, thus improving the quality of life for individuals affected by these conditions.

References

Amanollahi, M., Jameie, M., Heidari, A., & Rezaei, N. (2023). The Dialogue Between Neuroinflammation and Adult Neurogenesis: Mechanisms Involved and Alterations in Neurological Diseases. *Molecular neurobiology*, *60*(2), 923–959.

Athar, T., Al Balushi, K., & Khan, S. A. (2021). Recent advances on drug development and emerging therapeutic agents for Alzheimer's disease. *Molecular biology reports*, *48*(7), 5629–5645. https://doi.org/10.1007/s11033-021-06512-9.

Ayata, P., Amit, I., & Cuda, C. M. (2023). Editorial: Microglia in neuroinflammation. *Frontiers in immunology*, *14*, 1227095.

Benallegue, N., Kebir, H., & Alvarez, J. I. (2022). Neuroinflammation: Extinguishing a blaze of T cells. *Immunological reviews*, *311*(1), 151–176.

Bersano, A., Engele, J., & Schäfer, M. K. E. (2023). Neuroinflammation and Brain Disease. *BMC neurology*, *23*(1), 227.

Brandl, S., & Reindl, M. (2023). Blood-Brain Barrier Breakdown in Neuroinflammation: Current In Vitro Models. *International journal of molecular sciences*, *24*(16), 12699.

Candelario-Jalil, E., Dijkhuizen, R. M., & Magnus, T. (2022). Neuroinflammation, Stroke, Blood-Brain Barrier Dysfunction, and Imaging Modalities. *Stroke*, *53*(5), 1473–1486. https://doi.org/10.1161/STROKEAHA.122.036946.

Carter, B., Justin, H. S., Gulick, D., & Gamsby, J. J. (2021). The Molecular Clock and Neurodegenerative Disease: A Stressful Time. *Frontiers in molecular biosciences*, 8, 644747.

Cedernaes, J., Waldeck, N., & Bass, J. (2019). Neurogenetic basis for circadian regulation of metabolism by the hypothalamus. *Genes & development*, *33*(17-18), 1136–1158.

Cox, K. H., & Takahashi, J. S. (2019). Circadian clock genes and the transcriptional architecture of the clock mechanism. *Journal of molecular endocrinology*, 63(4), R93–R102.

Dhapola, R., Hota, S. S., Sarma, P., Bhattacharyya, A., Medhi, B., & Reddy, D. H. (2021). Recent advances in molecular pathways and therapeutic implications targeting neuroinflammation for Alzheimer's disease. *Inflammopharmacology*, *29*(6), 1669–1681.

Dong, D., Yang, D., Lin, L., Wang, S., & Wu, B. (2020). Circadian rhythm in pharmacokinetics and its relevance to chronotherapy. *Biochemical pharmacology*, *178*, 114045.

Federico, S., & Moro, S. (2022). Promising Targets and Strategies to Control Neuroinflammation (Part I). *Current medicinal chemistry*, *29*(27), 4630.

Federico, S., & Moro, S. (2022). Promising Targets and Strategies to Control Neuroinflammation (Part II). *Current medicinal chemistry*, *29*(28), 4779. https://doi.org/10.2174/092986732928220629152149.

Feldman R. A. (2022). Microglia orchestrate neuroinflammation. *eLife*, *11*, e81890. https://doi.org/10.7554/eLife.81890.

Fyfe I. (2022). Gene therapy protects against neuroinflammation. *Nature reviews. Neurology*, *18*(7), 381.

Gorji A. (2022). Neuroinflammation: The Pathogenic Mechanism of Neurological Disorders. *International journal of molecular sciences*, *23*(10), 5744.

Griffin, P., Dimitry, J. M., Sheehan, P. W., Lananna, B. V., Guo, C., Robinette, M. L., Hayes, M. E., Cedeño, M. R., Nadarajah, C. J., Ezerskiy, L. A., Colonna, M., Zhang, J., Bauer, A. Q., Burris, T. P., & Musiek, E. S. (2019). Circadian clock protein Rev-erbα regulates neuroinflammation. *Proceedings of the National Academy of Sciences of the United States of America*, *116*(11), 5102–5107.

Guo, S., Geng, X., Lee, H., & Ding, Y. (2021). Phenothiazine Inhibits Neuroinflammation and Inflammasome Activation Independent of Hypothermia After Ischemic Stroke. *Molecular neurobiology*, *58*(12), 6136–6152.

Hergenhan, S., Holtkamp, S., & Scheiermann, C. (2020). Molecular Interactions Between Components of the Circadian Clock and the Immune System. *Journal of molecular biology*, 432(12), 3700–3713.

Hou Y, Wei Y, Lautrup S, Yang B, Wang Y, Cordonnier S, Mattson MP, Croteau DL, Bohr VA. NAD$^+$supplementation reduces neuroinflammation and cell senescence in a transgenic mouse model of Alzheimer's disease via cGAS-STING. *Proc Natl Acad Sci USA*. 2021 Sep 14;118(37):e2011226118.

Huang, L., & Zhang, J. H. (2022). Introduction to Special Issue: Brain Immunity and Neuroinflammation. *Experimental neurology*, *349*, 113957.

Huang, Y., Xu, W., & Zhou, R. (2021). NLRP3 inflammasome activation and cell death. Cellular & molecular immunology, 18(9), 2114–2127.

Ingelfinger, F., Beltrán, E., Gerdes, L. A., & Becher, B. (2022). Single-cell multiomics in neuroinflammation. *Current opinion in immunology*, *76*, 102180.

Kölliker-Frers, R., Udovin, L., Otero-Losada, M., Kobiec, T., Herrera, M. I., Palacios, J., Razzitte, G., & Capani, F. (2021). Neuroinflammation: An Integrating Overview of Reactive-Neuroimmune Cell Interactions in Health and Disease. *Mediators of inflammation*, *2021*, 9999146.

Kumar V. (2019). Toll-like receptors in the pathogenesis of neuroinflammation. *Journal of neuroimmunology*, *332*, 16–30.

Kwon M. S. (2022). Advanced therapeutic strategies targeting microglia: beyond neuroinflammation. *Archives of pharmacal research*, *45*(9), 618–630.

Lananna, B. V., & Musiek, E. S. (2020). The wrinkling of time: Aging, inflammation, oxidative stress, and the circadian clock in neurodegeneration. *Neurobiology of disease*, *139*, 104832.

Lee, Y., Field, J. M., & Sehgal, A. (2021). Circadian Rhythms, Disease and Chronotherapy. *Journal of biological rhythms*, *36*(6), 503–531.

Lemprière S. (2023). Neuroinflammation predicts cognitive decline in FTD. *Nature reviews. Neurology*, *19*(5), 258.

Leng, F., & Edison, P. (2021). Neuroinflammation and microglial activation in Alzheimer disease: where do we go from here?. *Nature reviews. Neurology*, *17*(3), 157–172.

Lindahl, H., & Bryceson, Y. T. (2022). Neuroinflammation Associated With Inborn Errors of Immunity. *Frontiers in immunology*, *12*, 827815.

Lopez-Rodriguez, A. B., Hennessy, E., Murray, C. L., Nazmi, A., Delaney, H. J., Healy, D., Fagan, S. G., Rooney, M., Stewart, E., Lewis, A., de Barra, N., Scarry, P., Riggs-Miller, L., Boche, D., Cunningham, M. O., & Cunningham, C. (2021). Acute systemic inflammation exacerbates neuroinflammation in Alzheimer's disease: IL-1β drives amplified responses in primed astrocytes and neuronal network dysfunction. *Alzheimer's & dementia : the journal of the Alzheimer's Association*, *17*(10), 1735–1755.

Lovos, A., Bottrill, K., Sakhon, S., Nyhuis, C., Egleson, E., Luongo, A., Murphy, M., Thurman, A. J., Abbeduto, L., Lee, N. R., Hughes, K., & Edgin, J. (2021). Circadian Sleep-Activity Rhythm across Ages in Down Syndrome. Brain sciences, 11(11), 1403.

Mishra, A., Bandopadhyay, R., Singh, P. K., Mishra, P. S., Sharma, N., & Khurana, N. (2021). Neuroinflammation in neurological disorders: pharmacotherapeutic targets from bench to bedside. *Metabolic brain disease*, *36*(7), 1591–1626.

Mogi, A., Yomoda, R., Kimura, S., Tsushima, C., Takouda, J., Sawauchi, M., Maekawa, T., Ohta, H., Nishino, S., Kurita, M., Mano, N., Osumi, N., & Moriya, T. (2018). Entrainment of the Circadian Clock in Neural Stem Cells by Epidermal Growth Factor is Closely Associated with ERK1/2-mediated Induction of Multiple Clock-related Genes. *Neuroscience*, *379*, 45–66.

Monji, A., & Mizoguchi, Y. (2022). Neuroinflammation in Late-Onset Schizophrenia: Viewing from the Standpoint of the Microglia Hypothesis. *Neuropsychobiology*, *81*(2), 98–103.

Moradi, F., & Dashti, N. (2022). Targeting neuroinflammation by intranasal delivery of nanoparticles in neurological diseases: a comprehensive review. *Naunyn-Schmiedeberg's archives of pharmacology*, *395*(2), 133–148.

Muraro, N. I., Pírez, N., & Ceriani, M. F. (2013). The circadian system: plasticity at many levels. *Neuroscience*, *247*, 280–293.

Musiek, E. S., & Holtzman, D. M. (2016). Mechanisms linking circadian clocks, sleep, and neurodegeneration. *Science (New York, N.Y.)*, *354*(6315), 1004–1008.

Neves, A. R., Albuquerque, T., Quintela, T., & Costa, D. (2022). Circadian rhythm and disease: Relationship, new insights, and future perspectives. *Journal of cellular physiology*, *237*(8), 3239–3256.

Roenneberg, T., & Merrow, M. (2016). The Circadian Clock and Human Health. *Current biology : CB*, 26(10), R432–R443.

Saade-Lemus, S., & Videnovic, A. (2023). Sleep Disorders and Circadian Disruption in Huntington's Disease. *Journal of Huntington's disease*, *12*(2), 121–131.

Serna-Rodríguez, M. F., Bernal-Vega, S., de la Barquera, J. A. O., Camacho-Morales, A., & Pérez-Maya, A. A. (2022). The role of damage associated molecular pattern molecules (DAMPs) and permeability of the blood-brain barrier in depression and neuroinflammation. *Journal of neuroimmunology*, *371*, 577951.

Shimba, A., & Ikuta, K. (2020). Glucocorticoids Regulate Circadian Rhythm of Innate and Adaptive Immunity. *Frontiers in immunology*, *11*, 2143.

Srinivasan, M., & Walker, C. (2022). Circadian Clock, Glucocorticoids and NF-κB Signaling in Neuroinflammation- Implicating Glucocorticoid Induced Leucine Zipper as a Molecular Link. ASN neuro, 14, 17590914221120190.

Takahashi J. S. (2017). Transcriptional architecture of the mammalian circadian clock. Nature reviews. *Genetics,* 18(3), 164–179.

Tran, V. T. A., Lee, L. P., & Cho, H. (2022). Neuroinflammation in neurodegeneration *via*microbial infections. *Frontiers in immunology*, *13*, 907804.

Villasana-Salazar, B., & Vezzani, A. (2023). Neuroinflammation microenvironment sharpens seizure circuit. *Neurobiology of disease*, *178*, 106027.

Wang, X. L., & Li, L. (2021). Circadian Clock Regulates Inflammation and the Development of Neurodegeneration. *Frontiers in cellular and infection microbiology*, *11*, 696554.

Wilson, D. M., 3rd, Cookson, M. R., Van Den Bosch, L., Zetterberg, H., Holtzman, D. M., & Dewachter, I. (2023). Hallmarks of neurodegenerative diseases. *Cell*, *186*(4), 693–714.

Won, E., Na, K. S., & Kim, Y. K. (2021). Associations between Melatonin, Neuroinflammation, and Brain Alterations in Depression. *International journal of molecular sciences*, *23*(1), 305.

Yu, F., Liu, Y., Zhang, R., Zhu, L., Zhang, T., & Shi, Y. (2022). Recent advances in circadian-regulated pharmacokinetics and its implications for chronotherapy. *Biochemical pharmacology*, *203*, 115185.

Zhao, Y., Zhang, J., Zheng, Y., Zhang, Y., Zhang, X. J., Wang, H., Du, Y., Guan, J., Wang, X., & Fu, J. (2021). NAD^+ improves cognitive function and reduces neuroinflammation by ameliorating mitochondrial damage and decreasing ROS production in chronic cerebral hypoperfusion models through Sirt1/PGC-1α pathway. *Journal of neuroinflammation*, *18*(1), 207.

Zhu, H., Jian, Z., Zhong, Y., Ye, Y., Zhang, Y., Hu, X., Pu, B., Gu, L., & Xiong, X. (2021). Janus Kinase Inhibition Ameliorates Ischemic Stroke Injury and Neuroinflammation Through Reducing NLRP3 Inflammasome Activation *via*JAK2/STAT3 Pathway Inhibition. *Frontiers in immunology*, *12*, 714943.

Zielinski, M. R., & Gibbons, A. J. (2022). Neuroinflammation, Sleep, and Circadian Rhythms. *Frontiers in cellular and infection microbiology*, 12, 853096.

Chapter 12

Dysfunctional Circadian Clock and Mood Disorders

Mehmet Buğrahan Gürcan[1,*], MD
Zeynep Nur Demirok[1], MD
and Erdoğdu Akça[2], MD
[1]Department of Psychiatry, Kartal Lütfi Kırdar City Hospital, Istanbul, Turkiye
[2]Department of Psychiatry, Marmara University Pendik Training and Research Hospital, Istanbul, Turkiye

Abstract

Circadian rhythm refers to an approximately 24-hour process created by endogenous biological clocks and influenced by environmental stimuli (zeitgebers). The sleep-wake cycle of the human body, body temperature, feeding schedule, hormones, and many psychiatric disorders are closely related to the circadian clock. Optimal coordination of the circadian rhythm with the internal and external environment is essential for the environmental adaptation and optimal functioning of the organism. It has been supported by studies that hormonal mechanisms affecting circadian rhythm, environmental and genetic factors, and chronotypes of eveningness and morningness are effective in mood disorders. The relationship between mood disorders and the circadian clock will be examined in this section.

Keywords: biological clocks, circadian rhythm, mood disorders, zeitgeber

---

[*] Corresponding Author's Email: mbgurcan@gmail.com.

In: Human Health is a Matter of Timing
Editors: Sumeyya Deniz Aybek, Gonca Gulbay and Mucahit Secme
ISBN: 979-8-89113-467-6

Introduction

The circadian clock is a biological timing system that organizes daily events and physiological rhythmic changes to predict the 24-hour environmental light/dark cycle for organisms and to adapt to external conditions created by the Earth's daily rotation around its axis. Circadian rhythms have an impact on biological processes in many living beings from bacteria to humans (Takahashi et al., 2008). Functions regulated by circadian rhythms are, mainly the sleep-wake cycle, as follows: body temperature, feeding behaviors, hormone secretion, xenobiotic metabolism, glucose regulation, and cellular cycles (Takahashi et al., 2008; Hastings et al., 2003). If the circadian rhythm is disrupted by genetic or environmental factors, physiological deterioration is inevitable (Hastings et al., 2003). Chronobiology is a field of science investigating the biological rhythms associated with events that change with minute, hour, daily, monthly, seasonal, annual, or longer rhythms in animals and humans.

Two important scientists stand out in the history of chronobiology. The first of these was Aschoff (1913-1998), who served as director of the Max-Planck Institute. Aschoff conducted research on circadian rhythm in both humans and animals and introduced the term "zeitgeber" (Lemmer, 2009). This term is the name given to external factors that affect the biological rhythm. Another important name, Franz Halberg (1919), played an important role in the introduction of chronobiology into the scientific literature (Lemmer, 2009; Cornelissen et al., 2013). Halberg first introduced the term "circadian," which was defined as an "internal day," meaning slightly shorter or slightly longer than 24 hours under steady conditions (Lemmer, 2009; Cornelissen et al., 2013). In 1764, Medicus described the winter depression as "Dr. Helwig noticed a relapse of depression in one patient during the month of December each year. Geiger (1606–1671) drew attention to the sleep and wake cycles in melencholia and emphasized that being awake after midnight is not a pleasant situation in mental problems (Lemmer, 2009). Springel mentioned an increase in fatigue during the daytime compared to the evening hours in melancholia (Lemmer, 2009). Helmut Marx reported the effect of light on the physiological changes and winter depression of soldiers in the Arctic Circle (Lemmer, 2009; Marx, 1946). It is known that the disruption of circadian physiology has a broad effect on neural and neuroendocrine functions that cause mental illnesses (Kirlioglu & Balcıoğlu, 2020). Many studies have shown that many factors related to the human circadian clock at the hormonal and molecular level are effective in mood disorders. In this section, the relationship between the circadian clock and mood disorders will be explained.

Mood Disorders

Circadian rhythm disturbance is an important feature of mood disorders. The effects of zeitgebers on morningness-eveningness, hormonal rhythms, and circadian rhythm are crucial in major depressive disorder (MDD) and bipolar disorder (Alloy et al., 2017; Kirlioglu & Balcioglu, 2020). Various body functions were found to differ between patients with mood disorders compared to healthy individuals, such as body temperature, blood pressure, pulse rate, plasma cortisol levels, hormones such as thyroid stimulating hormone, and melatonin. (Kirlioglu & Balcioglu, 2020; Novakova et al., 2015; Souêtre et al., 1989). Hypersomnia and insomnia are the diagnostic criteria for mood disorders. It is thought that insomnia may be a predictor of the development of the first depression episode, the relapse of depressed patients in remission, and the development of manic episodes (Plante & Winkelman, 2008; Ohayon, & Roth, 2003). The association between circadian rhythms and mood disorders has been mainly based on a seasonal characteristic of mood episodes, the role of drug treatments on circadian rhythm, and the link of daylight to mood (Benedetti et al., 2015; Kirlioglu & Balcioglu, 2020; Faedda et al., 1993). The role and mechanisms of the human biological clock in bipolar disorder and depression, which are the main mood disorders, will be addressed in this section.

Bipolar Mood Disorders

Bipolar Disorder (BD), with recurrent episodes of depression and mania, is defined as a mental disorder with deterioration of behavior, cognition, sleep, and functionality. BD encompasses a variety of diseases, including cyclothymic disorder characterized by periods of mood elevation and depression in which symptoms of mania and depression are not fully met, bipolar II disorder consisting of hypomania and depression periods, and bipolar I disorder with fully developed manic episodes (Alloy et al., 2012). 4.4% of the US population has bipolar spectrum disorder, resulting in low functionality, comorbid diseases, and a risk of suicide (Alloy et al., 2017;

Merikangas et al., 2007). It is clear that we still need to better understand the disease.

Sleep problems are one of the most common problems in bipolar mood disorder. (Alloy et al., 2017). Insomnia (40-45%) and hypersomnia (23-78%) are seen in depressive episodes, whereas a decrease in the need for sleep (66-99%) is observed especially in manic episodes (Takaesu, 2018). The frequent appearance of sleep problems in euthymic periods suggests that sleep is closely related to the pathophysiology of bipolar disorder. (Chung et al., 2012; Ng et al., 2015). The sleep-wake cycle, which is one of the circadian rhythms, is regulated by the suprachiasmatic nucleus (SCN) located in the anterior hypothalamus, which is known as the main biological clock. (Alloy et al., 2017; Schulz & Steimer, 2009). The sleep-wake cycle is mainly driven by genetic predisposition, chronotype, and melatonin secretion. Although the SCN functions autonomously, it can be influenced by external factors called zeitgeber (rhythm regulator) (Alloy et al., 2017). Although the strongest zeitgeber is light, there are zeitgebers that vary from auditory stimuli to daily activities (Grandin et al., 2006). Daily schedules such as bedtime and mealtime may have an effect on the circadian rhythm in healthy people, as well as in people with mood disorders (Alloy et al., 2017; Stetler et al., 2004). These changes are explained by the social rhythm hypothesis. Social rhythms such as eating and working seem to operate the circadian rhythm, and individuals with mood disorders have a more disrupted social rhythm than healthy individuals (Malkoff-Schwartz et al., 2000). It can be noted that both endogenous and external circadian factors play a role in the mood episodes in patients with bipolar spectrum disorders. In this context, the relationship between mood disorders and biological clock sources such as melatonin, genetics, chronotype, social factors, and life events will be discussed in this section.

Biological Clock and Endogenous Disruptions

Melatonin, which is released from the pineal gland, has one of the most prominent roles in the circadian rhythm. A substantial body of research had focused on melatonin levels, sleep cycles, and depression. Lerner was the first to evaluate of the effect of melatonin on human behavior (Lerner & Nordlund, 1978). Melatonin secretion begins about a few hours before sleep, contributes to the onset of sleep by activating GABA in the SCN. The level of melatonin increases with the transition to sleep and decreases close to awakening

(Srinivasan et al., 2009, Kirlioglu & Balcioglu, 2020). Melatonin was shown to have both direct hypnotic effects and sleep-related circadian rhythm regulatory effects (Srinivasan et al., 2009). There are studies showing changes in melatonin secretion in mood episodes (Novakova et al., 2015; Takaesu, 2018). The effect of lithium and valproic acid on the level and release of melatonin provides a better understanding of their mechanisms related to mood disorders (Manchia et al., 2019). Lewy et al. showed that melatonin was suppressed more in bipolar patients than in healthy individuals in light exposure (Lewy et al., 1980). Kennedy et al. suggested that there was no difference in serum melatonin levels between mood episodes and euthymic periods in patients with bipolar disorder, although the serum melatonin levels in all periods (manic, depressive and euthymic) were lower in patients with bipolar disorder than those in healthy groups (Kennedy, 1996). The difference in melatonin levels in people with bipolar disorder appears to be a feature of the disease, independent of thc mood episode (Kennedy, 1996). Given the effect of melatonin levels on circadian rhythm and some neurotransmitters, more studies are needed in the spectrum of bipolar disorder.

Recent genetic studies have gained importance, especially in circadian rhythm irregularity, revealing a relationship between bipolar disorder and certain circadian genes such as CLOCK, TIMELESS, ARNTL2, GSK3-β, PER3, DBP, and NR1D1 ROR. The relationship established between these genes and bipolar disorder also indicates the existence of a polygenetic structure. (Alloy et al., 2017; Murray & Harvey, 2014). Nováková et al., measured melatonin levels in the saliva of bipolar patients in manic and depressive episodes and healthy controls and reported no difference between melatonin levels. However, they found an increase in the Per 1 and Nrd 1 gene expressions in the samples they took from the buccal mucosa of the patients with manic episodes compared to the patients with depression (Nováková et al., 2015). The risk of suicide was found to be higher in depressive patients with bipolar spectrum disorder who have the Rs1801260*C CLOCK gene variant (Benedetti et al., 2015). The CLOCK rs1801260 gene modulated the association between early life stress, adult suicide attempt history, and current suicidal ideation. This study shows that biological clock-related factors may affect the basic psychopathological features of mood disorders rather than the circadian clock. (Benedetti et al., 2015).

It has been shown that there are interesting relationships between Glycolene Synthase Kinase 3-b (GSK3-b), which is found in drosphilias, and its ortholog in humans (Mansour et al., 2005). GSK3-b is located on chromosome 3q21.1 and plays an important role in the regulation of the molecular clock in the SCN (Hansen et al., 1997). It was proposed that lithium inhibits the activation of this gene and plays a role in the treatment of Bipolar Mood disorder (Benedetti et al., 2015). Similarly, family studies and gene expression studies show that there is a relationship between circadian clock gene expressions and mood disorders (Alloy et al., 2017; Murray & Harvey, 2014, Mansour et al., 2005, 18). Since there is substantial evidence of circadian dysfunction in patients with mood disorders, it has been emphasized that it is important to investigate the role of circadian gene variation in the pathogenesis of mood disorders (Mansour et al., 2005).

The chronotype is the behavioral appearance underlying the biological clock, which is formed by the effects of physical and genetic factors. People have different chronotypes such as "morningness" and "eveningness" in terms of differences in biological and behavioral rhythms including sleep-wake cycle, body temperature, cortisol, and melatonin secretion time (Bullock et al., 2014). This reflects a person's 24-hour ultradian predisposition to the waking or sleeping state. Three different chronotypes have been defined: morningness type, eveningness type, and intermediate type (Benedetti, 2015 et al., 2015). While 40% of the population is of the morning or evening-type, 60% is intermediate type that is not included in these two types (Selvi et al., 2011). The evening chronotype has been associated with physiological measures of circadian phase latency, such as a later circadian temperature phase and a later melatonin secretion phase compared to the morning chronotype. (Selvi et al., 2011; Adan et al., 2012). Studies show that the evening type has a stronger association with bipolar disorder (Melo et al., 2017). In a study by Seleem et al., which included 257 bipolar I and II patients, it was shown that patients with bipolar disorder had a delayed sleep onset regardless of their current mood (Seleem et al., 2015). In their study with 200 patients, Baek et al. revealed that patients with bipolar II had higher evening scores than those with bipolar I, in the euthymic period (Baek et al., 2016). Chung et al. reported that bipolar II patients showed more eveningness than bipolar I, while major depression patients showed less morningness than bipolar I patients (Chung et al., 2012). In another study, the rate of eveningness was found to be higher in patients with rapid cycling compared to non-rapid cycling bipolar patients. (Mansour et al., 2005). Some studies have revealed findings suggesting that eveningness is a feature that can be associated with bipolar disorder and may be a risk factor rather than an outcome of the disease (Etain et al., 2014; Bullock et al., 2014). Although many studies show that evening sleepiness is more common in bipolar disorder, more studies are needed for a better understanding in this area.

Social Cues and life events that affect biological rhythms such as bedtime, mealtime, starting and finishing work, and exercises play an important role in driving the sleep-wake rhythm. One of the theories in the etiology of mood disorder is the social zeitgeber theory. (Ng et al., 2015). According to social rhythm theory, life events initiate biological changes that will trigger mood episodes such as mania and depression. (Grandin et al., 2006; Malkoff-Schwartz et al., 2000). Social rhythm changes can also affect biological rhythms through exposure to light and the release of melatonin (Alloy et al., 2017, Stetler et al., 2004). It was suggested that the regularity of the social zeitgeber can provide synchronization of social rhythms and thus stabilize mood (Takaesu, 2018). On the contrary, irregularities in the social zeitgeber may cause circadian rhythm disorders and mood episodes (Takaesu, 2018). Additionally, some studies have indicated that there are significant worsening in social zeitgebers in the euthymic periods of bipolar disorder patients. (Shen et al., 2008). Malkoff-Schwartz et al., also found that life events associated with social rhythm disorder may be associated with the onset of manic episodes (Malkoff-Schwartz et al., 2000). Howland and these suggested that individuals who organize their daily lives can control their biological rhythms (Howland & Thase, 1999). Considering the potential of social zeitgebers to adapt biological rhythms to the external environment, the regularity of social rhythm may be effective in regulating the circadian rhythms of individuals at risk of developing Bipolar I and II disorders (Shen et al., 2008). In a study conducted in patients with rapid cycling bipolar disorder, "social rhythm metrics" scores and activity markers (eating, watching TV, going to bed, going out, work, first human contact, etc.) were found to be lower than in healthy volunteers (Ashman et al., 1999). In the same study, it was observed that rapid-cycling bipolar patients started their morning activities later than healthy individuals (Ashman et al., 1999).

As a result, an organized and regular lifestyle may be beneficial in preventing depressive, manic, or hypomanic episodes, and it should be considered that daily schedules may affect mood episodes (delaying or inhibiting the onset). It is recommended to design studies to examine the longitudinal effects of lifestyle change in patients with bipolar disorder (Shen et al., 2008).

Major Depressive Disorder

Major depressive disorder (MDD) is one of the most common psychiatric disorders worldwide and is the second leading cause of disability (Gutiérrez-Rojas et al., 2020). Depression is a complex phenomenon that can be explained by multilayered biopsychosocial factors. While MDD continues to be studied from various directions in the current scientific paradigm, the neurobiological foundations of its heterogeneous nature have received increasingly more attention in recent years. Chronobiology is a topic that remains highly relevant among the noteworthy neurobiological etiology targets for various psychiatric disorders, including Major Depressive Disorder (MDD). Circadian rhythm disorders have been frequently studied in depression, with their different aspects in both physiological and psychological dimensions. Our initial knowledge in this domain indicated that chronobiological variables are in particular related to bipolar spectrum disorders and seasonal depression. However, increasing evidence suggests that differences in circadian rhythms may form the basis for a new classification of depression that can be distinguished by objective markers in mood disorders (MD) (Carpenter et al., 2021). Chronobiology provides MD with a new definition from a transdiagnostic perspective. Although current international classifications make it difficult to directly examine the relationship between chronobiology and MD, this section will examine only the relationship between chronobiology and MDD.

The relationship between circadian rhythm and sleep disturbance in MDD

The basic information obtained in the clinical evaluation about chronobiology will be related to individuals' sleep behavior and sleep disorders. The close relationship between sleep habits and mood will facilitate our understanding of the chronobiological basis of depression. Most people with depressive disorders report sleep abnormalities that can include abnormally short or long sleep duration, insomnia (early, middle, or late types), poor sleep quality, non-restful sleep, or daytime sleepiness (Carpenter et al., 2021). Specific patterns of the sleep-wake cycle can commonly appear in depressive disorders (Smagula et al., 2018, Glozier et al., 2014). For example, a delayed sleep phase has been associated with a significant increase in depressive symptoms (Glozier et al., 2014; Sivertsen et al., 2015). On the other hand, the relationship between chronotype and depression is well-known. Individuals with an eveningness chronotype who have more severe depressive symptoms are a consistent finding (Haraden et al., 2018; Au & Reece 2017). The genetic studies where these clinical relationships are also found confirm the place of chronotype in the nature of MDD. A recent genome-wide association study has shown that morning chronotype individuals are less prone to depression (Jones et al., 2019). Data on motor activity patterns, an objective measurement method for chronotype, can provide information about the clinical course of MDD. It is interesting to note that individuals with depressive disorders have a lower average mobility (Burton et al., 2013), and there is an increase in daytime mobility and a decrease in evening mobility during treatment (Burton et al., 2013). The close link of melatonin with circadian rhythm is also important in depressive disorder. The low melatonin nocturnal levels of individuals with depressive disorder have been consistently shown to be associated with a delay in its onset and offset (Dc Bcrardis et al., 2015). Although the pattern of change in melatonin levels in MDD patients who frequently have difficulty falling asleep and staying asleep is expected, it would be appropriate to say that the level of evidence to establish a causal link in this relationship is inadequate. As a matter of fact, there have been studies that found nocturnal melatonin levels to be higher in depression (Shafii et al., 1996). It is possible to explain the conflict in a way that the heterogeneous nature of MDD and the biases arising from the study sample. Above all, it is known that the risk of mood disturbance increases even in healthy people when the endogenous clock is affected by environmental conditions such as jet-lag, work shifts, etc. There has been evidence suggesting that circadian misalignment may influence mood beyond sleep disturbance. For instance, individuals diagnosed with delayed sleep phase disorder who also have circadian misalignment have been found to exhibit greater depressive symptoms than subjects with delayed sleep phase disorder without circadian misalignment (Murray et al., 2017). Body temperature is another physiological marker of chronobiology, and study results in depressive patients seem to be inconsistent (Carpenter et al., 2021).

The chronobiologic role of Hypothalamus-Pituitary-Adrenal Axis in MDD

Cortisol, another hormone with a circadian release pattern, also shows marked differences in mood changes. Hypothalamus-Pituitary-Adrenal axis (HHA) is a well-known circuit that plays an important role in the interplay between the elements of the circadian rhythm. Chronic elevation of cortisol and disruption of HPA rhythm is an important clinical manifestation of a depressive episode (Keller et al., 2017). The disturbance in circadian rhythmicity of the HPA axis activity was shown to be related to the initial phase of depression-like behavior in a rat model (Christiansen et al., 2012). Given the close network of circadian rhythm with sleep disorder, the relationship of sleep deprivation with the diurnal rhythm of cortisol and dysfunction in HPA elements would not be puzzling. For example, severe sleep loss was found to be associated with a dampened morning cortisol awakening response and an increased afternoon/evening cortisol level (Guyon et al., 2014; Omisade et al., 2010). On the other hand, 35-hour sleep deprivation with sleep phase advance has been shown to improve treatment-resistant depression and reduce cortisol levels (Kurczewska et al., 2021). Conflicting results on sleep deprivation and cortisol release suggest that circadian and ultradian rhythms on HPA and sleep pressure may also be related to subtle associations therein. The junctional role of HPA for both the inflammatory systems and the MD makes it inevitable to examine the effect of circadian rhythm on depression from the perspective of inflammation (Rhen et al., 2019). Indeed, it has been shown that the disrupted circadian system by the clock gene deletion causes not only alteration in inflammation but also metabolic syndrome (Maury, 2019) and depression (Germain & Kupfer, 2008). For instance, the signal pathway of Nuclear Factor-Cappa B is activated in circadian rhythm disruptions as one of the key instruments of inflammation (Narasimamurthy et al., 2012). It should be noted that the well-established association of sleep-wake and circadian disorders with elevation in inflammatory markers (Irwin et al., 2016) is bidirectional (Morris et al., 2018).

Circadian Rhythm in the Depression Spectrum: Individual Differences

Granted the complexity of the relationships discussed so far, it can be noticed that circadian rhythm-related parameters have been studied at a broad level. Heterogeneity also holds true for depressive disorder. a deeper insight into chronobiology can give us information about its etiologic potential in the spectrum of depressive disorders. It can be suggested that the examination of age and gender characteristics, symptomatology, and biological overlaps will also differ for therapeutic modalities.

Age would be one of the important targets in the relationship between depression and circadian rhythm differences, considering that the early onset age in many psychiatric disorders evokes the biological fundamentals more. In younger individuals, delayed sleep-wake patterns are more frequent (Robillard et al., 2013), and the lower level of melatonin was found to be associated with severe depression (Sundberg et al., 2016). The early onset age of atypical depression in a closer relationship with circadian rhythm disorders is another supporting evidence (Ratheesh et al., 2017).

Some sex differences in circadian rhythm also appear in depression. Sleep phase misalignment was reported to display sex differences in the association of depressive symptoms and antidepressant response (Swanson et al., 2017). It was found that gender has a moderation effect on the relationship between total sleep time, mean activity level, both amplitude and peak of rest-activity rhythm, and depression level (White et al., 2017).

Atypical depression features also apply to circadian rhythm disturbances such as hypersomnia, fatigue, psychomotor retardation, etc. (Carpenter et al., 2021). Furthermore, women who exhibit phase-delayed sleep characteristics were found to have increased levels of hypersomnia, appetite, and BMI (Meliska et al., 2011). Similarly, a disrupted circadian rhythm confers risks for seasonal affective disorder and/or bipolar depression displays. Clinical manifestations of the bipolar depressive spectrum suggest that they share a common susceptibility to an impaired internal clock.

Conclusion

In conclusion, it can be said that there is a relationship between mood disorders and melatonin, genes, chronotype, and zeitgebers, which affect the circadian clock. However, we can say that this relationship still carries an uncertainty regarding the onset, type, and even treatment of mood disorders. The mystery of whether the disruption in the circadian clock is a marker or situational variability for mood disorders still remains. As this mystery between mood and the circadian clock decreases, it will contribute to the diagnosis and treatment systems for mood disorders. Conducting more extensive studies in this area will facilitate our understanding of mood disorders.

References

Adan, A., Archer, S. N., Hidalgo, M. P., Di Milia, L., Natale, V., & Randler, C. (2012). Circadian typology: a comprehensive review. *Chronobiology international*, *29*(9), 1153–1175. https://doi.org/10.3109/07420528.2012.719971.

Alloy, L. B., Urošević, S., Abramson, L. Y., Jager-Hyman, S., Nusslock, R., Whitehouse, W. G., & Hogan, M. (2012). Progression along the bipolar spectrum: a longitudinal study of predictors of conversion from bipolar spectrum conditions to bipolar I and II disorders. *Journal of abnormal psychology*, *121*(1), 16–27. https://doi.org/10.1037/a0023973.

Alloy, L. B., Ng, T. H., Titone, M. K., & Boland, E. M. (2017). Circadian Rhythm Dysregulation in Bipolar Spectrum Disorders. *Current psychiatry reports*, *19*(4), 21. https://doi.org/10.1007/s11920-017-0772-z.

Ashman, S. B., Monk, T. H., Kupfer, D. J., Clark, C. H., Myers, F. S., Frank, E., & Leibenluft (1999). Relationship between social rhythms and mood in patients with rapid cycling bipolar disorder. *Psychiatry research*, *86*(1), 1–8. https://doi.org/10.1016/s0165-1781(99)00019-0.

Au, J., & Reece, J. (2017). The relationship between chronotype and depressive symptoms: A meta-analysis. *Journal of affective disorders*, *218*, 93–104. https://doi.org/10.1016/j.jad.2017.04.021.

Baek, J. H., Kim, J. S., Kim, M. J., Ryu, S., Lee, K., Ha, K., & Hong, K. S. (2016). Lifetime Characteristics of Evening-Preference and Irregular Bed-Rise Time Are Associated with Lifetime Seasonal Variation of Mood and Behavior: Comparison Between Individuals with Bipolar Disorder and Healthy Controls. *Behavioral sleep medicine*, *14*(2), 155–168. https://doi.org/10.1080/15402002.2014.974179.

Benedetti, F., Riccaboni, R., Dallaspezia, S., Locatelli, C., Smeraldi, E., & Colombo, C. (2015). Effects of CLOCK gene variants and early stress on hopelessness and suicide in bipolar depression. *Chronobiology international*, *32*(8), 1156–1161. https://doi.org/10.3109/07420528.2015.1060603.

Bullock, B., Corlass-Brown, J. & Murray, G. Eveningness and Seasonality are Associated with the Bipolar Disorder Vulnerability Trait. J Psychopathol Behav Assess 36, 443–451 (2014). https://doi.org/10.1007/s10862-014-9414-5.

Burton, C., McKinstry, B., Szentagotai Tătar, A., Serrano-Blanco, A., Pagliari, C., & Wolters, M. (2013). Activity monitoring in patients with depression: a systematic review. *Journal of affective disorders*, *145*(1), 21–28. https://doi.org/10.1016/j.jad.2012.07.001.

Carpenter, J. S., Crouse, J. J., Scott, E. M., Naismith, S. L., Wilson, C., Scott, J., Merikangas, K. R., & Hickie, I. B. (2021). Circadian depression: A mood disorder phenotype. *Neuroscience and biobehavioral reviews*, *126*, 79–101. https://doi.org/10.1016/j.neubiorev.2021.02.045.

Christiansen, S., Bouzinova, E. V., Palme, R., & Wiborg, O. (2012). Circadian activity of the hypothalamic-pituitary-adrenal axis is differentially affected in the rat chronic mild stress model of depression. *Stress (Amsterdam, Netherlands)*, *15*(6), 647–657. https://doi.org/10.3109/10253890.2011.654370.

Chung, J. K., Lee, K. Y., Kim, S. H., Kim, E. J., Jeong, S. H., Jung, H. Y., Choi, J. E., Ahn, Y. M., Kim, Y. S., & Joo, E. J. (2012). Circadian Rhythm Characteristics in Mood Disorders: Comparison among Bipolar I Disorder, Bipolar II Disorder and Recurrent Major Depressive Disorder. *Clinical psychopharmacology and neuroscience : the official scientific journal of the Korean College of Neuropsychopharmacology*, *10*(2), 110–116. https://doi.org/10.9758/cpn.2012.10.2.110.

Cornelissen, G., Halberg, F., Halberg, J., Schwartzkopff, O. (2013). Franz Halberg, MD (5 July 1919–9 June 2013) – In Appreciation. Chronobiology International, *30*(10), 1205-1207. https://doi.org/10.3109/07420528.2013.841628.

De Berardis, D., Orsolini, L., Serroni, N., Girinelli, G., Iasevoli, F., Tomasetti, C., Mazza, M., Valchera, A., Fornaro, M., Perna, G., Piersanti, M., Di Nicola, M., Cavuto, M., Martinotti, G., & Di Giannantonio, M. (2015). The role of melatonin in mood disorders. *ChronoPhysiology and Therapy*, *5*, 65. https://doi.org/10.2147/CPT.S41761.

Etain, B., Jamain, S., Milhiet, V., Lajnef, M., Boudebesse, C., Dumaine, A., Mathieu, F., Gombert, A., Ledudal, K., Gard, S., Kahn, J. P., Henry, C., Boland, A., Zelenika, D., Lechner, D., Lathrop, M., Leboyer, M., & Bellivier, F. (2014). Association between circadian genes, bipolar disorders and chronotypes. *Chronobiology international*, *31*(7), 807–814. https://doi.org/10.3109/07420528.2014.906445.

Faedda, G. L., Tondo, L., Teicher, M. H., Baldessarini, R. J., Gelbard, H. A., & Floris, G. F. (1993). Seasonal mood disorders. Patterns of seasonal recurrence in mania and depression. *Archives of general psychiatry*, *50*(1), 17–23. https://doi.org/10.1001/archpsyc.1993.01820130019004.

Germain, A., & Kupfer, D. J. (2008). Circadian rhythm disturbances in depression. *Human psychopharmacology*, *23*(7), 571–585. https://doi.org/10.1002/hup.964.

Glozier, N., O'Dea, B., McGorry, P. D., Pantelis, C., Amminger, G. P., Hermens, D. F., Purcell, R., Scott, E., & Hickie, I. B. (2014). Delayed sleep onset in depressed young people. *BMC psychiatry*, *14*, 33. https://doi.org/10.1186/1471-244X-14-33

Gold, A. K., & Kinrys, G. (2019). Treating Circadian Rhythm Disruption in Bipolar Disorder. *Current psychiatry reports*, *21*(3), 14. https://doi.org/10.1007/s11920-019-1001-8

Grandin, L. D., Alloy, L. B., & Abramson, L. Y. (2006). The social zeitgeber theory, circadian rhythms, and mood disorders: review and evaluation. *Clinical psychology review*, *26*(6), 679–694. https://doi.org/10.1016/j.cpr.2006.07.001.

Gutiérrez-Rojas, L., Porras-Segovia, A., Dunne, H., Andrade-González, N., & Cervilla, J. A. (2020). Prevalence and correlates of major depressive disorder: a systematic review. *Revista brasileira de psiquiatria (Sao Paulo, Brazil : 1999)*, *42*(6), 657–672. https://doi.org/10.1590/1516-4446-2020-0650.

Guyon, A., Balbo, M., Morselli, L. L., Tasali, E., Leproult, R., L'Hermite-Balériaux, M., Van Cauter, E., & Spiegel, K. (2014). Adverse effects of two nights of sleep restriction on the hypothalamic-pituitary-adrenal axis in healthy men. *The Journal of clinical endocrinology and metabolism*, *99*(8), 2861–2868. https://doi.org/10.1210/jc.2013-4254.

Hansen, L., Arden, K. C., Rasmussen, S. B., Viars, C. S., Vestergaard, H., Hansen, T., Møller, A. M., Woodgett, J. R., & Pedersen, O. (1997). Chromosomal mapping and mutational analysis of the coding region of the glycogen synthase kinase-3alpha and beta isoforms in patients with NIDDM. *Diabetologia*, *40*(8), 940–946. https://doi.org/10.1007/s001250050771.

Haraden, D. A., Mullin, B. C., & Hankin, B. L. (2019). Internalizing symptoms and chronotype in youth: A longitudinal assessment of anxiety, depression and tripartite model. *Psychiatry research*, *272*, 797–805. https://doi.org/10.1016/j.psychres.2018.12.117.

Hastings, M. H., Reddy, A. B., & Maywood, E. S. (2003). A clockwork web: circadian timing in brain and periphery, in health and disease. *Nature reviews. Neuroscience*, *4*(8), 649–661. https://doi.org/10.1038/nrn1177.

Howland, R. H., Thase, M. E. (1999). Affective disorders: biological aspects. In: Millon, T., Blaney, P. H., Davis, R. D. (eds), *Oxford Textbook of Psychopathology* (pp. 166-202). New York: Oxford University Press.

Irwin, M. R., Olmstead, R., & Carroll, J. E. (2016). Sleep Disturbance, Sleep Duration, and Inflammation: A Systematic Review and Meta-Analysis of Cohort Studies and Experimental Sleep Deprivation. *Biological psychiatry*, *80*(1), 40–52. https://doi.org/10.1016/j.biopsych.2015.05.014.

Jones, S. E., Lane, J. M., Wood, A. R., van Hees, V. T., Tyrrell, J., Beaumont, R. N., Jeffries, A. R., Dashti, H. S., Hillsdon, M., Ruth, K. S., Tuke, M. A., Yaghootkar, H., Sharp, S. A., Jie, Y., Thompson, W. D., Harrison, J. W., Dawes, A., Byrne, E. M., Tiemeier, H., Allebrandt, K. V., Bowden, J., Ray, D. W., Freathy, R. M., Murray, A., Mazzotti, D. R., Gehrman, P. R., Lawlor, D. A., Frayling, T. M., Rutter, M. K., Hinds, D. A., Saxena, R. & Weedon, M. N. (2019). Genome-wide association analyses of chronotype in 697,828 individuals provides insights into circadian rhythms. *Nature communications*, *10*(1), 343. https://doi.org/10.1038/s41467-018-08259-7.

Keller, J., Gomez, R., Williams, G., Lembke, A., Lazzeroni, L., Murphy, G. M., Jr, & Schatzberg, A. F. (2017). HPA axis in major depression: cortisol, clinical symptomatology and genetic variation predict cognition. *Molecular psychiatry*, *22*(4), 527–536. https://doi.org/10.1038/mp.2016.120.

Kennedy, S. H., Kutcher, S. P., Ralevski, E., & Brown, G. M. (1996). Nocturnal melatonin and 24-hour 6-sulphatoxymelatonin levels in various phases of bipolar affective disorder. *Psychiatry research*, *63*(2-3), 219–222. https://doi.org/10.1016/0165-1781(96)02910-1.

Kirlioglu, S. S., & Balcioglu, Y. H. (2020). Chronobiology Revisited in Psychiatric Disorders: From a Translational Perspective. *Psychiatry investigation*, *17*(8), 725–743. https://doi.org/10.30773/pi.2020.0129.

Kurczewska, E., Ferensztajn-Rochowiak, E., Rybakowski, F., Michalak, M., & Rybakowski, J. (2021). Treatment-resistant depression: Neurobiological correlates and the effect of sleep deprivation with sleep phase advance for the augmentation of pharmacotherapy. *The world journal of biological psychiatry : the official journal of the World Federation of Societies of Biological Psychiatry*, *22*(1), 58–69. https://doi.org/10.1080/15622975.2020.1755449.

Lemmer B. (2009). Discoveries of rhythms in human biological functions: a historical review. *Chronobiology international*, *26*(6), 1019–1068. https://doi.org/10.3109/07420520903237984.

Lerner, A. B., & Nordlund, J. J. (1978). Melatonin: clinical pharmacology. *Journal of neural transmission. Supplementum*, (13), 339–347. doi: 10.1007/978-3-7091-4427-5_25.

Lewy, A. J., Wehr, T. A., Goodwin, F. K., Newsome, D. A., & Markey, S. P. (1980). Light suppresses melatonin secretion in humans. *Science (New York, N.Y.)*, *210*(4475), 1267–1269. https://doi.org/10.1126/science.7434030.

Malkoff-Schwartz, S., Frank, E., Anderson, B. P., Hlastala, S. A., Luther, J. F., Sherrill, J. T., Houck, P. R., & Kupfer, D. J. (2000). Social rhythm disruption and stressful life events in the onset of bipolar and unipolar episodes. *Psychological medicine*, *30*(5), 1005–1016. https://doi.org/10.1017/s0033291799002706.

Manchia, M., Squassina, A., Pisanu, C., Congiu, D., Garzilli, M., Guiso, B., Suprani, F., Paribello, P., Pulcinelli, V., Iaselli, M. N., Pinna, F., Valtorta, F., Carpiniello, B., & Comai, S. (2019). Investigating the relationship between melatonin levels, melatonin system, microbiota composition and bipolar disorder psychopathology across the different phases of the disease. *International journal of bipolar disorders*, *7*(1), 27. https://doi.org/10.1186/s40345-019-0163-y.

Mansour, H. A., Monk, T. H., & Nimgaonkar, V. L. (2005). Circadian genes and bipolar disorder. *Annals of medicine*, *37*(3), 196–205. https://doi.org/10.1080/07853890510007377.

Marx, H. (1946). Zur Klinik des Hypophysen zwischenhirn systems: 2. Mitteilung "Hypophysa¨re Insuffizienz" bei Lichtmangel [On the clinic of the interbrain pituitary system: 2nd communication "pituitary insufficiency" in the case of a lack of light]. *Klin. Wochenschr, 24,*18–21.

Maury, E. (2019). Off the Clock: From Circadian Disruption to Metabolic Disease. *International journal of molecular sciences*, *20*(7), 1597. https://doi.org/10.3390/ijms20071597.

Meliska, C. J., Martínez, L. F., López, A. M., Sorenson, D. L., Nowakowski, S., & Parry, B. L. (2011). Relationship of morningness-eveningness questionnaire score to melatonin and sleep timing, body mass index and atypical depressive symptoms in peri- and post-menopausal women. *Psychiatry Research*, *188*(1), 88–95. https://doi.org/10.1016/j.psychres.2010.12.010.

Melo, M. C. A., Abreu, R. L. C., Linhares Neto, V. B., de Bruin, P. F. C., & de Bruin, V. M. S. (2017). Chronotype and circadian rhythm in bipolar disorder: A systematic review. *Sleep medicine reviews*, *34*, 46–58. https://doi.org/10.1016/j.smrv.2016.06.007.

Merikangas, K. R., Akiskal, H. S., Angst, J., Greenberg, P. E., Hirschfeld, R. M., Petukhova, M., & Kessler, R. C. (2007). Lifetime and 12-month prevalence of bipolar spectrum disorder in the National Comorbidity Survey replication. *Archives of general psychiatry*, *64*(5), 543–552. https://doi.org/10.1001/archpsyc.64.5.543.

Morris, G., Stubbs, B., Köhler, C. A., Walder, K., Slyepchenko, A., Berk, M., & Carvalho, A. F. (2018). The putative role of oxidative stress and inflammation in the pathophysiology of sleep dysfunction across neuropsychiatric disorders: Focus on chronic fatigue syndrome, bipolar disorder and multiple sclerosis. *Sleep medicine reviews*, *41*, 255–265. https://doi.org/10.1016/j.smrv.2018.03.007.

Murray, G., & Harvey, A. (2010). Circadian rhythms and sleep in bipolar disorder. *Bipolar disorders*, *12*(5), 459–472. https://doi.org/10.1111/j.1399-5618.2010.00843.x.

Murray, J. M., Sletten, T. L., Magee, M., Gordon, C., Lovato, N., Bartlett, D. J., Kennaway, D. J., Lack, L. C., Grunstein, R. R., Lockley, S. W., Rajaratnam, S. M., & Delayed Sleep on Melatonin (DelSoM) Study Group (2017). Prevalence of Circadian Misalignment and Its Association with Depressive Symptoms in Delayed Sleep Phase Disorder. *Sleep*, *40*(1), 10.1093/sleep/zsw002. https://doi.org/10.1093/sleep/zsw002.

Narasimamurthy, R., Hatori, M., Nayak, S. K., Liu, F., Panda, S., & Verma, I. M. (2012). Circadian clock protein cryptochrome regulates the expression of proinflammatory cytokines. *Proceedings of the National Academy of Sciences of the United States of America*, *109*(31), 12662–12667. https://doi.org/10.1073/pnas.1209965109.

Ng, T. H., Chung, K. F., Ho, F. Y., Yeung, W. F., Yung, K. P., & Lam, T. H. (2015). Sleep-wake disturbance in interepisode bipolar disorder and high-risk individuals: a systematic review and meta-analysis. *Sleep medicine reviews*, *20*, 46–58. https://doi.org/10.1016/j.smrv.2014.06.006.

Nováková, M., Praško, J., Látalová, K., Sládek, M., & Sumová, A. (2015). The circadian system of patients with bipolar disorder differs in episodes of mania and depression. *Bipolar disorders*, *17*(3), 303–314. https://doi.org/10.1111/bdi.12270.

Ohayon, M. M., & Roth, T. (2003). Place of chronic insomnia in the course of depressive and anxiety disorders. *Journal of psychiatric research*, *37*(1), 9–15. https://doi.org/10.1016/s0022-3956(02)00052-3.

Omisade, A., Buxton, O. M., & Rusak, B. (2010). Impact of acute sleep restriction on cortisol and leptin levels in young women. *Physiology & behavior*, *99*(5), 651-656.

Plante, D. T., & Winkelman, J. W. (2008). Sleep disturbance in bipolar disorder: therapeutic implications. *The American journal of psychiatry*, *165*(7), 830–843. https://doi.org/10.1176/appi.ajp.2008.08010077.

Ratheesh, A., Davey, C., Hetrick, S., Alvarez-Jimenez, M., Voutier, C., Bechdolf, A., McGorry, P. D., Scott, J., Berk, M., & Cotton, S. M. (2017). A systematic review and meta-analysis of prospective transition from major depression to bipolar disorder. *Acta psychiatrica Scandinavica*, *135*(4), 273–284. https://doi.org/10.1111/acps.12686.

Rhen, T., & Cidlowski, J. A. (2005). Antiinflammatory action of glucocorticoids--new mechanisms for old drugs. *The New England journal of medicine*, *353*(16), 1711–1723. https://doi.org/10.1056/NEJMra050541.

Robillard, R., Naismith, S. L., Rogers, N. L., Ip, T. K., Hermens, D. F., Scott, E. M., & Hickie, I. B. (2013). Delayed sleep phase in young people with unipolar or bipolar affective disorders. *Journal of affective disorders*, *145*(2), 260–263. https://doi.org/10.1016/j.jad.2012.06.006.

Schulz, P., & Steimer, T. (2009). Neurobiology of circadian systems. *CNS drugs*, *23 Suppl 2*, 3–13. https://doi.org/10.2165/11318620-000000000-00000.

Selvi, Y., Beşiroğlu, L., Aydın, A. (2011) Kronobiyoloji ve Duygudurum Bozuklukları [Chronobiology and Mood Disorders]. *Psikiyatride Güncel Yaklaşımlar. 3*(3): 368-386. https://doi.org/10.5455/cap.20110317.

Seleem, M. A., Merranko, J. A., Goldstein, T. R., Goldstein, B. I., Axelson, D. A., Brent, D. A., Nimgaonkar, V. L., Diler, R. S., Sakolsky, D. J., Kupfer, D. J., & Birmaher, B. (2015). The longitudinal course of sleep timing and circadian preferences in adults with bipolar disorder. *Bipolar disorders*, *17*(4), 392–402. https://doi.org/10.1111/bdi.12286.

Shafii, M., MacMillan, D. R., Key, M. P., Derrick, A. M., Kaufman, N., & Nahinsky, I. D. (1996). Nocturnal serum melatonin profile in major depression in children and adolescents. *Archives of general psychiatry*, *53*(11), 1009–1013. https://doi.org/10.1001/archpsyc.1996.01830110047006.

Shen, G. H., Alloy, L. B., Abramson, L. Y., & Sylvia, L. G. (2008). Social rhythm regularity and the onset of affective episodes in bipolar spectrum individuals. *Bipolar disorders*, *10*(4), 520–529. https://doi.org/10.1111/j.1399-5618.2008.00583.x.

Sivertsen, B., Harvey, A. G., Pallesen, S., & Hysing, M. (2015). Mental health problems in adolescents with delayed sleep phase: results from a large population-based study in Norway. *Journal of sleep research*, *24*(1), 11–18. https://doi.org/10.1111/jsr.12254.

Smagula, S. F., Krafty, R. T., Thayer, J. F., Buysse, D. J., & Hall, M. H. (2018). Rest-activity rhythm profiles associated with manic-hypomanic and depressive symptoms. *Journal of psychiatric research*, *102*, 238–244. https://doi.org/10.1016/j.jpsychires.2018.04.015.

Souêtre, E., Salvati, E., Belugou, J. L., Pringuey, D., Candito, M., Krebs, B., Ardisson, J. L., & Darcourt, G. (1989). Circadian rhythms in depression and recovery: evidence for blunted amplitude as the main chronobiological abnormality. *Psychiatry research*, *28*(3), 263–278. https://doi.org/10.1016/0165-1781(89)90207-2.

Srinivasan, V., Pandi-Perumal, S. R., Trakht, I., Spence, D. W., Hardeland, R., Poeggeler, B., & Cardinali, D. P. (2009). Pathophysiology of depression: role of sleep and the melatonergic system. *Psychiatry research*, *165*(3), 201–214. https://doi.org/10.1016/j.psychres.2007.11.020.

Stetler, C., Dickerson, S. S., & Miller, G. E. (2004). Uncoupling of social zeitgebers and diurnal cortisol secretion in clinical depression. *Psychoneuroendocrinology*, *29*(10), 1250–1259. https://doi.org/10.1016/j.psyneuen.2004.03.003.

Sundberg, I., Ramklint, M., Stridsberg, M., Papadopoulos, F. C., Ekselius, L., & Cunningham, J. L. (2016). Salivary Melatonin in Relation to Depressive Symptom Severity in Young Adults. *PloS one*, *11*(4), e0152814. https://doi.org/10.1371/journal.pone.0152814.

Swanson, L. M., Burgess, H. J., Huntley, E. D., Bertram, H., Mooney, A., Zollars, J., Dopp, R., Hoffmann, R., Armitage, R., & Todd Arnedt, J. (2017). Relationships between circadian measures, depression, and response to antidepressant treatment: A preliminary investigation. *Psychiatry research*, *252*, 262–269. https://doi.org/10.1016/j.psychres.2017.03.010.

Takaesu Y. (2018). Circadian rhythm in bipolar disorder: A review of the literature. *Psychiatry and clinical neurosciences*, *72*(9), 673–682. https://doi.org/10.1111/pcn.12688.

Takahashi, J. S., Hong, H. K., Ko, C. H., & McDearmon, E. L. (2008). The genetics of mammalian circadian order and disorder: implications for physiology and disease. *Nature reviews. Genetics*, *9*(10), 764–775. https://doi.org/10.1038/nrg2430.

White, K. H., Rumble, M. E., & Benca, R. M. (2017). Sex Differences in the Relationship Between Depressive Symptoms and Actigraphic Assessments of Sleep and Rest-Activity Rhythms in a Population-Based Sample. *Psychosomatic medicine*, *79*(4), 479–484. https://doi.org/10.1097/PSY.0000000000000434.

Chapter 13

The Connection of Circadian Clock to Gastrointestinal Diseases

Serdar Tanas*, MD
Clinic of Gastroenterology, Etlik City Hospital, University of Health Sciences, Ankara, Turkiye

Abstract

The circadian clock is a system of molecular and physiological rhythms that regulate various biological functions over a 24-hour cycle. The circadian clock is found in the central nervous system and also in peripheral tissues, including the gastrointestinal system and accessory organs. The circadian clock coordinates digestive processes such as mobility, secretion, absorption, hormone release, barrier function, and microbiota composition in response to environmental signals such as light and food intake. Disruption of the circadian clock due to genetic mutations, sleep disorders, shift work, or jet lag can disrupt the normal functioning of the gastrointestinal system and increase the risk of various diseases, such as irritable bowel syndrome, gastroesophageal reflux disease, peptic ulcer disease, inflammatory bowel disease, and gastrointestinal cancers. Furthermore, as our understanding of the role of the circadian clock in the regulation of gastrointestinal physiology and pathophysiology increases and as our ability to regulate the circadian clock increases, it is evident that a new field will open in the future for the treatment of gastrointestinal diseases. In this chapter, the relationship between the circadian clock and the gastrointestinal system will be discussed in the literature.

---

* Corresponding Author's Email: stanas26@hotmail.com.

In: Human Health is a Matter of Timing
Editors: Sumeyya Deniz Aybek, Gonca Gulbay and Mucahit Secme
ISBN: 979-8-89113-467-6

Keywords: circadian clock, gastroenterology system, gastroenterology diseases

Introduction

The circadian clock is a biological system that generates approximately 24-hour self-sustained oscillations in various molecular and physiological processes that enable organisms to adapt to daily changes in their environment. The circadian clock consists of a central stimulator located in the suprachiasmatic nucleus (SCN) of the hypothalamus, which is stimulated by light entering the retina and synchronizes the light-dark cycle like an orchestra conductor. It also includes peripheral clocks found in almost every cell of the body, and these peripheral clocks use both the input from the central pacemaker and various stimuli, such as eating schedules, body temperature, and hormones, to generate autonomous responses. This sensitive clock, which can be affected by factors such as light, temperature, and nutrition, has changed according to modern lifestyles. Our internal rhythms have been disrupted due to the consequences of staying active and eating until late at night, sleep disorders, long-distance air travel, and jet lag (Mohawk et al., 2012; Voigt et al., 2019; Konturek et al., 2011; Vasey et al., 2021).

The circadian clock also has a molecular clock mechanism, which is regulated through a transcriptional and translational feedback loop regulated by a set of clock genes and the proteins they synthesize, and this mechanism can be referred to as the "Molecular Clock." Circadian clock genes are the genes that regulate the biological clock in the body. These genes are crucial in the cell cycle, the response to DNA damage, and tumor suppression. They control gene functions in many pathways, such as metabolism, immunity, cell cycle, and inflammation, with their rhythmic effects on the expression of other genes. The basic molecular mechanisms underlying the circadian rhythm are also composed of these clock genes. The system is basically formed of two transcription factors: Circadian Locomotor Output Cycles Kaput (CLOCK) and Aryl-Hydrocarbon receptor Nuclear Translocator-like 1 (ARNT1, also known as BMAL1/2), and their target genes, Period and Cryptochrome genes (Voigt et al., 2019; Konturek et al., 2011).

Circadian clock proteins (CLOCK and BMAL1/2) form dimers and bind to the promoter sequences of the target circadian clock genes, which are Period (Per 1, 2, and 3) and Cryptochrome (Cry 1 and Cry 2), in a cis-element regulatory region called the E-box. The Per and Cry proteins are formed with transcription and translation of these two clock genes, and these last products accumulate in the cytoplasm, form dimers, and then enter the nucleus to further inhibit Clock-BMAL1-mediated transcription. In summary, while Clock and Bmal1 are positive elements in the system, the Per and Cry proteins, which they promote the transcription of, are negative elements. In addition to this fundamental mechanism, there are some other mechanisms that adjust the circadian clock finely. The CLOCK-BMAL1 complex, respectively, activates the expression of genes, Retinoic acid-related Orphan Receptor (RORα), which activates BMAL1 expression, and also inhibits genes such as Reverse Transcript of Erythroblastosis (Rev-ERBα). Post-translational modifications (phosphorylation and acetylation) affect the half-lives of the CLOCK, BMAL1, CRY, and PER genes, increasing their stability (Voigt et al., 2019; Konturek et al., 2011).

The gastrointestinal system is one of the main peripheral organs that exhibits circadian rhythms in its structure and function. The gastrointestinal tract contains internal clocks that are affected by eating schedules and modulated by intestinal hormones, and it also communicates with the central clock through neural and hormonal signals. The circadian clock regulates various aspects of gastrointestinal physiology, such as digestion, absorption, motility, secretion, barrier function, and microbiota composition. These processes are coordinated by the circadian clock to optimize the utilization of nutrients and energy balance during the normal feeding period and to provide protection against pathogens and toxins during the fasting state (Mohawk et al., 2012; Lee, 2021; Konturek et al., 2011).

Disruption of the circadian clock can occur due to genetic mutations in clock genes or environmental factors that change the normal light-dark or eating-fasting cycles. This disruption can impair the normal functioning of the gastrointestinal system and increase the risk of various gastrointestinal diseases. For example, the disruption of circadian rhythms due to disturbances in sleep or shift work can lead to changes in the motility, secretion, and barrier function of the gastrointestinal system that cause symptoms such as abdominal pain, constipation, or diarrhea. Furthermore, the disruption of circadian rhythms can affect the composition and function of the gut microbiota, which can impact host metabolism and inflammation, and affect immunity. Additionally, the disruption of circadian rhythms can accelerate aging by affecting cell cycle regulation, DNA repair mechanisms, and oxidative stress responses, and it can also contribute to cancer development in the liver and gastrointestinal tract (Mohawk et al., 2012; Segers & Depoortere, 2021; Voigt et al., 2019; Kaczmarek et al., 2017).

Therefore, understanding the role of the circadian clock in the physiology and pathophysiology of the gastrointestinal is essential for the development of new diagnostic and therapeutic approaches for gastrointestinal diseases.

Circadian Clock on Liver Diseases

The liver is an important metabolic organ that exhibits strong circadian rhythms in gene expression and function. The liver includes internal clocks regulated by hormonal signals from the pancreas (insulin) and intestines (glucagon-like peptide-1) in response to the eating schedule. The liver also communicates with the central clock through neural and hormonal signals. The circadian clock regulates various aspects of liver physiology, such as glucose, lipid, and bile acid metabolism, detoxification, oxidative stress response, and cell cycle regulation. These processes are coordinated by the circadian clock to balance metabolic supply and demand during the eating and fasting cycles (Reinke & Asher, 2016; Kupfer & Northfield, 1983).

Disruption of the circadian clock can occur due to genetic mutations in clock genes or environmental factors that change the normal light-dark or eating-fasting cycles. Such a disruption can impair the normal functioning of the liver and increase the risk of various liver diseases such as fatty liver disease, cholestasis, hepatitis, cirrhosis, and liver cancer. For instance, disruption of circadian rhythms due to alcohol consumption or a high-fat diet can lead to changes in lipid metabolism and increased oxidative stress in the liver which causes steatosis, inflammation, and fibrosis. Furthermore, disruption of circadian rhythms can lead to cholestasis and liver damage by affecting the expression and activity of key enzymes and transporters involved in bile acid synthesis and secretion. Furthermore, disruption of circadian rhythms can lead to genomic instability and tumor formation by affecting cell cycle regulation and DNA repair mechanisms in the liver (Costa et al., 2023; Reinke & Asher, 2016; Kupfer & Northfield, 1983).

Circadian Clock on Gallbladder Diseases

The gallbladder is a small organ that stores and concentrates the bile produced by the liver. The gallbladder exhibits circadian rhythms in its motility and secretion in response to hormonal signals from the intestine (cholecystokinin) and brain (melatonin) (Vasey et al., 2016). The circadian clock regulates various aspects of gallbladder physiology, such as bile composition, gallbladder contraction and relaxation, gallstone formation, and gallbladder inflammation. These processes are coordinated by the circadian clock to optimize bile distribution and digestion during normal eating schedules and to prevent bile stasis and damage during fasting periods (Kupfer et al., 2019).

Disruption of the circadian clock in the gallbladder can occur due to genetic mutations in clock genes or environmental factors that alter the normal eating-fasting or light-dark cycles. This disruption can impair the normal functioning of the gallbladder and increase the risk of various gallbladder disorders, such as gallstone formation, cholecystitis, and gallbladder cancer. For instance, disruption of circadian rhythms due to irregular meal timing or a high-fat diet can lead to changes in bile composition and increased cholesterol saturation in the gallbladder, contributing to the formation of gallstones. Furthermore, disruption of circadian rhythms can affect the motility and secretion of the gallbladder, leading to gallbladder stasis and inflammation. Moreover, disruption of circadian rhythms can lead to genomic instability and tumor formation by affecting cell cycle regulation and DNA repair mechanisms in the gallbladder (Kupfer et al., 2019; Voigt et al., 2019).

Circadian Clock on Pancreatic Diseases

The pancreas is a dual-function organ that produces digestive enzymes and hormones. The pancreas exhibits circadian rhythms in its exocrine and endocrine functions in response to hormonal signals from the intestine (cholecystokinin, secretin, and incretins) and brain (melatonin). Circadian rhythms regulate various aspects of pancreatic physiology, such as enzyme secretion, insulin secretion, glucagon secretion, and pancreatic regeneration. These processes are coordinated by the circadian clock to optimize digestion and glucose homeostasis during normal eating schedules and prevent hypoglycemia and damage during fasting periods.

The impairment of the circadian clock in the pancreas can develop due to genetic mutations in clock genes or environmental factors that change normal eating-fasting or light-dark cycles. This disruption can impair the normal functioning of the pancreas and increase the risk of various pancreatic diseases, such as pancreatitis, diabetes, and pancreatic cancer. Disruption of circadian rhythms because of irregular eating habits or a high-fat diet can cause altered insulin secretion and glucose homeostasis, leading to insulin resistance and diabetes (Harris & Czaja, 2023). With the loss of the BMAL1 and Per1 clock genes in pancreatic beta cells, severe glucose intolerance and impairments in insulin production have been observed. Furthermore, the disruption of circadian rhythms can affect the secretion and activity of digestive enzymes in the pancreas, leading to pancreatitis and pancreatic damage. It can also contribute to cancer development by affecting cell cycle regulation and DNA repair mechanisms in the pancreas (Stenvers et al., 2019; Chan et al., 2022; Völkl & Poort1983; Kim et al., 2022; Brubaker & Martchenko, 2022).

Circadian Clock and Gut Microbiota

The intestinal microbiota is a complex community of microorganisms that colonizes the gastrointestinal system and has crucial roles in digestion, immunity, metabolism, and host-microbe interactions. The intestinal microbiota exhibits circadian rhythms in its composition, function, and interactions with the host. The circadian clock regulates various aspects of gut microbiota physiology, such as microbial diversity, metabolite production, immune modulation, and pathogen colonization. These processes are coordinated by the circadian clock to optimize the utilization of nutrients and energy balance during the normal eating schedule and to provide protection against pathogens and toxins during fasting periods (Paschos & FitzGerald, 2017; Kaczmarek et al., 2017; Voigt et al., 2016; Curtis et al., 2014).

The disruption of the circadian clock in the gut microbiota can occur due to genetic mutations in clock genes or environmental factors that alter the normal eating-fasting or light-dark cycles. This disruption can impair the normal functioning of the gut microbiota and increase the risk of various microbiota-related diseases, including obesity, diabetes, inflammatory bowel disease, and colorectal cancer. Irregular eating habits and a high-fat diet can disrupt circadian rhythms, leading to changes in microbial diversity and metabolite production, resulting in dysbiosis and metabolic syndrome. Disruption of circadian rhythms can affect immune modulation and pathogen colonization by the gut microbiota, leading to inflammation and infection. Furthermore, disruption of circadian rhythms can lead to a vicious cycle by affecting the interaction between the host's circadian clock and the gut microbiota, resulting in metabolic dysfunction (Paschos & FitzGerald, 2017; Kaczmarek et al., 2017; Voigt, et al., 2016; Curtis et al., 2014).

Circadian Clock and Inflammatory Bowel Diseases

Inflammatory bowel disease (IBD) is a chronic inflammatory disorder of the gastrointestinal system, including conditions such as Crohn's disease and ulcerative colitis. The etiology of IBD is complex and multifactorial, involving factors such as genetic susceptibility, environmental influences, immune dysregulation, and alterations in the gut microbiota. The circadian clock has a significant role in the pathogenesis of IBD, with regulatory effects on immune responses, cell proliferation, barrier function, oxidative stress, gastric acid production, nutrient absorption, hormone production, and gut microbiota composition. These processes are coordinated by the circadian clock to maintain intestinal homeostasis during regular eating and prevent excessive inflammation, as well as to promote tissue repair during fasting periods (Gombert et al., 2019; Kaczmarek et al., 2017; Konturek et al., 2011; Voigt et al., 2019; Sobolewska-Włodarczyk et al., 2016).

Disruption of the circadian clock in IBD can occur due to genetic mutations in clock genes or environmental factors that alter normal eating-fasting or light-dark cycles. This disruption can impair the normal functioning of the inflammatory processes in the intestines and increase the risk of IBD. Disruption of circadian rhythms due to sleep disorders or shift work can increase susceptibility to inflammation and infections by impairing the immune response and barrier function in the intestines. The chronotype refers to an individual's sleep behavior, with morningness (being active in the early hours of the day) and eveningness (being active in the later hours of the day) representing the two extremes. In patients with IBD, those in the eveningness group tend to have a more aggressive course of the disease. With polymorphisms in the circadian clock gene, Per3 has been shown to be a greater need for immunosuppressive treatment and a higher incidence of the fistulizing/stricturing phenotype in Crohn's disease. However, disruption of circadian rhythms resulting in dysbiosis can exacerbate inflammation (Gombert et al., 2019; Kaczmarek et al., 2017; Konturek et al., 2011; Voigt et al., 2019).

The disruption of circadian rhythms can, at the molecular level, affect the expression and activity of key inflammatory mediators such as cytokines, chemokines, and nuclear factor kappa B (NF-κB), leading to chronic inflammation and tissue damage (Hong et al., 2018; Gombert et al., 2019; Kaczmarek et al., 2017; Konturek et al., 2011; Voigt et al., 2019; Sobolewska-Włodarczyk et al., 2016).

Circadian Clock and Gastrointestinal Cancers

Gastrointestinal cancers refer to a group of malignant tumors that originate in the gastrointestinal system or its accessory organs. The etiology of gastrointestinal cancers is complex and multifactorial, involving genetic mutations, environmental factors, chronic inflammation, and dysbiosis of the gut microbiota. The circadian clock has a significant role in cancer pathogenesis by modulating various aspects of cancer development, such as the cell cycle, DNA repair, apoptosis, angiogenesis, invasion, metastasis, and immune response. These processes are coordinated by the circadian clock to maintain genomic stability and cellular homeostasis, preventing excessive proliferation and malignancy (Voigt et al., 2019; Konturek et al., 2011; Yuan et al., 2023; Rao & Lin, 2022).

Disruption of the circadian clock in gastrointestinal cancers can occur due to genetic mutations in clock genes or environmental factors that alter normal eating-fasting or light-dark cycles. This disruption can impair the normal functioning of tumor formation and tumor progression, increasing the risk of gastrointestinal cancers. This kind of disruption can occur in gastrointestinal cancers due to genetic mutations in clock genes or changes in environmental factors that regulate normal eating-fasting or light-dark cycles. The BMAL1 clock gene has a central role in the cell cycle and the response to DNA damage in cancer cells. Downregulation of BMAL1 leads to an increased cancer development incidence and a decreased response to anticancer drugs. The clock gene Per1 provides a relation between the circadian system and the cell cycle; its overexpression can alter the expression of oncogenes such as c-MYC and p21. Increased levels of the CLOCK, BMAL1, and Per proteins have also been demonstrated in cancer tissues (Voigt et al., 2019; Konturek et al., 2011; Yuan et al., 2023; Rao & Lin, 2022; Liu et al., 2023; Rajendran et al., 2021). Disruption of circadian rhythms due to sleep disorders or shift work can lead to increased susceptibility to cancer development and growth. Disruption of circadian rhythms can also affect the pharmacokinetics and pharmacodynamics of anticancer drugs and cause reduced effectiveness and increased toxicity (Liu et al., 2023; Wang et al., 2022; Hofmeister et al., 2020).

Conclusion

The circadian clock is a vital system that regulates various aspects of gastrointestinal physiology and pathophysiology. The circadian clock coordinates the digestive processes in response to environmental signals such as light and food intake. Disruption of the circadian clock can disrupt the normal functioning of the gastrointestinal system and increase the risk of various diseases such as irritable bowel syndrome, gastroesophageal reflux disease, peptic ulcer disease, inflammatory bowel disease, and gastrointestinal cancers. Therefore, understanding the role of the circadian clock in gastrointestinal physiology and pathophysiology is essential for the development of new diagnostic and therapeutic approaches to gastrointestinal diseases. Some potential strategies to modulate the circadian clock to improve gastrointestinal health include time-restricted feeding (limiting daily food intake to eight hours or less), timed exercise, chronobiotics, melatonin supplementation, and gene therapy.

References

Brubaker, P. L., & Martchenko, A. (2022). Metabolic Homeostasis: It's All in the Timing. *Endocrinology*, *163*(1), bqab199. https://doi.org/10.1210/endocr/bqab199.

Chan, K., Wong, F. S., & Pearson, J. A. (2022). Circadian rhythms and pancreas physiology: A review. *Frontiers in endocrinology*, *13*, 920261. https://doi.org/10.3389/fendo.2022.920261.

Costa, R., Mangini, C., Domenie, E. D., Zarantonello, L., & Montagnese, S. (2023). Circadian rhythms and the liver. *Liver international : official journal of the International Association for the Study of the Liver*, *43*(3), 534–545. https://doi.org/10.1111/liv.15501.

Curtis, A. M., Bellet, M. M., Sassone-Corsi, P., & O'Neill, L. A. (2014). Circadian clock proteins and immunity. *Immunity*, *40*(2), 178–186. https://doi.org/10.1016/j.immuni.2014.02.002.

Garaulet, M., Gómez-Abellán, P., Alburquerque-Béjar, J. J., Lee, Y. C., Ordovás, J. M., & Scheer, F. A. (2013). Timing of food intake predicts weight loss effectiveness. *International journal of obesity (2005)*, *37*(4), 604–611. https://doi.org/10.1038/ijo.2012.229.

Gombert, M., Carrasco-Luna, J., Pin-Arboledas, G., & Codoñer-Franch, P. (2019). The connection of circadian rhythm to inflammatory bowel disease. *Translational research: the journal of laboratory and clinical medicine*, *206*, 107–118. https://doi.org/10.1016/j.trsl.2018.12.001.

Harris, C., & Czaja, K. (2023). Can Circadian Eating Pattern Adjustments Reduce Risk or Prevent Development of T2D?. *Nutrients*, *15*(7), 1762. https://doi.org/10.3390/nu15071762.

Hofmeister, E. N., Fisher, S., Palesh, O., & Innominato, P. F. (2020). Does circadian rhythm influence gastrointestinal toxicity?. *Current opinion in supportive and palliative care*, *14*(2), 120–126. https://doi.org/10.1097/SPC.0000000000000498.

Hong, H. K., Maury, E., Ramsey, K. M., Perelis, M., Marcheva, B., Omura, C., Kobayashi, Y., Guttridge, D. C., Barish, G. D., & Bass, J. (2018). Requirement for NF-κB in maintenance of molecular and behavioral circadian rhythms in mice. *Genes & development*, *32*(21-22), 1367–1379. https://doi.org/10.1101/gad.319228.118.

Kaczmarek, J. L., Thompson, S. V., & Holscher, H. D. (2017). Complex interactions of circadian rhythms, eating behaviors, and the gastrointestinal microbiota and their potential impact on health. *Nutrition reviews*, *75*(9), 673–682. https://doi.org/10.1093/nutrit/nux036.

Kim, H. K., Radak, Z., Takahashi, M., Inami, T., & Shibata, S. (2022). Chrono-exercise: Time-of-day-dependent physiological responses to exercise. *Sports medicine and health science*, *5*(1), 50–58. https://doi.org/10.1016/j.smhs.2022.11.003.

Konturek, P. C., Brzozowski, T., & Konturek, S. J. (2011). Gut clock: implication of circadian rhythms in the gastrointestinal tract. *Journal of physiology and pharmacology: an official journal of the Polish Physiological Society*, *62*(2), 139–150.

Kupfer, R. M., & Northfield, T. C. (1983). Diurnal variation in cholesterol saturation of gall-bladder bile. *Gut*, *24*(10), 950–953. https://doi.org/10.1136/gut.24.10.950.

Lee Y. (2021). Roles of circadian clocks in cancer pathogenesis and treatment. *Experimental & molecular medicine*, *53*(10), 1529–1538. https://doi.org/10.1038/s12276-021-00681-0.

Liu, Y., Wang, Z., Hao, H., Wang, Y., & Hua, L. (2023). Insight into immune checkpoint inhibitor therapy for colorectal cancer from the perspective of circadian clocks. *Immunology*, *170*(1), 13–27. https://doi.org/10.1111/imm.13647.

Mohawk, J. A., Green, C. B., & Takahashi, J. S. (2012). Central and peripheral circadian clocks in mammals. *Annual review of neuroscience*, *35*, 445–462. https://doi.org/10.1146/annurev-neuro-060909-153128.

Paschos, G. K., & FitzGerald, G. A. (2017). Circadian Clocks and Metabolism: Implications for Microbiome and Aging. *Trends in genetics : TIG*, *33*(10), 760–769. https://doi.org/10.1016/j.tig.2017.07.010.

Rajendran, S., Barbon, S., & Pucciarelli, S. (2021). Spotlight on Circadian Genes and Colorectal Cancer Crosstalk. *Endocrine, metabolic & immune disorders drug targets*, *21*(1), 4–11. https://doi.org/10.2174/1871530320666200624192517.

Rao, X., & Lin, L. (2022). Circadian clock as a possible control point in colorectal cancer progression (Review). *International journal of oncology*, *61*(6), 149. https://doi.org/10.3892/ijo.2022.5439.

Reinke, H., & Asher, G. (2016). Circadian Clock Control of Liver Metabolic Functions. *Gastroenterology*, *150*(3), 574–580. https://doi.org/10.1053/j.gastro.2015.11.043.

Segers, A., & Depoortere, I. (2021). Circadian clocks in the digestive system. *Nature reviews. Gastroenterology & hepatology*, *18*(4), 239–251. https://doi.org/10.1038/s41575-020-00401-5.

Sobolewska-Włodarczyk, A., Włodarczyk, M., Szemraj, J., Stec-Michalska, K., Fichna, J., & Wiśniewska-Jarosińska, M. (2016). Circadian rhythm abnormalities - Association with the course of inflammatory bowel disease. *Pharmacological reports : PR*, *68*(4), 847–851. https://doi.org/10.1016/j.pharep.2016.04.007.

Stenvers, D. J., Scheer, F. A. J. L., Schrauwen, P., la Fleur, S. E., & Kalsbeek, A. (2019). Circadian clocks and insulin resistance. *Nature reviews. Endocrinology*, *15*(2), 75–89. https://doi.org/10.1038/s41574-018-0122-1.

Vasey, C., McBride, J., & Penta, K. (2021). Circadian Rhythm Dysregulation and Restoration: The Role of Melatonin. *Nutrients*, *13*(10), 3480. https://doi.org/10.3390/nu13103480.

Voigt, R. M., Forsyth, C. B., & Keshavarzian, A. (2019). Circadian rhythms: a regulator of gastrointestinal health and dysfunction. *Expert review of gastroenterology & hepatology*, *13*(5), 411–424. https://doi.org/10.1080/17474124.2019.1595588.

Voigt, R. M., Forsyth, C. B., Green, S. J., Engen, P. A., & Keshavarzian, A. (2016). Circadian Rhythm and the Gut Microbiome. *International review of neurobiology*, *131*, 193–205. https://doi.org/10.1016/bs.irn.2016.07.002.

Völkl, A., & Poort, C. (1983). Circadian rhythm of protein synthesis activity in the exocrine pancreas of fed and starved rats. *Journal of cell science*, *61*, 467–473. https://doi.org/10.1242/jcs.61.1.467.

Wang, J., Huang, Q., Hu, X., Zhang, S., Jiang, Y., Yao, G., Hu, K., Xu, X., Liang, B., Wu, Q., Ma, Z., Wang, Y., Wang, C., Wu, Z., Rong, X., Liao, W., & Shi, M. (2022). Disrupting Circadian Rhythm via the PER1-HK2 Axis Reverses Trastuzumab Resistance in Gastric Cancer. *Cancer research*, *82*(8), 1503–1517. https://doi.org/10.1158/0008-5472.CAN-21-1820.

Yuan, S., Mason, A. M., Titova, O. E., Vithayathil, M., Kar, S., Chen, J., Li, X., Burgess, S., & Larsson, S. C. (2023). Morning chronotype and digestive tract cancers: Mendelian randomization study. *International journal of cancer*, *152*(4), 697–704. https://doi.org/10.1002/ijc.34284.

Chapter 14

Pediatric Circadian Clock Disorders

Emre Öztürk*, MD
Department of Pediatrics, Akkus State Hospital, Ordu, Turkiye

Abstract

The circadian rhythm (CR) is present in most organisms, from eubacteria to humans. It is known that many cells and tissues have autonomous clocks and that disruption of these clock genes leads to metabolic disorders. The central circadian clock, located in the suprachiasmatic nucleus (SCN) in the hypothalamus, regulates the secondary circadian clocks in the rest of the body by exposure to light. Changes in life patterns in industrialized societies lead to CR disorders. As a result of this, the incidence of various diseases, from mental illnesses to autoimmune diseases, from changes in quality of life to metabolic syndrome, has increased. CR in children begins from fetal life. With the change in this rhythm, it increased in pathological conditions such as obesity, asthma, changes in breast milk content, and autism. In this section, we have CR disorder; we tried to examine changes in breast milk content and its effect on infants, its place in allergic diseases, its association with febrile seizures, its position in autism spectrum disorder and obesity, and its changes in the intestinal microbiota. Early detection of CR disorder, which is a modifiable risk factor, is an important opportunity to prevent future health problems.

Keywords: circadian rhythm, pediatric diseases, breast milk, obesity, allergic diseases, febrile seizure

---

* Corresponding Author's Email: ozturk12emre@gmail.com.

In: Human Health is a Matter of Timing
Editors: Sumeyya Deniz Aybek, Gonca Gulbay and Mucahit Secme
ISBN: 979-8-89113-467-6

Introduction

The 24-hour cycle that occurs as a result of the Earth's rotation causes almost all organisms to develop CRs in approximately 24 hours (Dunlap, 1999). In mammals, including humans, the circadian system works in concert with a central pacemaker in the SCN of the hypothalamus region of the central nervous system (Levi & Schibler, 2007). The SCN synchronizes many physiological and behavioral CRs, including sleep-wake, temperature, nutritional, neuroendocrine, and autonomic effects, with 24-hour periods in accordance with the light-dark cycle of the environment and provides an optimized internal order (Zisapel, 2018). Cellular oscillators and peripheral tissues in the brain of humans and multicellular organisms are interconnected to form a circadian network that coordinates physiological and behavioral rhythms such as sleep-wake, hormone production, body temperature, blood pressure, immune and neural systems (Patke et al., 2020). Thanks to this binding, almost all kinds of molecular and cellular processes are managed.

Modern times have largely eliminated people's regular eating, sleeping, and working habits. The basis of the problems that occur with this disorder is the disruption of the circadian rhythm. With the deterioration of this rhythm, the incidence of many diseases such as cancer, cardio-metabolic, digestive, immune, and neuropsychiatric diseases has increased. Animal studies subjected to circadian desynchronization have demonstrated the relationship between circadian disorder and pathological conditions (Lee et al., 2021).

Main Body

Scientists wondering when the circadian rhythm begins in children have revealed that this rhythm begins in fetal life (Mirmiran et al., 2003). In studies based on the measurement of melatonin and its metabolites in urine and saliva, starting from the neonatal period, the highest values were measured especially in the hours from 24.00 at night to 08.00 in the morning. In light of these data, it is understood that the circadian melatonin rhythm emerges at the end of the neonatal period and continues after it (Ardura et al., 2003). The circadian rhythm of temperature first appears immediately after birth (McGraw et al., 1999). Results of rodent studies suggest that circadian disturbance during fetal development is associated with adult-onset reduced bone mass, insulin resistance, depression, cardiovascular disease, and glucose intolerance (Wong et al., 2021). There are many physiological processes in the body that oscillate around the clock. It is known that the changes that occur in these physiological processes with the disruption of the circadian rhythm are associated with many clinical conditions. The effect of CR causes problems in these physiological processes at certain hours and, accordingly, it is seen at the same hours in certain diseases (Allada & Bass, 2021). As a result of the change in the circadian rhythm, many problems such as the emergence of asthma attacks in children, the triggering of febrile seizures, the development of obesity, and the change in maternal milk content are seen. Identification of preventable factors in the early stages of their development provides an important opportunity to intervene in both existing and potential health problems (Wong et al., 2021).

Table 1 shows clinical links in humans associated with 24-hour oscillatory physiological processes in various tissues and circadian disruption during the day and night (Allada & Bass, 2021).

Table 1. Circadian timing of physiological processes and disease

Clocks	Clinical correlates	Circadian physiology
Wake	Asthma Attack	Hemoglobin Production
06.00	Epileptic Seizures	Oxygen Consumption
	Bronchitis	Insulin Release
	Epistaxis	Nutrient Absorption
	Rheumatoid Arthritis	Glucose Disposal
12.00	Myocardial İnfarction	Mitochondrial Respiration
	Allergic Rhinitis	Adrenal Stress Response
	Sickle Cell Anemia Crisis	
	Peptic Ulcer	
18.00	Alzheimer's	
Sleep	Osteoarthritis	Vascular Tone
18.00	Dermatosis	Atherogenesis
	Chronic Pain	Cardiac Metabolism
	Epileptic Seizures	Adipogenesis
	Exacerbation of Peptic Ulcer	Thermogenesis
24.00	İncontinence	Appetite, Sleep
	Congestive Heart Failure	Gluconeogenesis
	Sleep Apnea	Lipogenesis
	Asthma Attack	Steroidogenesis
06.00		Cytokine Release
		Bone Marrow Extravasation

Change in Breast Milk Content with CR and Its Effect on the Baby

Breast milk is the main source of nutrition for babies from birth. Breastfeeding has positive effects on mother-baby health in the near and distant future. The World Health Organization recommends exclusive breastfeeding for the first six months and then breastfeeding until the age of two. Breast milk contains all the nutrients necessary for growth and development and is responsible for the transmission of many factors such as hormones, immune factors, and the microbiota from mother to baby (Italianer et al., 2020). The circadian rhythm of the newborn depends on cues such as synchronization with the light/dark exposure, the external environment, and feeding timing. Circadian changes in the content of breast milk inform the newborn about the time of day. This makes breast milk a unique form of 'timed feeding' and possibly helps the newborn synchronize with its external environment. Improperly timed milk intake can impair infants' development of CR, reduce their physiological adaptation to their mothers and their environment, and potentially contribute to sleep problems (Hahn-Holbrook et al., 2019). Despite the limited study to date on the need to coordinate between the time of expression and the delivery of milk to the infant, it is a plausible fact that incorrectly timed milk can impair or delay the development of CRs.

Circadian Change in Breast Milk Components

In many studies, CRs also have an effect on the release of bioactive metabolites such as tryptophan, triacylglycerol, cholesterol, iron, melatonin, and cortisol. These oscillation differences related to the biological clock can play a serious role in the growth and development of the child (Italianer et al., 2020).

It has been shown statistically that there is a significant difference between morning and evening levels of adrenal steroids, which are responsible for the growth of infants and the regulation of stress, depending on the circadian rhythm, and it continues throughout the first year of life in infants starting from one month old (Ivars et al., 2015). In a recent study, milk was taken from 23 breastfeeding mothers 24 hours before and after each breastfeeding session, and daily significant changes were seen in cortisol levels in milk from all mothers. Cortisol levels were on average 330% higher in morning milk compared to afternoon and evening milk (Pundir et al., 2017). Many studies have shown that cortisol levels in both infants and breast milk differ during the day depending on CR. In addition, there are many data investigating the effectiveness of cortisol, which is secreted depending on the light-dark cycle, on growth, weight gain, and duration sleep. Mann et al. reported that providing a light/dark cycle in the neonatal intensive care unit decreased feeding time, increased weight gain, and increased sleep time compared to babies receiving continuous light (Mann et al., 1986). In this study, the importance of the baby's cortisol circadian rhythm, independent of breast milk, was demonstrated.

Of all the endocrine metabolites in human milk, melatonin has the best circadian rhythm. The increase in the level of melatonin is an important indicator of the night. At the same time, melatonin functions as an antioxidant, anti-inflammatory, and immune regulator. A study to investigate melatonin levels in day and night breast milk revealed significantly higher concentrations of melatonin in night milk (Katzer et al., 2016). Breast milk consisting of melatonin is likely to be effective in reducing infantile colic and regulating infant sleep. A questionnaire on irritability, infantile colic, and sleep characteristics was completed in 94 mothers of infants aged 2 to 4 months to evaluate the differences in severity of infantile colic and duration of nighttime sleep between breastfed and supplement-fed infants. As a result, the incidence of colic attacks was significantly lower in exclusively breastfed infants, irritability attacks were observed to be less severe, and longer duration of sleep was detected at night. Simultaneously, melatonin levels of breast milk and artificial formulas were measured. While a significant amount of melatonin was detected in breast milk at night, it was observed that artificial formulas did not contain melatonin (Engler et al., 2012). We can say that, especially the night sleep of the mother and increasing the level of melatonin in her milk are very important in reducing the incidence of infantile colic.

Apart from these two metabolites, there are many metabolites secreted by CR in breast milk. For example, there are studies showing that the leptin level in breast milk is higher at night than during the day, which prevents hunger and regulates energy balance (Langendonk et al., 1998). Similarly, it has been suggested that immune cell elements exhibit CRs in breast milk and are generally present in greater increased concentrations during the day, particularly in the early postnatal period. Mature breast milk contains more antibodies, C3, C4 proteins, and phagocytes during the day than at night. In line with these results, higher levels of interferon-γ were found in mature daytime milk than at night (Giachini et al., 2013).

A better understanding of the circadian rhythms of the components in breast milk may open up new possibilities for interventions to improve infant health. Infants, especially those fighting active infection or at high risk of infection, may benefit from milk that is selectively collected during the day because essential immune factors are generally higher in milk expressed during the day than at night (Giachini et al., 2013). Most infants in urban and industrialized societies are fed pre-expressed breast milk regardless of the time of milking. Considering the negative impact of this practice and the increase in the number of formula-fed infants on infant circadian biology, and the wide-ranging potential harmful effects on infant health, it is predicted that the impact of this field on preventive and therapeutic child health will gradually increase in the coming years (Hahn-Holbrook et al., 2019).

CR and Allergic Diseases in Children

Atopic dermatitis (AD) is a chronic inflammatory skin disease that affects 10-20% of children in the United States (USA) (Shaw et al., 2011). AD is characterized by intense nocturnal pruritus. This seriously affects the continuity and quality of sleep. 60% of children with AD experience sleep disturbance due to AD, and 83% reported sleep problems during the acute symptom period (Chamlin et al., 2005). It is thought that the most common cause of sleep-related problems in children with AD is itching (Chang & Chiang, 2016). Cortisol levels associated with CR are highest in the morning, decreasing during the day, and reaching their lowest levels in the evening after sleeping. This diurnal pattern has been suggested to contribute to itching in AD. Nocturnal cortisol has little anti-inflammatory effect (Patel et al., 2007). As a result, topical corticosteroid creams form the basis of treatment due to the decrease in cortisol secretion at night.

Asthma is a heterogeneous inflammatory airway disease that remains the most common chronic disease of in children in developed countries (Pavord et al., 2018). As a Greek doctor named Arataeus of Cappadocia observed observationally around 100 AD, the symptoms of patients with allergic asthma typically worsen at night, especially in the early morning hours (Smolensky et al., 2009). The airways are at their narrowest in the early morning, exactly between 2:00 and 5:00 am, when asthmatics are most likely to have respiratory symptoms (Clark, 1987). Disruption of CRs in the lung may contribute to the exacerbation of chronic diseases such as asthma by regulating the observed changes in airway resistance, airway inflammation, bronchial reactivity, and mucus production (Powell et al., 2022). The pathogenesis of asthma is multifactorial, but one of the most critical reasons for its development is susceptibility to respiratory viruses. In 80% of children with asthma and 60% of adults, the virus can be isolated from the respiratory tract during an attack (Rossi et al., 2016). In asthmatics, lower respiratory tract symptoms due to viral agents are longer and more severe than non-viral agents (Corne et al., 2002). In mammals, CRs are formed by regulatory proteins expressed as the circadian clock and a group of transcription factors. The core transcription factor is a heterodimer composed of BMAL1/CLOCK proteins carrying genes containing "E-Box" motifs in their promoters. Among the genes processed by BMAL1/CLOCK are other "clock genes" that provide positive or negative feedback to it. More importantly, lung parenchymal cells express clock genes and harbor an ongoing circadian clock. Data are emerging that clock genes may contribute to fibrosis, glucocorticoid responses, lung inflammation, and immunity (Green et al., 2008). Bmal1 deletion of circadian function resulted in a n exaggerated lung response during viral disease. Deletion of Bmal1 also induced high replication of the parainfluenza virus in tissue culture cells and mice. As a result, Bmal1-null animals had worse airway symptoms during an asthma attack (Ehlers et al., 2018). In light of these data, it is thought that disruption of the circadian rhythm plays a role in the more severe course of symptoms in asthma attacks due to viral agents (Nosal et al., 2020). Furthermore, CR plasma cortisol levels in the autonomic nervous system cause temporal differences in airway inflammation. It is known that this situation contributes to the worsening of lung function and asthma at night and in the morning (Smolensky et al., 1986).

Nasal congestion, runny nose, and sneezing, which are the main symptoms of allergic rhinitis, tend to worsen in the early morning and after waking up, but the mechanisms that cause these symptoms, which occur mostly in the morning, have not been fully elucidated (Aoyagi et al., 1999). Whatever the cause, the symptoms of rhinorrhea are thought to arise from tissue damage due to immunological reactions and the release of chemical mediators associated with inflammation of the upper airways. The causative processes of the pathophysiology of inflammation are regulated by certain circadian rhythmic processes (Smolensky et al., 2009). In a study conducted to demonstrate this, increased levels of inflammatory activation products were found in nasal secretions at 06:00 in the morning (Aoyagi et al., 1999). Topical nasal corticotherapy is used especially in the treatment of allergic rhinitis. Day and night drug administration times are chosen primarily to ensure patient compliance. Although the circadian dependence of nasal discharge is known, unfortunately, not much attention is paid to this situation in the planning of pharmacotherapy (Smolensky et al., 2009).

CR in Childhood Febrile Seizures

Febrile seizure (FS) is the most common type of seizure in children (Dubé et al., 2007). This type of seizure is defined as a seizure occurring after a febrile illness in children aged 6-60 months without metabolic disorders or a central nervous system infection. Body temperature should be at least 37.8 °C and there should be no history of febrile seizures. (Sharafi et al., 2017). Although the exact cause is not known, genetics are an important factor in the formation of this age-related seizure. A family history of febrile seizures has been reported in most of the patients (Patterson et al., 2014). CR can be said as another factor. CR has potential effects on secondary cyclical changes in hormones and sleep-wake cycles and the timing of seizures. Epileptic seizures often occur at a certain time of day. Studies have shown that FS occurs mostly in the evening hours. FS is seen 5-7 times more in the evening than in the morning (Sharafi et al., 2017) (Aoyagi et al., 1999). Therefore, due to the high prevalence of evening seizures, the administration of prophylactic oral diazepam in the appropriate time window may help prevent relapse (Manfredini et al., 2004).

The Relationship between Autism Spectrum Disorder and CR

Autism Spectrum Disorder (ASD) is a neurodevelopmental disorder that is detected most frequently in the first 3 years of life. Social interaction disorder, repetitive and restrictive behaviors, or stereotypical behavior patterns characterize different symptoms of ASD (Posar et al., 2015). ASD is likely to arise as a result of the complex interaction between the environment and genes, which gradually alters the development of brain functions and structures. Sleep disturbances and low melatonin levels are often seen in ASD. This raises the hypothesis that CRs may have an effect on the etiology of ASD (Geoffray et al., 2016). Studies conducted to investigate the etiology of ASD have shown that dysregulation of neurodevelopmental signals may be associated with the clinical presentation of ASD (Vallée et al., 2020). The WNT/β-catenin pathway is one of the main pathways involved in developmental cognitive disorders (Al-Harthi, 2012). Various molecular mechanisms, including the formation and development of synapses in the central nervous system, are modified by the WNT/β-catenin pathway (Ahmad-Annuar et al., 2006). The potential role of overactivation of the WNT/β-catenin pathway has been observed in patients with ASD. Dysregulation of CRs in ASD excessively increases the WNT/β-catenin pathway. This excessive increase contributes negatively to the progression of symptoms in ASD (Vallée et al., 2020). Evidence from clinical and basic studies suggests that disruption in the circadian system may be associated with the pathogenesis of ASD (Lorsung et al., 2021).

These children experience sleep problems at a higher rate than children with other developmental disorders and normally developing children (Johnson & Zarrinnegar, 2021). Prolonged sleep delay, frequent nocturnal awakenings, unusual morning awakenings, and a decrease in total sleep time are common in children with autism (Polimeni et al., 2005). Possible causes of sleep problems in ASD include abnormal levels of hormones such as melatonin and mutations in genes that regulate circadian rhythm. Disruption of circadian biomarkers such as melatonin and cortisol in biological samples such as blood, urine, and saliva is known to contribute to the progression of ASD symptoms. Apart from this, the relationship between circadian dysfunction and ASD may also be reciprocal. Just as the evidence that CR is effective in the etiology of ASD is increasing day by day, problems such as sleep disorders in ASD also disrupt the circadian rhythm. Being aware of the irregularity of the circadian clock in neurodevelopmental disorders and its importance in neurodevelopment may provide a new perspective for the treatment of ASD. Clinical treatments for children with ASD should consider physical, mental, and social strategies, while integrating approaches with daily rhythms (Lorsung et al., 2021).

Obesity and CR

All over the world, childhood obesity has increased more than 8 times in 40 years, causing enormous personal, social, and economic problems (Koletzko et al., 2020). Due to the increasing risk, the importance of the prevention and treatment of obesity is increasing day by day. When we look at the causes of obesity, we see that there are many factors. These include a high-calorie diet, low physical activity due to screen exposure, and under- or over-nutrition in the early years of life. In addition to these reasons, it has been clearly shown by clinical and epidemiological studies that impaired circadian rhythm causes obesity (Boege et al., 2021). In recent years, lifestyles that cause environmental rhythm and internal clock system imbalance have emerged in children. For example, disruptions in the sleep/wake and feeding/hunger cycles cause an irregularity between the environmental rhythm and the internal clock system, and CRs are adversely affected. As a result of this misalignment, the risk of obesity is increasing in the pediatric population (Kawai, 2022).

With the increasing use of smartphones and tablets, screen time before bed has increased among children. The light from the screens of these devices and the exposure time to this light before going to bed can mimic sunlight and transmit inappropriate signals to the hypothalamus through the retina (Khalsa et al., 2003). Therefore, light exposure before bedtime delays the circadian clock by causing melatonin levels to remain high for a shorter time or to rise later. This has also been shown to reduce the rate of deep sleep (Gooley et al., 2011). Exposure to light at night has been shown to increase daytime food intake in animal models. The increased food intake of mice during the light phase results in increased body weight, as they are less metabolically active. Similar findings have been reported in association with increases in obesity parameters in humans with increased exposure to night light. In light of these findings, it has been shown that exposure to light at night causes the development of obesity by disrupting the circadian rhythm (Obayashi et al., 2016).

Short duration of sleep in preschool children is a risk factor for the development of obesity (Miller et al., 2021). In a study examining the relationship between short sleep hours and obesity, when those who slept for 11 hours or more were compared with other groups, it was seen that those who slept 10-11 hours were 1.20 times more likely to be obese, those who slept 9-10 hours 1.34 times, and those who slept less than 9 hours were 1.57 times more likely to be obese (Sekine). et al., 2002). Short sleep time disrupts the circadian rhythm, reduces the level of peptide YY, which reduces food intake, and increases cortisol and growth hormone levels in the evening. Increased cortisol levels lead to the development of visceral obesity and increased food intake. These results show that reduced sleep duration in preschool children is a risk factor for obesity (Björntorp, 2001).

Not having breakfast has been identified by researchers as one of the causes of obesity in children. Many cross-sectional studies have shown an increased risk of obesity. A meta-analysis of cross-sectional studies revealed a 1.44-fold increase in the risk of obesity (Ardeshirlarijani et al., 2019). While explaining the molecular mechanisms of the role of skipping breakfast in the formation of obesity, it was shown that delayed meal time in mice fed with high cholesterol caused the expression of clock genes to be altered in liver gene expression, which is involved in lipid metabolism. According to this result, it was understood that skipping breakfast causes a chronic misalignment between the peripheral and central clock systems of metabolic pathways in peripheral tissues (Kim et al., 2021).

The lifestyle that disrupts the circadian clock system is associated with obesity and related problems. For this reason, pediatricians should make arrangements for a lifestyle that disrupts the circadian rhythm in the treatment of obese children. It is extremely important in the arrangements regarding meal times. Because it is possible to reduce weight without reducing calories by simply shifting meal times to daytime (Kawai, 2022).

Intestinal Microbiota and Metabolic Syndrome

It is known that the microbiota contributes to the mucosal integrity of the intestinal epithelium, food absorption, and digestion. Recent evidence has shown that the circadian rhythm of the host and the microbial rhythms are closely related. Due to this rhythm, the microbiome also changes during the day (Bishehsari et al., 2020). *BMAL1* is the gene encoding the core molecular clock component, and its deletion disrupts the circadian clock, thus eliminating the rhythmicity of the fecal microbiota (Liang et al., 2015).

The gut microbiome that is damaged as a result of CR disorder may lead to the development of metabolic syndrome. (Moossavi & Bishehsari, 2019). There is an ongoing interaction between the host and the microbiota in the gastrointestinal tract, and disruption of this can lead to metabolic dysfunction. Therefore, it is possible that interventions to circadian rhythm beneficially alter gut microbiome communities, resulting in the prevention of chronic metabolic disorders and increased host resistance.

First of all, the way to regulate the intestinal microbiome is through lifestyle changes. Optimizing food consumption time is one of the interventions to increase the robustness of CRs in the gut. Limiting food intake to daytime hours only (10-12 hours of food availability, 12-14 hours fasting) can optimize the host microbiota and circadian rhythm. These circadian-focused interventions are thought to have the capacity to prevent proinflammatory processes such as metabolic syndrome and cancer. Again, probiotic or prebiotic supplements may be considered to smoother the microbiota community and CRs in high-risk populations (Bishehsari et al., 2020).

Conclusion

Thanks to genetic research on CRs, it has been realized that the circadian system has a tight connection with the processes that control metabolism. In the results obtained from the studies, it has been shown that CR disorder is involved in the etiopathogenesis of multiple diseases. Again, the symptoms seen in diseases within the cause-effect relationship also affect the CR and cause the progression of the pathology. The impact of CR disruption on disease is clear, but the biggest barrier to applying this understanding in clinical life is the difficulty of diagnosing and detecting circadian disruption. A clear understanding of the deterioration in CR may lead to the development of successful chronopharmacotherapy strategies, resulting in improved treatment results. Understanding circadian pharmacokinetics will also lead to the development of new strategies for treatment timing in the future. The interaction between peripheral clocks and the brain and how this interaction affects metabolic processes throughout the sleep-wake cycle has not yet been fully elucidated. As these future molecular connections are understood, we think that new methods will emerge in the interventions of diseases.

References

Ahmad-Annuar, A., Ciani, L., Simeonidis, I., Herreros, J., Fredj, N. Ben, Rosso, S. B., Hall, A., Brickley, S., & Salinas, P. C. (2006). Signaling across the synapse: a role for Wnt and Dishevelled in presynaptic assembly and neurotransmitter release. *The Journal of cell biology*, *174*(1), 127–139. https://doi.org/10.1083/JCB.200511054.

Al-Harthi, L. (2012). Wnt/β-catenin and its diverse physiological cell signaling pathways in neurodegenerative and neuropsychiatric disorders. *Journal of neuroimmune pharmacology : the official journal of the Society on NeuroImmune Pharmacology*, 7(4), 725–730. https://doi.org/10.1007/S11481-012-9412-X.

Allada, R., & Bass, J. (2021). Circadian Mechanisms in Medicine. *The New England journal of medicine*, *384*(6), 550. https://doi.org/10.1056/NEJMRA1802337.

Aoyagi, M., Watanabe, H., Sekine, K., Nishimuta, T., Konno, A., Shimojo, N., & Kohno, Y. (1999). Circadian variation in nasal reactivity in children with allergic rhinitis: correlation with the activity of eosinophils and basophilic cells. *International archives of allergy and immunology*, *120 Suppl 1*(SUPPL. 1), 95–99. https://doi.org/10.1159/000053604.

Ardeshirlarijani, E., Namazi, N., Jabbari, M., Zeinali, M., Gerami, H., Jalili, R. B., Larijani, B., & Azadbakht, L. (2019). The link between breakfast skipping and overweigh/obesity in children and adolescents: a meta-analysis of observational studies. *Journal of Diabetes and Metabolic Disorders*, *18*(2), 657. https://doi.org/10.1007/S40200-019-00446-7.

Ardura, J., Gutierrez, R., Andres, J., & Agapito, T. (2003). Emergence and Evolution of the Circadian Rhythm of Melatonin in Children. *Hormone Research in Paediatrics*, *59*(2), 66–72. https://doi.org/10.1159/000068571.

Bishehsari, F., Voigt, R. M., & Keshavarzian, A. (2020). Circadian rhythms and the gut microbiota: from the metabolic syndrome to cancer. *Nature reviews. Endocrinology*, *16*(12), 731. https://doi.org/10.1038/S41574-020-00427-4.

Björntorp, P. (2001). Do stress reactions cause abdominal obesity and comorbidities? *Obesity Reviews*, *2*(2), 73–86. https://doi.org/10.1046/J.1467-789X.2001.00027.X.

Boege, H. L., Bhatti, M. Z., & St-Onge, M. P. (2021). Circadian rhythms and meal timing: impact on energy balance and body weight. *Current opinion in biotechnology*, *70*, 1. https://doi.org/10.1016/J.COPBIO.2020.08.009.

Chamlin, S. L., Mattson, C. L., Frieden, I. J., Williams, M. L., Mancini, A. J., Cella, D., & Chren, M. M. (2005). The price of pruritus: sleep disturbance and cosleeping in atopic dermatitis. *Archives of pediatrics & adolescent medicine*, *159*(8), 745–750. https://doi.org/10.1001/ARCHPEDI.159.8.745.

Chang, Y. Sen, & Chiang, B. L. (2016). Mechanism of Sleep Disturbance in Children with Atopic Dermatitis and the Role of the Circadian Rhythm and Melatonin. *International Journal of Molecular Sciences*, *17*(4). https://doi.org/10.3390/IJMS17040462.

Clark, T. J. (1987). Diurnal rhythm of asthma. *Chest*, *91*(6 Suppl), 137S-141S. https://doi.org/10.1378/CHEST.91.6_SUPPLEMENT.137S.

Corne, J. M., Marshall, C., Smith, S., Schreiber, J., Sanderson, G., Holgate, S. T., & Johnston, S. L. (2002). Frequency, severity, and duration of rhinovirus infections in asthmatic and non-asthmatic individuals: a longitudinal cohort study. *The Lancet*, *359*(9309), 831-834. https://doi.org/10.1016/S0140-6736(02)07953-9.

Dubé, C. M., Brewster, A. L., Richichi, C., Zha, Q., & Baram, T. Z. (2007). Fever, febrile seizures and epilepsy. *Trends in neurosciences*, *30*(10), 490–496. https://doi.org/10.1016/J.TINS.2007.07.006.

Dunlap, J. C. (1999). Molecular Bases for Circadian Clocks. *Cell*, *96*(2), 271–290. https://doi.org/10.1016/S0092-8674(00)80566-8.

Ehlers, A., Xie, W., Agapov, E., Brown, S., Steinberg, D., Tidwell, R., Sajol, G., Schutz, R., Weaver, R., Yu, H., Castro, M., Bacharier, L. B., Wang, X., Holtzman, M. J., & Haspel, J. A. (2018). BMAL1 links the circadian clock to viral airway pathology and asthma phenotypes. *Mucosal immunology*, *11*(1), 97–111. https://doi.org/10.1038/MI.2017.24.

Engler, A. C., Hadash, A., Shehadeh, N., & Pillar, G. (2012). Breastfeeding may improve nocturnal sleep and reduce infantile colic: Potential role of breast milk melatonin. *European Journal of Pediatrics*, *171*(4), 729–732. https://doi.org/10.1007/S00431-011-1659-3.

Geoffray, M. M., Nicolas, A., Speranza, M., & Georgieff, N. (2016). Are circadian rhythms new pathways to understand Autism Spectrum Disorder? *Journal of physiology, Paris*, *110*(4 Pt B), 434–438. https://doi.org/10.1016/J.JPHYSPARIS.2017.06.002.

Giachini, F. R., França, E. L., Silva, N. A., Honorio-Franca, C., Mores, L., Goncalves De Souza, E., & Luzia Franca, E. (2013). Bioactive factors of colostrum and human milk exhibits a day-night variation. *Article in American Journal of Immunology*, *9*(2), 68–74. https://doi.org/10.3844/ajisp.2013.68.74.

Gooley, J. J., Chamberlain, K., Smith, K. A., Khalsa, S. B. S., Rajaratnam, S. M. W., Van Reen, E., Zeitzer, J. M., Czeisler, C. A., & Lockley, S. W. (2011). Exposure to room light before bedtime suppresses melatonin onset and shortens melatonin duration in humans. *The Journal of clinical endocrinology and metabolism, 96*(3). https://doi.org/10.1210/JC.2010-2098.

Green, C. B., Takahashi, J. S., & Bass, J. (2008). The meter of metabolism. *Cell*, *134*(5), 728–742. https://doi.org/10.1016/J.CELL.2008.08.022.

Hahn-Holbrook, J., Saxbe, D., Bixby, C., Steele, C., & Glynn, L. (2019). Human milk as "chrononutrition": implications for child health and development. *Pediatric Research 2019 85:7*, *85*(7), 936–942. https://doi.org/10.1038/s41390-019-0368-x.

Italianer, M. F., Naninck, E. F. G., Roelants, J. A., van der Horst, G. T. J., Reiss, I. K. M., van Goudoever, J. B., Joosten, K. F. M., Chaves, I., & Vermeulen, M. J. (2020). Circadian Variation in Human Milk Composition, a Systematic Review. *Nutrients*, *12*(8), 1–16. https://doi.org/10.3390/NU12082328.

Ivars, K., Nelson, N., Theodorsson, A., Theodorsson, E., Ström, J. O., & Mörelius, E. (2015). Development of Salivary Cortisol Circadian Rhythm and Reference Intervals in Full-Term Infants. *PLoS ONE*, *10*(6). https://doi.org/10.1371/JOURNAL.PONE.0129502.

Johnson, K. P., & Zarrinnegar, P. (2021). Autism Spectrum Disorder and Sleep. *Child and adolescent psychiatric clinics of North America*, *30*(1), 195–208. https://doi.org/10.1016/J.CHC.2020.08.012.

Katzer, D., Pauli, L., Mueller, A., Reutter, H., Reinsberg, J., Fimmers, R., Bartmann, P., & Bagci, S. (2016). Melatonin Concentrations and Antioxidative Capacity of Human Breast Milk According to Gestational Age and the Time of Day. *Journal of human lactation : official journal of International Lactation Consultant Association*, *32*(4), NP105–NP110. https://doi.org/10.1177/0890334415625217.

Kawai, M. (2022). Disruption of the circadian rhythms and its relationship with pediatric obesity. *Pediatrics international : official journal of the Japan Pediatric Society*, *64*(1). https://doi.org/10.1111/PED.14992.

Khalsa, S. B. S., Jewett, M. E., Cajochen, C., & Czeisler, C. A. (2003). A phase response curve to single bright light pulses in human subjects. *The Journal of physiology*, *549*(Pt 3), 945–952. https://doi.org/10.1113/JPHYSIOL.2003.040477.

Kim, D., Hanzawa, F., Sun, S., Laurent, T., Ikeda, S., Umeki, M., Mochizuki, S., & Oda, H. (2021). Delayed Meal Timing, a Breakfast Skipping Model, Increased Hepatic Lipid Accumulation and Adipose Tissue Weight by Disintegrating Circadian Oscillation in Rats Fed a High-Cholesterol Diet. *Frontiers in Nutrition*, *8*, 681436. https://doi.org/10.3389/FNUT.2021.681436/FULL.

Koletzko, B., Fishbein, M., Lee, W. S., Moreno, L., Mouane, N., Mouzaki, M., & Verduci, E. (2020). Prevention of Childhood Obesity: A Position Paper of the Global Federation of International Societies of Paediatric Gastroenterology, Hepatology and Nutrition (FISPGHAN). *Journal of pediatric gastroenterology and nutrition*, *70*(5), 702–710. https://doi.org/10.1097/MPG.0000000000002708.

Langendonk, J. G., Pijl, H., Toornvliet, A. C., Burggraaf, J., Frölich, M., Schoemaker, R. C., Doornbos, J., Cohen, A. F., & Meinders, A. E. (1998). Circadian rhythm of plasma leptin levels in upper and lower body obese women: influence of body fat distribution and weight loss. *The Journal of clinical endocrinology and metabolism*, *83*(5), 1706–1712. https://doi.org/10.1210/JCEM.83.5.4717.

Lee, Y., Field, J. M., & Sehgal, A. (2021). Circadian Rhythms, Disease and Chronotherapy. *Journal of biological rhythms*, *36*(6), 503. https://doi.org/10.1177/0748730 4211044301.

Levi, F., & Schibler, U. (2007). Circadian Rhythms: Mechanisms and Therapeutic Implications. *https://doi.org/10.1146/annurev.pharmtox.47.120505.105208*, *47*, 593–628. https://doi.org/10.1146/ANNUREV.PHARMTOX.47.120505.105208.

Liang, X., Bushman, F. D., & FitzGerald, G. A. (2015). Rhythmicity of the intestinal microbiota is regulated by gender and the host circadian clock. *Proceedings of the National Academy of Sciences of the United States of America*, *112*(33), 10479–10484. https://doi.org/10.1073/PNAS.1501305112.

Lorsung, E., Karthikeyan, R., & Cao, R. (2021). Biological Timing and Neurodevelopmental Disorders: A Role for Circadian Dysfunction in Autism Spectrum Disorders. *Frontiers in Neuroscience*, *15*. https://doi.org/10.3389/FNINS.2021.642745.

Manfredini, R., Vergine, G., Boari, B., Faggioli, R., & Borgna-Pignatti, C. (2004). Circadian and seasonal variation of first febrile seizures. *The Journal of pediatrics*, *145*(6), 838–839. https://doi.org/10.1016/J.JPEDS.2004.06.079.

Mann, N. P., Haddow, R., Stokes, L., Goodley, S., & Rutter, N. (1986). Effect of night and day on preterm infants in a newborn nursery: randomised trial. *British Medical Journal (Clinical research ed.)*, *293*(6557), 1265. https://doi.org/10.1136/BMJ.293.6557.1265.

McGraw, K., Hoffmann, R., Harker, C., & Herman, J. H. (1999). The development of circadian rhythms in a human infant. *Sleep*, *22*(3), 303–310. https://doi.org/10.1093/SLEEP/22.3.303.

Miller, M. A., Bates, S., Ji, C., & Cappuccio, F. P. (2021). Systematic review and meta-analyses of the relationship between short sleep and incidence of obesity and effectiveness of sleep interventions on weight gain in preschool children. *Obesity reviews : an official journal of the International Association for the Study of Obesity*, *22*(2). https://doi.org/10.1111/OBR.13113.

Mirmiran, M., Maas, Y. G. H., & Ariagno, R. L. (2003). Development of fetal and neonatal sleep and circadian rhythms. *Sleep Medicine Reviews*, *7*(4), 321–334. https://doi.org/10.1053/SMRV.2002.0243.

Moossavi, S., & Bishehsari, F. (2019). Microbes: possible link between modern lifestyle transition and the rise of metabolic syndrome. *Obesity reviews : an official journal of the International Association for the Study of Obesity*, *20*(3), 407–419. https://doi.org/10.1111/OBR.12784.

Nosal, C., Ehlers, A., & Haspel, J. A. (2020). Why Lungs Keep Time: Circadian Rhythms and Lung Immunity. *Annual review of physiology*, *82*, 391. https://doi.org/10.1146/ANNUREV-PHYSIOL-021119-034602.

Obayashi, K., Saeki, K., & Kurumatani, N. (2016). Ambient Light Exposure and Changes in Obesity Parameters: A Longitudinal Study of the HEIJO-KYO Cohort. *The Journal of clinical endocrinology and metabolism*, *101*(9), 3539–3547. https://doi.org/10.1210/JC.2015-4123.

Patel, T., Ishiuji, Y., & Yosipovitch, G. (2007). Nocturnal itch: why do we itch at night? *Acta dermato-venereologica*, *87*(4), 295–298. https://doi.org/10.2340/00015555-0280.

Patke, A., Young, M. W., & Axelrod, S. (2020). Molecular mechanisms and physiological importance of circadian rhythms. *Nature reviews. Molecular cell biology*, *21*(2), 67–84. https://doi.org/10.1038/S41580-019-0179-2.

Patterson, K. P., Baram, T. Z., & Shinnar, S. (2014). Origins of temporal lobe epilepsy: febrile seizures and febrile status epilepticus. *Neurotherapeutics : the journal of the American Society for Experimental NeuroTherapeutics*, *11*(2), 242–250. https://doi.org/10.1007/S13311-014-0263-4.

Pavord, I. D., Beasley, R., Agusti, A., Anderson, G. P., Bel, E., Brusselle, G., Cullinan, P., Custovic, A., Ducharme, F. M., Fahy, J. V., Frey, U., Gibson, P., Heaney, L. G., Holt, P. G., Humbert, M., Lloyd, C. M., Marks, G., Martinez, F. D., Sly, P. D., Bush, A. (2018). After asthma: redefining airways diseases. *Lancet (London, England)*, *391*(10118), 350–400. https://doi.org/10.1016/S0140-6736(17)30879-6.

Polimeni, M. A., Richdale, A. L., & Francis, A. J. P. (2005). A survey of sleep problems in autism, Asperger's disorder and typically developing children. *Journal of intellectual disability research : JIDR*, *49*(Pt 4), 260–268. https://doi.org/10.1111/J.1365-2788.2005.00642.X.

Posar, A., Resca, F., & Visconti, P. (2015). Autism according to diagnostic and statistical manual of mental disorders 5(th) edition: The need for further improvements. *Journal of pediatric neurosciences*, *10*(2), 146–148. https://doi.org/10.4103/1817-1745.159195.

Powell, W. T., Rich, L. M., Vanderwall, E. R., White, M. P., & Debley, J. S. (2022). Temperature synchronisation of circadian rhythms in primary human airway epithelial cells from children. *BMJ Open Respiratory Research*, *9*(1). https://doi.org/10.1136/BMJRESP-2022-001319.

Pundir, S., Wall, C. R., Mitchell, C. J., Thorstensen, E. B., Lai, C. T., Geddes, D. T., & Cameron-Smith, D. (2017). Variation of Human Milk Glucocorticoids over 24 hour Period. *Journal of Mammary Gland Biology and Neoplasia*, *22*(1), 85–92. https://doi.org/10.1007/S10911-017-9375-X/METRICS.

Rossi, G. A., Silvestri, M., & Colin, A. A. (2016). Viral Bronchiolitis in Children. *The New England journal of medicine*, *374*(18), 1792–1793. https://doi.org/10.1056/NEJMc1601509.

Sekine, M., Yamagami, T., Hamanishi, S., Handa, K., Saito, T., Nanri, S., Kawaminami, K., Tokui, N., Yoshida, K., & Kagamimori, S. (2002). Parental obesity, lifestyle factors and obesity in preschool children: results of the Toyama Birth Cohort study. *Journal of epidemiology*, *12*(1), 33–39. https://doi.org/10.2188/JEA.12.33.

Sharafi, R., Hassanzadeh Rad, A., & Aminzadeh, V. (2017). Circadian Rhythm and the Seasonal Variation in Childhood Febrile Seizure. *Iranian Journal of Child Neurology*, *11*(3), 27. https://doi.org/10.22037/ijcn.v11i3.10865.

Shaw, T. E., Currie, G. P., Koudelka, C. W., & Simpson, E. L. (2011). Eczema prevalence in the United States: Data from the 2003 National Survey of Children's Health. *The Journal of investigative dermatology*, *131*(1), 67. https://doi.org/10.1038/JID.2010.251.

Smolensky, M. H., Barnes, P. J., Reinberg, A., & Mcgovern, J. P. (1986). Chronobiology and asthma. I. Day-night differences in bronchial patency and dyspnea and circadian rhythm dependencies. *The Journal of asthma : official journal of the Association for the Care of Asthma*, *23*(6), 321–343. https://doi.org/10.3109/02770908609073179.

Vallée, A., Lecarpentier, Y., Guillevin, R., & Vallée, J. N. (2020). The influence of circadian rhythms and aerobic glycolysis in autism spectrum disorder. *Translational Psychiatry*, *10*(1). https://doi.org/10.1038/S41398-020-01086-9.

Wong, S. D., Wright, K. P., Spencer, R. L., Vetter, C., Hicks, L. M., Jenni, O. G., & Lebourgeois, M. K. (2021). Is the use of high correlated color temperature light at night related to delay of sleep timing in university students? A cross-country study in Japan and China. *Journal of Physiological Anthropology*, *41*, 22. https://doi.org/10.1186/s40101-022-00294-0.

Zisapel, N. (2018). New perspectives on the role of melatonin in human sleep, circadian rhythms and their regulation. *British Journal of Pharmacology*, *175*(16), 3190. https://doi.org/10.1111/BPH.14116.

Chapter 15

Impact of Light and Circadian Clock on the Reproductive Health

Sena Özcan Yıldırım*, MD
and Merve Kavak Balgetir, MD
Department of Histology and Embriology, Elazığ Fethi Sekin City Hospital, Elazığ, Turkiye

Abstract

The circadian clock is an internal timing mechanism that regulates various physiological processes, including reproductive function in females and males. Recent research has found that circadian disruption, caused by shift work or jet lag, can negatively impact reproductive health by altering hormone levels which culminates in damaging the normal timing of the menstrual cycle in women and impairing spermatogenesis in men. Furthermore, preterm delivery and low birth weight are two complications of pregnancy that are more likely to occur when the circadian clock is disrupted. Additionally, irregularities in the circadian clock affect negatively sperm quality and quantity, increasing the risk of male infertility. The impact of the circadian clock on melatonin is assumed to be the mechanism that influences reproductive health in both females and males. Melatonin receptors are present in the uterus, placenta, and ovaries, indicating that they have a direct influence on female reproductive health, as well as the expression of melatonin receptors in the testes demonstrates its importance on male reproductive function. This book chapter thoroughly examines the intricate relationship between circadian rhythms and fertility, exploring the

* Corresponding Author's Email: senaozcan23@hotmail.com

In: Human Health is a Matter of Timing
Editors: Sumeyya Deniz Aybek, Gonca Gulbay and Mucahit Secme
ISBN: 979-8-89113-467-6

impact of circadian disruption on reproductive health and the potential for future therapeutic interventions to mitigate these effects.

Keywords: circadian clock, reproductive health, melatonin, fertility

Introduction

The sleep-wake cycle, hormone secretion, and gene expression are the various body's biological rhythms that are regulated by the circadian clock which is governed by a network of clock genes and proteins that collaborate to form a self-sustaining feedback loop that oscillates 24 hours a day. This mechanism involves multiple essential clock genes, including the circadian locomotor output cycle kaput (CLOCK), brain and muscle ARNT-like protein 1 (BMAL1), Period (PER1, PER2, and PER3), Cryptochrome (CRY1 and CRY2), and relevant clock-controlled genes (CCGs), which are present in numerous tissues across the body (Boden & Kennaway, 2006; Sen & Sellix, 2016).

CLOCK and BMAL1 promote the expression of additional clock genes, such as PER and CRY, which subsequently interact with CLOCK and BMAL1 to form a negative feedback loop. Other clock genes and proteins, such as REV-ERBs and RORs, also help regulate the circadian clock (Boden & Kennaway, 2006; Sen & Sellix, 2016).

These genes work together with other proteins to control the body's reaction to environmental influences, especially light and temperature. Light is one of the major external variables regulating the circadian clock since it serves as a reset clock in a daily period. The retina of the eye has specialized cells that can sense light and transfer the relevant data to the brain through the retinohypothalamic tract (RHT) which links the retina where light enters to the suprachiasmatic nucleus (SCN) that controls the circadian clock in animals. Intrinsically photosensitive retinal ganglion cells (ipRGCs), specialized photosensitive cells that carry the photopigment melanopsin and react to light directly, constitute the RHT (Pilorz et al., 2018).

SCN of the hypothalamus houses the brain's primary clock, which is essential for controlling the endocrine system and the timing of hormone release. The SCN synchronizes the timing of numerous physiological processes by receiving input from photoreceptors in the eye, which recognize variations in light and dark cycles (Mills & Kuohung, 2019).

The circadian clock mechanism consists of three fundamental components: the primary oscillator, the input pathway, and the output pathway. External light is detected by retinal ganglion cells coated with melanopsin, which transmit an electrical signal to a central oscillator through the retinohypothalamic tract (Li et al., 2022; Pilorz et al., 2018). Central clocks, typically found in the SCN of the hypothalamus, control and transmit rhythmic signals to peripheral tissues and organs, producing distinct biochemistry, physiology, and behavior (Shao et al., 2021). Human circadian rhythm is a sequential transcriptional and translational feedback loop (TTFL) that is incorporated by light and exhibits internal rhythmicity due to clock gene transcription factors in the SCN (Kennaway et al., 2012; Pilorz et al., 2018; Sletten et al., 2020). Dimerized transcription factors (CLOCK, BMAL1) aggregate in the nucleus during the main loop, and dimerized transcription factors (PER and CRY) attach and move to the nucleus to silence their genes and actions. The nuclear receptors of the orphan nuclear receptor (REV-ERBa/b) and retinoic acid-related orphan receptor alpha (RORa/b) create a second feedback loop, performing a suppressive and activating function in transcription. A different loop is formed by the REV-ERB and ROR target genes NFIL3 and the CLOCK-BMAL1 target genes D-site albumin promoter-binding protein (DBP) and E4 promoter-binding protein 4 (E4BP4). The feedback loop serves as the basis for the physiologic function of many tissues and organs, causing cyclical changes in the expression of genes and functions of tissues (Boden & Kennaway, 2006; Li et al., 2022; Pilorz et al., 2018; Shao et al., 2021, Yalcin et al., 2022). Abnormal clock genes or environmental factors can disrupt this feedback loop, leading to various illnesses, including infertility (Mills & Kuohung, 2019; Shao et al., 2021; Sen & Sellix, 2016).

The circadian clock is fundamental for health and well-being, since alterations in this process may result in a number of health issues. Accordingly, sleep has a profound connection to the circadian clock, and disruptions associated with this rhythm might result in complications, including insomnia, sleep apnea, and other sleep disorders (Lateef & Akintubosun, 2020; Mills & Kuohung, 2019). Sleep-related problems are related to a variety of health issues in both men and women, including depression, high blood pressure, diabetes problems, cardiovascular disease, and anxiety-related conditions. It has also been noted that sleep issues in women are linked to premenstrual dysphoria, pregnancy, menopause, and postpartum depression (Fishbein et al., 2021; Lateef & Akintubosun, 2020).

The circadian clock also regulates hormone secretion, which emerges in a periodic manner in the course of the day in the body. Systemic disruptions in the circadian rhythm can result in hormonal imbalances, which may have a wide range of adverse health consequences. Moreover, the circadian clock has been associated with various biological processes, including immunological functions, metabolism, and cognitive well-being. In order to promote a general state of health and wellness, it is necessary to comprehend what processes of the circadian clock and implement actions to maintain its normal function (Lateef & Akintubosun, 2020, Yalcin et al., 2022).

The Role of the Circadian Clock in Regulating Reproductive Health and Fertility

Fertility is tightly controlled by the HPG axis as well as other neuron groups of hypothalamus, known as gonadotropin-releasing hormone (GnRH) neurons and Kisspeptin neurons. The anterior ventral periventricular Kisspeptin neuron group is participating to the luteinizing hormone (LH) increase, whereas the hypothalamic Kisspeptin neuron group in the nucleus of arcuate delivers metabolical status data via the HPG axis and releases GnRH. The hypothalamus releases GnRH in a pulsatory way, and it affects the anterior pituitary lobe (Adeno-Hypophysis), controlling gonadotropin synthesis, and eventually secreting follicle-stimulating hormone (FSH) and LH to the circulation (Goldstein & Smith, 2016; Mills & Kuohung, 2019; Sciarra et al., 2020; Shechter et al., 2008). LH is required for testosterone synthesis in males, whereas FSH is essential for sperm formation. FSH signaling dysfunction leads to poor spermatogenesis and male infertility. FSH and LH participate in the generation of steroid hormones (estrogens) by follicles in the ovaries in females. A relationship between circadian rhythms and estrogen has been strongly confirmed, and recent research found that the majority of female reproductive hormones exhibit circadian rhythmicity. FSH, LH, estrogen, progesterone, and sex hormone binding-globulin (SHBG) all have unusual rhythms throughout the follicular period. Within the luteal phase, paricularly FSH and SHBG show that rhythmicity. Estrogens increase the level of LH and impact the emergence of secondary sexual traits in females. Estrogens are demonstrated to influence the expression of both PER1 and PER2. A detailed investigation further reveals that the Clock gene can regulate the function of the estrogen receptor alpha (ER) by altering its transcriptional functions. Additionally, finding that ER receptors are present in the SCN supports the connection across the circadian cycle and synthesis of estrogen. In experimental mouse models and in women who work shifts, clock genes impact infertility by generating low amounts of sex hormones, leading to failure in embryo implantation, and reduced sizes of newborns. Overall, a complicated network is defined by highly connected interactors, the most important of which are clock genes and hormones (Mills & Kuohung, 2019; Sciarra et al., 2020; Shechter et al., 2008).

While the SCN, or central pacemaker, is important in controlling rhythmicity via temporal cues, other clocks located in various central structures and organs also contribute to regulating reproduction timing. Melatonin, glucocorticoids, autonomic inputs, body temperature, and peripheral clocks are examples of other central clocks that serve as circadian oscillators (Sen & Sellix, 2016).

Investigations have demonstrated that shift work, jet lag, or sleep disorders that alter circadian rhythms can have detrimental effects on reproductive health, which may involve adversely affected fertility in both females and males. Disruption of the circadian clock is initiated with an irregular sleep schedule where both men's and women's reproductive health would be significantly impacted (Lateef & Akintubosun, 2020; Shechter et al., 2008). In studies with animals, sleep deprivation altered sexual hormones by decreasing testosterone concentrations while increasing progesterone and glucocorticoid concentrations in male rats (Lateef & Akintubosun, 2020).

Low libido, irregular menstruation, and poor sperm quality have all been related to inadequate sleep. Chronic sleep deprivation can also cause hormone abnormalities that may make reproductive health problems even worse. According to a study, women who worked night shifts were more likely to experience menstrual abnormalities and infertility than those who worked conventional daytime hours. Men who worked night shifts also had lower testosterone levels and worse sperm quality. This emphasizes the significance of maintaining a consistent sleep-wake cycle to sustain a good circadian rhythm (Chau et al., 2014; Shechter et al., 2008).

Sleep disorders, such as insomnia and sleep apnea, can potentially affect reproductive health. According to one research, women with sleep apnea had a greater risk of infertility than those experiencing no sleep apnea. Furthermore, insufficient sleep can result in elevated cortisol and reduced melatonin levels, which may have a severe influence on reproductive function (Lateef & Akintubosun, 2020; Shechter et al., 2008).

Hormones such as melatonin and cortisol are released under the control of the circadian clock. It has been demonstrated that melatonin has antioxidant capabilities and can be useful in preventing oxidative stress, which may harm reproductive cells. The pineal gland releases melatonin at night, which has been stated to enhance the quality of sleep and modulate sleep-wake cycles. Melatonin, which has receptors in the SCN, has a significant impact on neuronal firing and clock gene expression in the central pacemaker. Melatonin regulates TSH production in the pars tuberalis of the adenohypophysis (Lee, 2022; Mills & Kuohung, 2019; Shechter et al., 2008). Cortisol, which the adrenal gland releases in reaction to stress, can interfene with sleep and have a detrimental effect on reproductive health that has been associated with both male and female fertility deduction (Yalcin et al., 2022).

Disrupting the Circadian Rhythm: Effects on Fertility and Pregnancy in Women

Recent findings implicated that issues with female fertility might result from a disruption of the circadian clock, which can cause hormonal imbalances that are required for ovulation, increasing the risk of infertility. The expression of genes involved in reproductive function can also change as a result of circadian clock disruption, which can impair fertility. Numerous studies have demonstrated that working shifts appear to be linked to menstruation abnormalities, that it reduces women's fertility, and that working longer shifts increases the chance of infertility (Boden & Kennaway, 2006; Chau et al., 2014; Shechter et al., 2008). Additionally, research has shown that women who work night rotation shifts are more likely to have miscarriages and give birth prematurely. Rapid time zone changes that result in jet lag might affect ovulation timing and reduce fertility. Several studies have revealed that increased night shiftwork, excessive workload, poor sleep quality, and the widespread use of mobile devices damage the circadian rhythm, impairing female fertility by influencing the menstrual cycle and changing hormone production, ultimately increasing the incidence of preterm birth, spontaneous abortion, and membrane rupture, and decreasing breastfeeding success (Boden & Kennaway, 2006; Li et al., 2022; Mills & Kuohung, 2019; Shechter et al., 2008).

Although the exact processes by which circadian abnormalities could impact reproductive function remain unclear, it is believed that alterations in hormone control, inflammation, and oxidative stress can be involved. Melatonin, cortisol, and reproductive hormones, including FSH and LH, are among the hormones whose timing and magnitude are altered when the circadian clock is disrupted. In women's reproductive health, including ovulation, menstrual cycle management, and pregnancy maintenance, hormones including LH, FSH, and estradiol play a critical role. Because of this, alterations in the control of hormones may directly affect reproductive function (Figure 1). Women may experience irregular menstruation and decreased fertility as a result of changes in the control of these hormones (Goldstein & Smith, 2016; Mills & Kuohung, 2019).

The HPG axis regulates the whole female reproductive system in a based-on time. Numerous types of activities on the HPG axis and its auxiliary organs exhibit a biological rhythm, which is often mirrored by menstrual hormones. The hypothalamus regulates the ovulatory cycle by secreting GnRH, which leads the pituitary to produce and secrete LH and FSH. (Shao et al., 2021). Several studies have identified potential clock gene effects on reproduction, including insufficient LH secretion and stimulation of the ovary at ovulation to modified luteal progesterone synthesis and events resulting in implantation (Kennaway et al., 2012; Mills & Kuohung, 2019).

The first is estrogen synthesis, which is triggered by FSH, and the second is postovulatory progesterone release from the corpus luteum. The circadian clock mechanism regulates both steroid hormones, and its disruption can result in ovarian malfunction and infertility (Mills & Kuohung, 2019; Shao et al., 2021).

TSH levels increase during sleep, and acute sleep loss in healthy young women in their follicular period causes a substantial increase in TSH levels. Menstrual abnormalities, anovulation, amenorrhea, and recurrent miscarriages are all linked to high TSH secretion. TSH levels that are abnormally elevated might cause prolactin production, which can contribute to female infertility (Lateef & Akintubosun, 2020). LH increases steroid production from the ovaries, ovulation, and the corpus luteum's secretion of progesterone following ovulation (Shao et al., 2021). The SCN is critical in coordinating the steroid rhythm, leading to irregular estrus cycles through neural projections to endocrine targets. SCN efferents target neuroendocrine cells in the brain and stimulate the synthesis of hypothalamic-releasing hormones. This is consistent with increased GnRH neuron activity and SCN FOS (FBJ osteosarcoma oncogene) expression in the SCN. The ultimate output of a neural network that governs the precise time of the pre-ovulatory LH surge and ovulation is SCN-coordinated GnRH neurons (Figure 1) (Goldstein & Smith, 2016; Pilorz et al., 2018; Sen & Sellix, 2016).

Circadian irregularities can lead to elevated inflammation and oxidative stress in addition to alterations in hormone regulation, which can further harm reproductive function. It has been demonstrated that shift work and disrupted sleep raise levels of pro-inflammatory cytokines and signs of oxidative stress, which can harm the reproductive system and cause infertility. A variety of reproductive diseases, including endometriosis and polycystic ovarian syndrome (PCOS), have been associated with inflammation and oxidative stress. PCOS is characterized by an imbalance in neuroendocrine and endocrine function, which results in inconsistent amounts and timing of ovarian steroid hormone release. The fluctuating hormones linked to these illnesses may cause or contribute to a modified timing of clock gene expression in peripheral organs, including the ovary (Sen & Sellix, 2016).

PCOS is a prevalent condition associated with hyperandrogenism, insulin resistance, and oligo anovulation. Three of these features are associated with the development of PCOS. Increased insulin is commonly associated with hyperandrogenism, and it is commonly recognized that insulin resistance inhibits liver sex hormone-binding globulin (SHBG) production while increasing androgen production, reducing follicular maturity, and decreasing the chances of ovulation. The latest research has proven that biorhythm abnormalities cause PCOS's metabolic and reproductive features. Continuous light exposure may cause PCOS-like ovarian alterations as well as glucose metabolism issues due to impaired islet beta-cell activity. Similarly, persistent darkness produced consistent outcomes, as did arrhythmic BMAL1 expression, which enhanced insulin resistance through GLUT4. PCOS causes ovulatory infertility and early loss of pregnancy in women. PCOS is related to a risk of obstructive sleep apnea that is up to 30 times higher than in healthy individuals. Obstructive sleep apnea is a risk factor for insulin resistance, glucose intolerance, and type 2 diabetes in PCOS. Additionally, treating obstructive sleep apnea increases insulin sensitivity in PCOS women. Resistance to insulin can lead to infertility and recurrent loss of pregnancy in women with or without PCOS. As a result, evaluating and treating sleep-disordered breathing may have the potential to increase fertility in these women. Furthermore, because sleep deprivation disrupts glucose homeostasis, adequate sleep duration may be critical in this situation (Shao et al., 2021).

Circadian irregularities may also affect reproductive function by causing inflammation. Increases in pro-inflammatory cytokines, such as tumor necrosis factor-alpha (TNF-alpha) and interleukin-6 (IL-6), and indicators of inflammation, such as C-reactive protein (CRP), have been linked to shift work and sleep disturbance. Fertility reduction and a higher possibility of pregnancy problems including preterm labor and preeclampsia have been linked to an elevated level of these inflammatory markers.

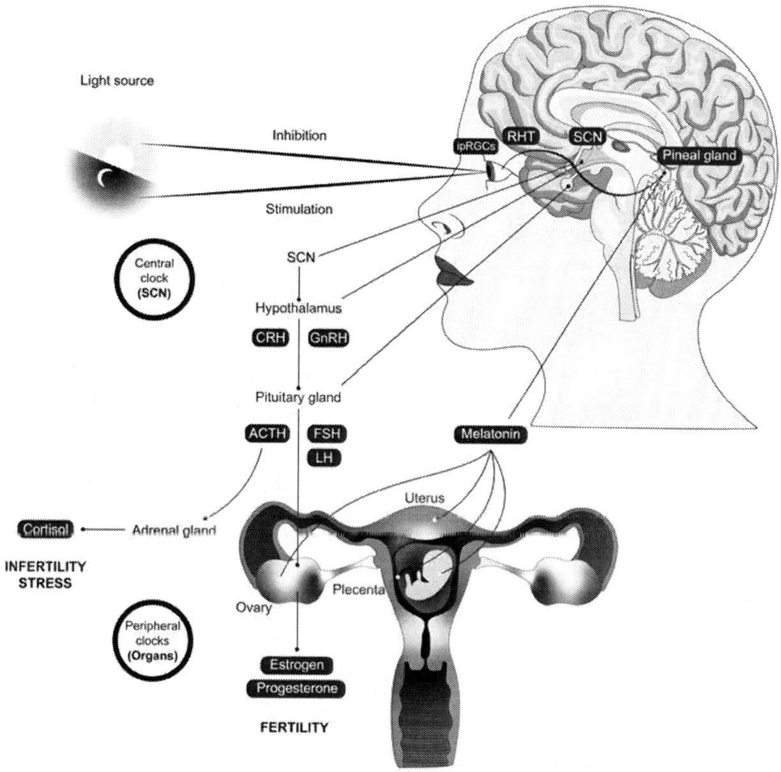

Figure 1. Schematic representation of the circadian clock in female reproduction regulation. The circadian clock regulates reproductive organs and hormone secretion through a central clock and a peripheral clock where light serves as a main modulator. The light signal at ipRGCs is transported to the SCN through RHT. SCN initiated signals in the brain mediate GnRH release from hypothalamus that triggers FSH and LH secretion from the pituitary gland. When the circadian clock is disrupted by irregular timing of light, cortisol release is stimulated by ACTH secretion from the pituitary gland that is triggered by CRH. Melatonin release from the pineal gland is directly regulated by the timing of the light, in which it incorporates several mechanisms in female reproductive organs. ipRGCs, intrinsically photosensitive retinal ganglion cells; RHT, retinohypothalamic tract; SCN, suprachiasmatic nucleus; GnRH, gonadotropin-releasing hormone; CRH, corticotropin-releasing hormone; FSH, follicle-stimulating hormone; LH, luteinizing hormone; ACTH, adrenocorticotropic hormone.

The detrimental consequences of circadian disturbances on reproductive health are also linked to oxidative stress. Reactive oxygen species (ROS), which could damage cells and impede reproductive function, have been demonstrated to be produced in greater amounts when the circadian rhythm is disturbed. In oocytes, ROS can damage DNA, which affects fertility and increases the chance of complications during pregnancy. Melatonin levels are high in human ovarian follicular fluid, which is released by the pineal gland and ovaries. Melatonin in the ovarian follicles is important during ovulation because it protects the oocyte from oxidative damage. Reduced levels of follicular melatonin have been revealed to be related to greater levels of reactive oxygen species (ROS) and worse oocyte quality in infertile women. Sleep deprivation disrupts the natural release of melatonin and has a negative impact on reproductive health (Goldstein & Smith, 2016; Lateef & Akintubosun, 2020; Shao et al., 2021).

According to some findings, lifestyle changes, such as increasing exposure to natural light during the day and reducing exposure to artificial light at night, may be useful in enhancing reproductive results. Several investigations on the molecular mechanisms behind circadian clock failure and its consequences on female fertility are required to discover novel therapeutics for treating infertility caused by circadian clock dysfunction (Shechter et al., 2008).

Disrupting the Circadian Rhythm: Effects on Fertility of Man

Circadian rhythm disruptions, those caused by shift work or jet lag, have been proven to have a detrimental impact on men's reproductive health and fertility. According to the research, the condition may be triggered by disruptions in hormone control, inflammation, and oxidative stress. Studies have revealed a link between shift employment and sperm DNA damage, as well as reduced sperm motility and concentration. Another study revealed that prolonged exposure to light causes male infertility by lowering testosterone levels and increasing oxidative stress. Artificial light persistently disrupted the wake/sleep cycle and the circadian rhythm, ultimately reducing male fertility by lowering melatonin levels (Li et al., 2022). Long-term exposure to light enhanced sperm counts and motility, but extending darkness decreased the prevalence of sperm aberrations. In the meantime, both prolonged light and darkness modified the release of hormones and decreased the production of estradiol while raising FSH, LH, testosterone, and prolactin. Additionally, extended exposure to light elevated PER1/2 expression while decreasing BMAL1, whereas darkness boosted PER1/2, CLOCK, and RER-ERAB expression. Gene mutations in major circadian clock genes, such as BMAL1, are linked to male infertility. Male BMAL1 null mice, on the other hand, are infertile, having reduced testes and seminal vesicles, decreased seminiferous tubule size, and 70% lower sperm counts than normal males. In Bmal1 null mice, LH and testosterone levels were lowered by around 50% and 70%, respectively, although FSH levels were about 3.5-fold greater than in wild-type mice. (Li et al., 2022; Peterlin et al., 2019). The altered testicular function was also observed in CRY1 knockout animals. CRY1 deficiency, in particular, enhanced testicular germ cell death and lowered sperm count, and was related to differential expression of more than 300 testicular genes (Peterlin et al., 2019).

According to studies, men who work rotational or night shifts had lower sperm counts and less active sperm than those who work normal daytime hours. Additionally, jet lag can alter the rhythm of the secretion of hormones and damage reproductive capacity. Multiple time zone travel has been linked in studies to a decline in testosterone levels, which can affect sperm production and fertility.

Although the particular processes remain unclear, it is thought that the brain's central clock may be involved in controlling the endocrine system and regulating the levels of hormones. Furthermore, reduced levels of testosterone may be associated with stimulation of the hypothalamus-pituitary-adrenal (HPA) axis, which increases corticosteroid concentrations in the blood. Sleep deprivation lowers testosterone levels by inhibiting the HPG axis, which promotes corticosteroid secretion. Corticosterone levels rise as a result of a negative feedback loop that activates the HPA axis (Choi et al., 2016; Lateef & Akintubosun, 2020; Li et al., 2022; Rizk et al., 2020). The pituitary gland generates pituitary gonadotropins such as LH and FSH under the control of the hypothalamus. LH activates the Leydig cells, which contain LH receptors on their surface; the stimulated Leydig cells make and release testosterone. (Goldstein & Smith, 2016; Lateef & Akintubosun, 2020). Being sleep-deprived boosts the release of serotonin and Leydig cell death, both of which disrupt testosterone production. Those complicated interactions between many physiological systems eventually result in a decline in testosterone production, which may lead to male infertility (Figure 2) (Lateef & Akintubosun, 2020).

A complicated feedback loop that includes numerous hormones, such as testosterone, FSH, and LH, controls the endocrine system in males. GnRH, which is released by the hypothalamus, triggers the pituitary gland to produce LH and FSH. The testes are subsequently stimulated to make testosterone by these hormones (Lateef & Akintubosun, 2020).

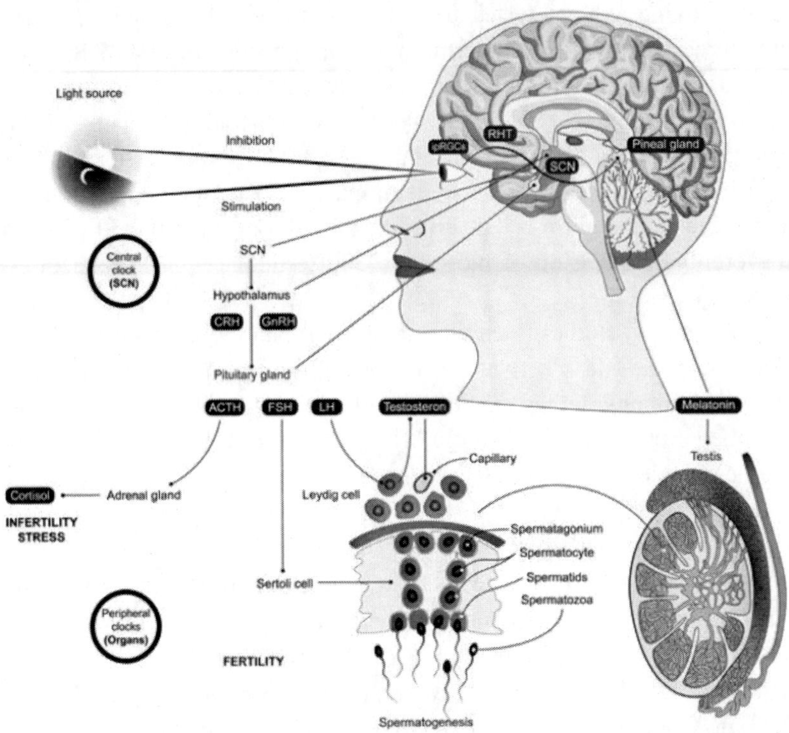

Figure 2. Schematic representation of the circadian clock in male reproduction regulation. The circadiam clock regulates reproductive organs and hormone secretion through a central clock and a peripheral clock where light serves as a main modulator. The light signal at ipRGCs is transported to the SCN through RHT. SCN initiated signals in the brain mediate GnRH release from the hypothalamus that triggers FSH and LH secretion from the pituitary gland, which affect Sertoli cells and Leyding cells in the testes, respectively. When the circadian clock is disrupted by irregular timing of light, cortisol release is stimulated by ACTH secretion from the pituitary gland that is triggered by CRH. Melatonin release from the pineal gland is directly regulated by the timing of the light, in which it incorporates several mechanisms in male reproductive organs. ipRGCs, intrinsically photosensitive retinal ganglion cells; RHT, retinohypothalamic tract; SCN, suprachiasmatic nucleus; GnRH, gonadotropin-releasing hormone; CRH, corticotropin-releasing hormone; FSH, follicle-stimulating hormone; LH, luteinizing hormone; ACTH, adrenocorticotropic hormone.

The frequency and magnitude of the secretion of hormones can be impacted by circadian rhythm dysregulation, and this can result in modifications to the levels of testosterone, FSH, and LH. For instance, compared to males who work conventional daytime hours, men who work rotating shifts or nights had lower testosterone levels and changed LH and FSH cycles (Figure 2) (Li et al., 2022).

The circadian clock regulates its production of hormones, including melatonin and cortisol, which have been shown to have a significant influence on reproductive function. Melatonin's antioxidant features are effective in avoiding oxidative stress which can damage reproductive cells (Goldstein & Smith, 2016; Lateef & Akintubosun, 2020; Shechter et al., 2008).

Additionally, inflammation and oxidative stress may cause circadian problems and might reduce sperm production and quality. The way the body responds to damage or illness is defined as inflammation, which is characterized by the production of cytokines and other inflammatory mediators. Immune cells that have been activated by chronic inflammation can harm sperm cells and hinder their synthesis. Moreover, inflammation can harm the testicles and damage the hormone balance that controls sperm production. According to studies, men who have chronic prostatitis, a disorder marked by inflammation of the prostate gland, have lower sperm counts and worse-quality sperm than men who do not have the disease (Li et al., 2022).

ROS are produced in excess amounts compared to the body's capacity to eliminate them using antioxidants, which causes oxidative stress. Through generating DNA damage, lipid peroxidation, and protein oxidation, ROS may affect sperm cells and limit their ability to function. Additionally, the synthesis of testosterone and other hormones required for the generation of sperm could be hampered by oxidative stress (Li et al., 2022).

The Impact of Light Exposure on Reproductive Health

Recent research indicates that exposure to light is critical for the control of the circadian clock and may possess a big impact on reproductive health. The female menstrual cycle and male reproductive function are two biological processes that are regulated by the circadian clock, an internal timing system. Fertility issues can result from disruptions in the circadian clock because they change the hormone levels required for ovulation and conception.

Daytime exposure to natural light has been reported to improve reproductive health and control the circadian cycle. The regular release of hormones required for reproductive function can, however, be disturbed by exposure to artificial light sources, including electronic devices. Both men's and women's reproductive health may be significantly impacted by these changes (Yaw et al., 2020).

A clinic survey found a higher frequency of PCOS among night-shift employees, stating the challenge of artificial light. According to the findings, exposure to the artificial light when sleeping during night increased the likelihood of developing overweight or obese, which is known as a feature of PCOS. As the SCN's primary input, light modulation may therefore reset circadian timing and is a potential treatment option for PCOS (Shao et al., 2021).

Further study is required to completely understand the complicated effects of light exposure on reproductive health. Researchers are investigating potential risks connected with specific forms of light exposure, such as blue light generated by electronic devices, as well as looking into the possible long-term impacts of light exposure over time. Exposure to this kind of light at night has been associated with reduced melatonin secretion and an increased risk of reproductive abnormalities, and it has been demonstrated that these devices are particularly disrupting the circadian cycle (Goldstein & Smith, 2016).

Additionally, scientists continue to investigate the various processes through which light exposure may affect reproductive health. Notably, research points to the potential importance of melatonin, a hormone involved in controlling the circadian rhythm, in this context. Melatonin may be used as a therapeutic intervention for people with problems of the circadian clock that affect reproductive function (Goldstein & Smith, 2016; Mills & Kuohung, 2019; Yaw et al., 2020).

Resetting the Circadian Clock: Implications for Improving Reproductive Health

Resetting the circadian clock may have a major impact on enhancing reproductive health outcomes. Changes in the hormone levels required for ovulation and fertilization driven by circadian clock disruptions might result in problems with fertility. On the other hand, the circadian clock can be reprogrammed using a variety of techniques, such as light therapy, pharmaceutical medications, chronotherapy, and behavioral treatment options. In order to optimize the body's normal sleep-wake cycle and restored the circadian clock, light therapy entails morning exposure to bright light. Utilizing melatonin, a hormone made by the pineal gland that is essential in controlling the circadian rhythm is one possible strategy (Goldstein & Smith, 2016; Roenneberg et al., 2016; Yalcin et al., 2022; Yaw et al., 2020).

Chronotherapy includes timing the delivery of medications to coincide with the body's circadian cycle, which can significantly affect the success of treatment. Supplementing with melatonin has been found to increase menstrual regularity in women with irregular periods and may enhance the success of reproductive therapies in couples. Furthermore, the hormone melatonin can influence clock timing, and novel agonists with higher potency and selectivity for the melatonin 2 receptor have been created (Sen & Sellix, 2016). Leuprolide acetate and goserelin acetate are two other pharmaceuticals that have been applied to inhibit GnRH and control menstrual periods in women with irregular cycles.

Resetting the circadian clock and enhancing reproductive health outcomes can both be significantly influenced by the timing of pharmaceutical delivery. The effectiveness of the therapy may be influenced by the timing of the administration of GnRH analogs, which are used to trigger ovulation in women undergoing assisted reproductive technology.

Additionally, behavioral treatments can help to reset the circadian rhythm and enhance reproductive health outcomes. It may be possible to improve reproductive outcomes by making lifestyle changes such as increasing physical activity and exposure to natural light during the day and reducing exposure to artificial light at night. Examples of these interventions include keeping a regular sleep-wake pattern and minimizing too much light at night (Li et al., 2022; Yalcin et al., 2022).

The chances of getting pregnant may be improved by interventions that restore hormonal balance and normal menstruation in women with irregular periods. Studies have revealed that treatments for the circadian rhythm, such as light therapy, behavioral modulations, and exercise, can help women with PCOS, a disorder that frequently results in infertility (Shao et al., 2021). Resetting the circadian rhythm in males may help to produce more and higher-quality sperm, which will eventually result in more successful fertilization.

Thus, melatonin supplementation, drug administration, light exposure optimization, and behavioral changes are the techniques to reset the circadian clock that have the potential to enhance reproductive health outcomes. Techniques such as chronotherapy and light therapy may be used to reduce the impacts and enhance reproductive health. A regular sleep schedule and other approaches to enhance sleep quality and sustain a normal circadian rhythm may also be used to lessen the harmful effects of circadian disruptions on reproductive health. The best strategies to reset the circadian clock and how this affects reproductive health require additional research. However, the prospective advantages of this technique for people seeking fertility preservation or dealing with infertility are encouraging. Resetting the circadian clock may be a useful strategy for enhancing reproductive health outcomes by increasing the control of menstrual cycle hormones and sperm quality and quantity (Yalcin et al., 2022).

Conclusion

In conclusion, it should be noted that the circadian clock is an essential system that controls a variety of physiological activities in the body. It is mostly regulated by a network of clock genes and proteins and is extremely responsive to environmental signals including light, temperature, and feeding cycles. The circadian clock is essential for general health and well-being, and it has been shown that disruptions to the circadian clock are associated with a number of health problems (Mills & Kuohung, 2019).

Alterations in hormone regulation, inflammation, and oxidative stress can all be involved a role in the detrimental consequences that circadian rhythm disruptions may have on both men's and women's reproductive health and fertility. Therapies such as chronotherapy and light therapy may be used to reduce the impacts and enhance reproductive health. A consistent sleep schedule and other methods to enhance sleep quality and maintain a normal circadian rhythm may also be used to reduce the harmful effects of circadian disturbances on reproductive health. To completely comprehend the processes through which circadian disturbances impair reproductive health and to create efficient therapies, more study is required (Goldstein & Smith, 2016; Roenneberg et al., 2016; Yalcin et al., 2022).

References

Boden, M. J., & Kennaway, D. J. (2006). Circadian rhythms and reproduction. *Reproduction (Cambridge, England)*, *132*(3), 379–392. https://doi.org/10.1530/REP.1.00614.

Chau, Y. M., West, S., & Mapedzahama, V. (2014). Night work and the reproductive health of women: an integrated literature review. *Journal of Midwifery & Women's Health*, *59*(2), 113–126. https://doi.org/10.1111/JMWH.12052.

Choi, J. H., Lee, S. H., Bae, J. H., Shim, J. S., Park, H. S., Kim, Y. S., & Shin, C. (2016). Effect of Sleep Deprivation on the Male Reproductive System in Rats. *Journal of Korean Medical Science*, *31*(10), 1624. https://doi.org/10.3346/JKMS.2016.31.10.1624.

Fishbein, A. B., Knutson, K. L., & Zee, P. C. (2021). Circadian disruption and human health. *The Journal of Clinical Investigation, 131*(19). https://doi.org/10.1172/JCI148286.

Goldstein, C. A., & Smith, Y. R. (2016). Sleep, Circadian Rhythms, and Fertility. *Current Sleep Medicine Reports 2016 2:4, 2*(4), 206–217. https://doi.org/10.1007/S40675-016-0057-9.

Kennaway, D. J., Boden, M. J., & Varcoe, T. J. (2012). Circadian rhythms and fertility. *Molecular and Cellular Endocrinology, 349*(1), 56–61. https://doi.org/10.1016/J.MCE.2011.08.013.

Lateef, O. M., & Akintubosun, M. O. (2020). Sleep and reproductive health. *Journal of Circadian Rhythms, 18*(1), 1–11. https://doi.org/https://doi.org/10.5334/jcr.190.

Lee, Y. (2022). Circadian Timing of the Female Reproductive System. *Chronobiology in Medicine, 4*(2), 58–64. https://doi.org/10.33069/CIM.2022.0017.

Li, T., Bai, Y., Jiang, Y., Jiang, K., Tian, Y., Gu, J., & Sun, F. (2022). The potential impacts of circadian rhythm disturbances on male fertility. *Frontiers in Endocrinology, 13*, 2473. https://doi.org/10.3389/FENDO.2022.1001316/BIBTEX.

Mills, J., & Kuohung, W. (2019). Impact of circadian rhythms on female reproduction and infertility treatment success. *Current Opinion in Endocrinology, Diabetes and Obesity, 26*(6), 317–321. https://doi.org/10.1097/MED.0000000000000511.

Peterlin, A., Kunej, T., & Peterlin, B. (2019). The role of circadian rhythm in male reproduction. *Current Opinion in Endocrinology, Diabetes, and Obesity, 26*(6), 313–316. https://doi.org/10.1097/MED.0000000000000512.

Pilorz, V., Helfrich-Förster, C., & Oster, H. (2018). The role of the circadian clock system in physiology. *Pflügers Archiv - European Journal of Physiology 2018 470:2, 470*(2), 227–239. https://doi.org/10.1007/S00424-017-2103-Y.

Rizk, N. I., Rizk, M. S., Mohamed, A. S., & Naguib, Y. M. (2020). Attenuation of sleep deprivation dependent deterioration in male fertility parameters by vitamin C. *Reproductive Biology and Endocrinology: RB&E, 18*(1). https://doi.org/10.1186/S12958-020-0563-Y.

Roenneberg, T., & Merrow, M. (2016). The Circadian Clock and Human Health. Current biology : CB, 26(10), R432–R443. https://doi.org/10.1016/j.cub.2016.04.011.

Sciarra, F., Franceschini, E., Campolo, F., Gianfrilli, D., Pallotti, F., Paoli, D., Isidori, A. M., & Venneri, M. A. (2020). Disruption of Circadian Rhythms: A Crucial Factor in the Etiology of Infertility. *International Journal of Molecular Sciences 2020, Vol. 21, Page 3943, 21*(11), 3943. https://doi.org/10.3390/IJMS21113943.

Sen, A., & Sellix, M. T. (2016). The Circadian Timing System and Environmental Circadian Disruption: From Follicles to Fertility. *Endocrinology, 157*(9), 3366–3373. https://doi.org/10.1210/EN.2016-1450.

Shao, S., Zhao, H., Lu, Z., Lei, X., & Zhang, Y. (2021). Circadian Rhythms Within the Female HPG Axis: From Physiology to Etiology. *Endocrinology, 162*(8). https://doi.org/10.1210/ENDOCR/BQAB117.

Shechter, A., James, F. O., & Boivin, D. B. (2008). Circadian Rhythms and Shift Working Women. *Sleep Medicine Clinics, 3*(1), 13–24. https://doi.org/10.1016/J.JSMC.2007.10.008.

Sletten, T. L., Cappuccio, F. P., Davidson, A. J., Van Cauter, E., Rajaratnam, S. M. W., & Scheer, F. A. J. L. (2020). Health consequences of circadian disruption. *Sleep*, *43*(1). https://doi.org/10.1093/SLEEP/ZSZ194.

Yalçin, M., Mundorf, A., Thiel, F., Amatriain-Fernández, S., Kalthoff, I. S., Beucke, J. C., Budde, H., Garthus-Niegel, S., Peterburs, J., & Relógio, A. (2022). It's About Time: The Circadian Network as Time-Keeper for Cognitive Functioning, Locomotor Activity and Mental Health. Frontiers in physiology, 13, 873237. https://doi.org/10.3389/fphys.2022.873237.

Yaw, A. M., McLane-Svoboda, A. K., & Hoffmann, H. M. (2020). Shiftwork and Light at Night Negatively Impact Molecular and Endocrine Timekeeping in the Female Reproductive Axis in Humans and Rodents. *International Journal of Molecular Sciences 2021, Vol. 22, Page 324*, *22*(1), 324. https://doi.org/10.3390/IJMS22010324.

Chapter 16

The Retinal Circadian Clock: Retinal Health and Retinal Disorders

Mahmut Doğan*, MD
Department of Ophthalmology, Yuksek Ihtisas University Faculty of Medicine, Ankara, Turkiye

Abstract

Circadian clocks are molecular pacemakers that regulate various behavioral and physiological processes according to the 24-hour light/dark cycle. Ocular clocks, which were first identified in the retina of the eye, have also been determined in the cornea, the retinal pigment epithelium (RPE), and the ciliary body. The retina represents a complex structure consisting of three layers and containing various cell types. Many studies have been conducted to determine which cell types in the retina have real clock properties. As a result of these studies, it has been determined that inner retinal neurons, as well as photoreceptors, also exhibit clock properties. However, clock properties are thought to be widely distributed among different retinal cell types. In mammals, only the cornea and retina maintain direct light-dependent phase regulation, which distinguishes the retina and probably other ocular clocks from peripheral oscillators, the phases of which depend on the rate-determining characteristics of the suprachiasmatic nuclei (SCN), the hypothalamic central brain clock. Dopamine and melatonin are used as light- and dark-adapting neuromodulators, respectively, by retinal circadian regulation in mammals and non-mammalian vertebrates, and the circadian phase can be regulated by light in an indirect manner via dopamine signaling. Circadian clocks in the eye are crucial for optimal

* Corresponding Author's Email: mahmutdogan13@gmail.com

In: Human Health is a Matter of Timing
Editors: Sumeyya Deniz Aybek, Gonca Gulbay and Mucahit Secme
ISBN: 979-8-89113-467-6

visual function, in which they are involved in fine-tuning visual sensitivity. The disrupted circadian rhythm in the retina through genetic or environmental stressors produces a state of circadian deviation associated with the development of different diseases, e.g., glaucoma, myopia, and RPE degeneration. The protective activity of molecules produced by the circadian rhythm in the retina against retinal inflammation, angiogenesis, apoptosis, and oxidative stress has been determined. This chapter presents the current knowledge about the retinal circadian clock, its molecular mechanism, and its potential role in eye diseases.

Keywords: circadian clocks, retina, melatonin, dopamine

Introduction

The enviromental changes that take place during the day/night cycle on a daily basis stimulate the life of the majority of living beings on the Earth. As a result, a daily rhythm occurs in living things. The rhythms mentioned above are not merely passive results of cyclical variations in the environment but arise from within the organism. An internal timing system called the circadian clock has been formed in living beings to predict changes brought by life and adjust physiology and behavior in accordance with the various requirements of day and night. In mammals, the main clock that controls 24-hour rhythms is located in the suprachiasmatic nuclei of the hypothalamus (SCN). The circadian clock in question temporally organizes various functions, such as sleep and food intake, and physiological events, including body temperature, hormone secretion, and heart rate. Experimental studies have demonstrated that the mammalian retina involves a complete circadian clock system. Additionally, a pathway that synchronizes the cycle of light with the environmental light/dark cycle of the retinal clock has been identified. The retinal circadian clock directs numerous processes in the retina, such as synaptic communication, gene expression, and metabolism, which restructure retinal circuits and shape retinal functioning according to the time of day. The circadian clock system in the retina enables predicting the normal cycle of scotopic and photopic visual conditions alternating with the day and night cycle. Acting as a gate for sensory information represents another essential function of the circadian clock. The above-mentioned function is a primary feature of sensory organs and systems across various types. This section of the book examines the mammalian retinal circadian clock, although reviews published before have included research on circadian rhythms in non-mammalian retinas (Besharse, 1982; Besharse et al., 1988; Cahill and Besharse, 1995).

A number of researches have demonstrated that the retinal circadian clock controls different features of mammalian retinal physiology and function. Some of these functions are as follows: dopamine synthesis (Nir et al., 2000; Doyle et al., 2002a; Doyle et al., 2002b), melatonin release (Besharse and Iuvone, 1983; Tosini and Menaker, 1996; Tosini and Menaker, 1998a; Tosini and Menaker, 1998b), gamma-aminobutyric acid (GABA) turnover and release (Jaliffa et al., 2001), UV opsin and rhodopsin gene expression (von Schantz et al., 1999), and electroretinogram (ERG) b-wave amplitude (Barnard et al., 2006; Storch et al., 2007). The mammalian retinal clock impacts the survival and development of retinal cells, including photoreceptor survival in animal retinal degeneration models (Ogilvie and Speck, 2002). Studies have shown that circadian signals arising from the retina influence rhythms in the hypothalamic biological clock, even when light/dark cycles are absent (Lee et al., 2003).

Molecules Involved in the Retinal Circadian Clock

Autoregulatory transcription/translation feedback loops creating near-24-hour cycles in gene expression produce circadian rhythms in the mammalian retina (Takahashi et al., 2008). The core circadian clock comprises an autoregulatory transcriptional-translational feedback loop (TTFL). In this cycle, the transcription factors CLOCK and BMAL1 heterodimerize to direct the expression of the Per and Cry genes through E-box response elements (Reppert et al., 2002). Then, CRY and PER proteins in a protein complex provide feedback to repress their transcription as a result of inhibiting the CLOCK:BMAL1 activity (Baba et al., 2022). The said inhibition is reversed by the disruption of PER and CRY, and TTFL restarts, resulting in an approximately 24-hour (hour) oscillation in PER/CRY generation and degradation. Figure 1 shows a scheme of the molecular circadian clock. Consequently, the core TTFL is known to be at the center of a complex network of additional feedback loops interacting to regulate the sensitivity and stability of the circadian clock (Cox et al., 2019).

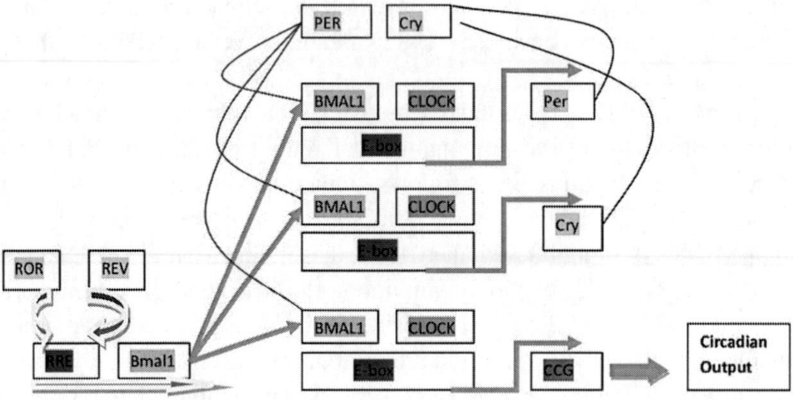

Figure 1. Scheme of the molecular circadian clock. The BMAL1:CLOCK heterodimer binds to the E-box in the promoter region of the Per and Cry genes. Afterward, PERs, along with CRYs, inhibit their transcription as a result of blocking the BMAL1:CLOCK action. The second feedback loop includes transactivating the Rev-Erb and Ror genes. There is a competition between REV-ERB and ROR for binding to RRE elements on the Bmal1 promoter, which drives a daily rhythm of Bmal1 transcription. A 24-hour rhythmic oscillation is produced by the feedback loops mentioned above.

Expression of Clock Genes

Many studies have primarily concentrated on the general expression of the essential molecular components of circadian oscillators in the retina (Peirson et al., 2006; Khampuis et al., 2005; Tosini et al., 2007a; Sandu et al., 2011; Schneider et al., 2010). When examined, the retina appears to be a heterogeneous tissue with circadian clocks in various subcell types. As shown by in situ hybridization research, the expression of clock genes in various cell types and phases is possible (Tosini et al., 2008).

One of the studies examined the expression of circadian clock proteins in the mouse retina (Liu et al., 2012). The said study reports that the core circadian clock proteins (PERIOD2, CRYPTOCHROME 2, CLOCK, NPAS2, PERIOD1, and BMAL1) are expressed in the inner and outer retina. However, the proteins in question display a diurnal and circadian variation only in cone photoreceptors. Nevertheless, we do not have precise information on the types of retinal cells that contain the circadian clock in the mammalian retina.

Clock Gene Reporters

Some research has utilized mice in which clock gene promoters are related to fluorescence or luminescence reporters providing an optical signal to quantify the gene. The said experimental studies have shown that it is successful in real-time reading of the circadian clock cycle in living tissues (Hastings et al., 2005).

Retinal Circadian Rhythms Are Disrupted by the Genetic Disruption of the Clock Gene Network

Studies have first approached the molecular organization of circadian clocks by knocking out clock genes in mice and then by behavioral tissue rhythmic analysis. Individual clock genes have been revealed to be crucial for clock function, with circadian rhythmicity lost after knockout. Such experimental studies have shown that the duties of individual clock genes differ across tissues, which suggests the possibility for tissue-specific variants of the basic circadian clock (Liu et al., 2007; Pendergast et al., 2010).

Neurochemical Organization

As mentioned previously, research into the molecular organization of the retinal circadian clock has demonstrated that more than one cell type can genetically produce and express circadian rhythms. Neurochemical communication between cell types has been identified for the formation of retinal rhythms. It is known that GABA, glutamate, acetylcholine, melatonin, and dopamine, which are the main neuromodulators and neurotransmitters in the retina, are secreted in a circadian rhythm (Tosini and Menaker, 1996; Jaliffa et al., 2001; Doyle et al., 2001; Doyle et al., 2002a; Doyle et al., 2002b) and may function as synchronization signals across the retina.

Furthermore, there is a need for spike-mediated neurotransmission and the neuropeptide vasoactive intestinal polypeptide (VIP) for the purpose of maintaining cellular synchronization and tissue-level rhythms in the SCN neural clock (Yamaguchi et al., 2003; Aton et al., 2005; Maywood et al., 2006). It has been found that the generation of molecular rhythms in all explanted retinas is not blocked by neurotransmitters such as GABA, acetylcholine, and melatonin. All of the findings mentioned above indicate that, differently from the SCN neural clock, where cellular coupling is crucial for maintaining rhythms at the cellular and tissue levels, cellular coupling between clock cells in the retina can be at a minimal level. Because the retina is directly exposed to a daily light-dark cycle under normal conditions, the strong external synchronization input in question is adequate to maintain the rhythmic organization of individual cell oscillators when strong cellular coupling mechanisms are absent. In this way, the retinal clock as a tissue is thought to ensure cell synchronization.

Neurotransmitters

It is known that none of the main neurotransmitters in the retina are required for rhythm production. However, two neurotransmitters have remarkable impacts on the other key features of the retinal circadian clock: The circadian clock of the retinal is reset by changing dopamine levels, whereas the rhythm amplitude is changed by altering GABA levels.

Dopamine secretion occurs in the retina in a circadian rhythm, at high levels during the daytime part of the circadian cycle. However, dopamine is also released in the retina as a reaction to light in the mammalian retina. Studies have found that the dopaminergic amacrine cells of the inner nuclear layer represent the dopamine source in the retina. These cells receive light input from cones and rods via bipolar cells and from ipRGCs via retrograde intra-retinal transmission (Zhang et al., 2008; Zhang et al., 2012). The dopamine that amacrine cells release affects many dopaminergic cells of the retina, bipolar cells, horizontal cells, and photoreceptor terminals of the outer retinal layers (Witkovsky, 2004). The role of retinal dopamine in the light resetting of the retinal clock was demonstrated for the first time in Xenopus, where the blocking of dopaminergic transmission through D2-like receptors was demonstrated to block phase shifts of melatonin secretion induced by light (Cahill and Besharse, 1991). Consequently, although the exact circuit has not been formed, it is evident that dopamine serves as a crucial input to clock neurons in the retina by mediating the impacts of light on the clock phase.

GABA is the main inhibitory neurotransmitter in the retina, and horizontal and amacrine cells constitute the main source of GABA secretion. There are two types: GABA1 receptors that are ionotropic Clion channels and GABA2 receptors which are metabotropic G-protein coupled receptors. There are fluctuations in GABA levels in the retina in the circadian rhythm, and high

GABA levels are seen in the night part of the circadian cycle (Jaliffa et al., 2001). The function of GABAergic impacts on the retinal clock gene cycle is less obvious compared to dopamine, suggesting that although dopamine represents a circadian signal for the day phase in the retina, GABA can be a circadian signal potentiating the night phase. Peaks in retinal GABA levels are observed at night (McMahon et al., 2014).

Signal Transmission between Clocks

The daily light-dark cycle is signaled to the hypothalamic SCN circadian clock by the retina through a specialized subset of intrinsically photosensitive retinal ganglion cells expressing the photopigment melanopsin (Berson 2003). Furthermore, apart from the said light-driven circadian signals, there are pieces of evidence indicating that retinal circadian signaling can take place without light:dark stimulation. For instance, in constant darkness, there are subregions of the SCN clock nuclei expressing retina-driven circadian rhythms (Lee et al., 2003). The retina receptor region of the mouse SCN clock displays circadian rhythms in the phosphorylation of the signaling kinase ERKα molecule, which is activated by the retinal ganglion cell entry into the retina under normal conditions (Besharse et al., 2016).

It has been demonstrated that clock genes are expressed by ipRGCs (Liu et al., 2012), and circadian rhythm and dopamine modulate their light responses (Weng et al., 2009; Van Hook et al., 2012). It has been revealed that the retina-driven rhythms in the SCN arise from ipRGCs themselves or from retinal neurons with synaptic input to ipRGCs that express melanopsin. Additionally, ipRGCs may take part in regulating circadian rhythm at the beginning of the postnatal period (Chew et al., 2017).

In conclusion, evidence from many experimental studies shows that ocular rhythms do not depend on the presence of SCN. Additionally, if the 24-hour rhythm persists after the removal of the SCN, this rhythm cannot be dragged into a novel light:dark schedule, indicating that the SCN or other brain region can play a role in regulating the aforesaid rhythm (Teirstein et al., 1980).

Potential Role of the Retinal Clock in Eye Diseases

Myopia and Refractive Development of the Eye

Considering its pathophysiology, myopia represents a complex disease that arises due to genetic and environmental factors. In the past, insufficient lighting or inadequate exposure to the outdoors was indicated as the etiology of myopia (Hobday, 2016). Later studies found that children were protected against myopia by exposure to the outdoors or natural light early in their life (French et al., 2013). Nowadays, light-induced retinal signaling has been revealed to be an essential factor for refractive error in myopia (Tedja et al., 2018; Wallman and Winawer, 2004; Zhou et al., 2017). A recent meta-analysis has proven that refractive errors are related to "circadian rhythms" and "circadian regulation of gene expression" (Hysi et al., 2020). However, artificial lighting in dark hours and computer usage for long hours make a contribution to the disease development and progression (Chakraborty et al., 2018). Studies have found that eye sizes fluctuate daily in both animal models and human eyes (Burfield et al., 2018; Chakraborty et al., 2011; Stone et al., 2013; Nickla, 2013). These changes occur in three layers: axial length, choroidal thickness, and vitreous cavity (Chakraborty et al., 2018). As a result of these studies, it has been determined that eye sizes and even changes during the day change in response to the applied optical defocus (Chakraborty et al., 2012; Nickla, 2013). Moreover, it has been observed that the applied optical focusing disrupts the rhythmic expression patterns of a number of clock genes in the retina/RPE and choroid (Stone et al., 2020). The data obtained from these studies confirm the possible connection between circadian clock mechanisms, refraction, and the retina. The mentioned connection can also be essential for the development of eyes. In the retina-specific Bmal1 KO mouse, a longer axial length and an elongated vitreous chamber developed in the eyes (Stone et al., 2019). Accordingly, KO mice were considerably more myopic compared to the control ones. However, similar anatomical variations have been stated in chicks raised under continuous light, which reveals the necessity of an appropriate day/night rhythm for the optimal growth of eyes (Stone et al., 1995). It is an interesting fact that brief bright light has also been reported to inhibit the growth of myopic eyes in case of exposure at a certain time of the day (evening) (Sarfare et al., 2020). In light of all these data, it has been seen that the effects of illumination on refraction development support the idea that it is linked to the circadian clock.

Diabetic Retinopathy

In diabetic retinopathy (DR), retinal vessels are damaged due to hyperglycemia, which leads to the occurrence of ischemic areas and exudation from capillaries, contributing to macular edema. Some studies have asserted a robust connection between the circadian clock and DR. First, DR was linked to decreased clock gene expression in the rat retina (Busik et al., 2009). On the contrary, another study showed that in mice, circadian disruption due to the Per2 mutation triggered DR, possibly via a retinal microvasculature phenotype (Bhatwadekar et al., 2013; Jadhav et al., 2016). In other studies supporting this result, it was observed that in the mouse retina, disorders in the circadian and dopamine-related regulation of fatty acid oxidation enzymes, which are necessary for the adaptation of energy metabolism on a daily basis, cause DR pathology (Vancura et al., 2016). In addition, research in patients with diabetes has determined that diabetes can disrupt circadian clock genes and, therefore, circadian rhythms. As a result, the retinal self-repair is weakened by the damage to the biological clock, leading to the progression of diabetic retinopathy (Liu et al., 2023). Furthermore, a study has found that the circadian rhythm is disrupted in several steps in diabetic retinopathy. These can be listed as follows: a decrease in melatonin, metabolic dysfunction, dysfunctional clock genes, and the changing rhythm of retinal thickness (Bhatwadekar et al., 2020).

Anterior Eye Segment: Cornea and Cataract

Some researches used Bmal1 and Clock KO mice. A study determined that the clear lens of mice became cloudy and cataracts developed. It has been suggested that this may be related to an acceleration in aging in the Bmal1 KO case (Dubrovsky et al., 2010; Kondratov et al., 2006). Recent studies have shown that Bmal1 depletion impairs antioxidant defense pathways in lens epithelial cells and derived cell lines, causing their vulnerability to reactive oxygen species (ROS) accumulation and apoptosis (Chhunchha et al., 2020).

Initial research on mice has shown that ocular abnormalities caused by Bmal1 or Clock deficiency also involve corneal inflammation (Dubrovsky et al., 2010; Kondratov et al., 2006; Yang et al., 2016). Signals coming from the retina drift these rhythms, the lights measured in all corneas. It has been determined that the healing process of the corneal epithelium is disrupted, i.e., wound healing and mitosis are impaired in case of the replacement of normal environmental lighting cycles with modified light programs (constant light and darkness, reverse LD, and jet-lag conditions) (Xue et al., 2017).

Age-Related Macular Degeneration (AMD)

AMD represents a progressive and chronic disease of the central retina that may progress with subretinal drusen formation and neovascularization (Bergen et al., 2019). Despite the unknown exact cause, it is known that oxidative stress, lipid metabolism, complement system, and local extracellular matrix variations play a role in the disease pathophysiology. Although there are not many studies showing the possible duty of the clock in AMD development, it is thought that clock dysfunction can lead to phenotypic variability in AMD due to the great significance of oxidative stress in AMD and the fact that circadian clocks constitute the main regulators of metabolism and the cellular redox state (Fanjul-Moles and Lopez-Riquelme, 2016; Ruan et al., 2021). In addition, it is known that the circadian rhythm controls the biosynthesis and transformation of the oxidative stress-protective melanin pigment in the RPE (Bergen, 2012). Finally, genetic, translation, and transduction research has found that genetic variants in the Rora CLOCK gene impact neovascular AMD (Jun et al., 2011; Silveira et al., 2010).

Glaucoma

Glaucoma is a multifactorial disease characterized by RGC degeneration leading to optic nerve damage and causing permanent vision defects in the visual field. Although the etiology of glaucoma is unclear, the most important risk factor is high intraocular pressure. It is known that IOP shows diurnal variation throughout the 24-hour circadian cycle (Aihara et al., 2003; Lozano et al., 2015; Nickla et al., 1998; Read et al., 2008). Studies have found that the intraocular pressure rhythm is at least partially linked to the circadian clock (Maeda et al., 2006) and have stated that clock genes are rhythmically expressed in the iris-ciliary body complex (Dalvin and Fautsch, 2015; Tsuchiya et al., 2017). This rhythmic expression is thought to depend on signals coming from the SCN through sympathetic pathway activation (Ikegami et al., 2020). IOP peaks at night (Liu et al., 1998). It has been suggested that the translaminar pressure on the optic nerve head, not the IOP alone, determines RGC damage in the pathophysiology of glaucoma. This may explain the vision loss in subjects with normal-tension glaucoma. Hence, it is possible to define translaminar pressure as the difference in pressure between IOP and intracerebral pressure (ICP) (Janssen et al., 2013). Additionally, the choroid plexus, which is involved in cerebrospinal fluid production in the brain, houses a circadian clock (Myung et al., 2018). Finally, differently from IOP and ICP, systemic blood pressure is at a minimum level at night (Bowe et al., 2015), which may raise the risk of decreased perfusion of eye and brain tissues during the night and make a possible contribution to the progression of glaucoma (Ciulla et al., 2020). In conclusion, the association between the fluid pressure controlled by the circadian rhythm in the related body parts within the framework of glaucoma development is complicated and requires more research to become clear.

Conclusion

Numerous recent studies have shown that it enhances the effect of the retinal circadian clock on numerous retinal functions. The melatonin-dopamine system represents the signaling pathway, which ensures that the retinal circadian clock rewires retinal circuits to improve light-adapted cone-mediated visual function in the daytime and dark-adapted rod-mediated visual signaling at night. Furthermore, circadian rhythms are also controlled by the retinal circadian clock in disc shedding, phagocytosis, and probably IOP. Moreover, the circadian clock plays a role in the pathogenesis of eye diseases, and data from experimental studies show that the dysfunction of the retinal circadian system adversely affects photoreceptors, RGCs, RPE, and probably the lens and cornea.

There are still issues that should be clarified concerning the circadian system functioning. There is a need for more research with more information on these issues.

References

Aihara, M., Lindsey, J. D., & Weinreb, R. N. (2003). Twenty-four-hour pattern of mouse intraocular pressure. *Experimental eye research*, 77(6), 681–686. https://doi.org/10.1016/j.exer.2003.08.011.

Aton, S. J., Colwell, C. S., Harmar, A. J., Waschek, J., & Herzog, E. D. (2005). Vasoactive intestinal polypeptide mediates circadian rhythmicity and synchrony in mammalian clock neurons. *Nature neuroscience*, *8*(4), 476–483. https://doi.org/10.1038/nn1419.

Aung, M. H., Park, H. N., Han, M. K., Obertone, T. S., Abey, J., Aseem, F., Thule, P. M., Iuvone, P. M., & Pardue, M. T. (2014). Dopamine deficiency contributes to early visual dysfunction in a rodent model of type 1 diabetes. *The Journal of neuroscience: the official journal of the Society for Neuroscience*, *34*(3), 726–736. https://doi.org/10.1523/JNEUROSCI.3483-13.2014.

Baba, K., Goyal, V., & Tosini, G. (2022). Circadian Regulation of Retinal Pigment Epithelium Function. *International journal of molecular sciences*, *23*(5), 2699. https://doi.org/10.3390/ijms23052699.

Barnard, A. R., Hattar, S., Hankins, M. W., & Lucas, R. J. (2006). Melanopsin regulates visual processing in the mouse retina. *Current biology: CB*, *16*(4), 389–395. https://doi.org/10.1016/j.cub.2005.12.045.

Bergen, A. A., Arya, S., Koster, C., Pilgrim, M. G., Wiatrek-Moumoulidis, D., van der Spek, P. J., Hauck, S. M., Boon, C. J. F., Emri, E., Stewart, A. J., & Lengyel, I. (2019). On the origin of proteins in human drusen: The meet, greet and stick hypothesis. *Progress in retinal and eye research*, *70*, 55–84. https://doi.org/10.1016/j.preteyeres.2018.12.003.

Bergen, A. A., Arya, S., Koster, C., Pilgrim, M. G., Wiatrek-Moumoulidis, D., van der Spek, P. J., Hauck, S. M., Boon, C. J. F., Emri, E., Stewart, A. J., & Lengyel, I. (2019). On the origin of proteins in human drusen: The meet, greet and stick hypothesis. *Progress in retinal and eye research*, *70*, 55–84. https://doi.org/10.1016/j.preteyeres.2018.12.003.

Berson D. M. (2003). Strange vision: ganglion cells as circadian photoreceptors. *Trends in neurosciences*, *26*(6), 314–320. https://doi.org/10.1016/S0166-2236(03)00130-9.

Besharse JC. *The daily light-dark cycle and rhythmic metabolism in the photoreceptor—Pigment epithelial complex. Progress in Retinal Research.* 1982; 1:81–124. https://doi.org/10.1007/BF00966866.

Besharse, J. C., & Iuvone, P. M. (1983). Circadian clock in Xenopus eye controlling retinal serotonin N-acetyltransferase. *Nature*, *305*(5930), 133–135. https://doi.org/10.1038/305133a0.

Besharse, J. C., & McMahon, D. G. (2016). The Retina and Other Light-sensitive Ocular Clocks. *Journal of biological rhythms*, *31*(3), 223–243. https://doi.org/10.1177/0748730416642657.

Bhatwadekar, A. D., Yan, Y., Qi, X., Thinschmidt, J. S., Neu, M. B., Li Calzi, S., Shaw, L. C., Dominiguez, J. M., Busik, J. V., Lee, C., Boulton, M. E., & Grant, M. B. (2013). Per2 mutation recapitulates the vascular phenotype of diabetes in the retina and bone marrow. *Diabetes*, *62*(1), 273–282. https://doi.org/10.2337/db12-0172.

Bhatwadekar, A. D., & Rameswara, V. (2020). Circadian rhythms in diabetic retinopathy: an overview of pathogenesis and investigational drugs. *Expert opinion on investigational drugs*, *29*(12), 1431–1442. https://doi.org/10.1080/13543784.2020.1842872.

Bowe, A., Grünig, M., Schubert, J., Demir, M., Hoffmann, V., Kütting, F., Pelc, A., & Steffen, H. M. (2015). Circadian Variation in Arterial Blood Pressure and

Glaucomatous Optic Neuropathy--A Systematic Review and Meta-Analysis. *American journal of hypertension*, *28*(9), 1077–1082. https://doi.org/10.1093/ajh/hpv016.

Burfield, H. J., Patel, N. B., & Ostrin, L. A. (2018). Ocular Biometric Diurnal Rhythms in Emmetropic and Myopic Adults. *Investigative ophthalmology & visual science*, *59*(12), 5176–5187. https://doi.org/10.1167/iovs.18-25389.

Busik, J. V., Tikhonenko, M., Bhatwadekar, A., Opreanu, M., Yakubova, N., Caballero, S., Player, D., Nakagawa, T., Afzal, A., Kielczewski, J., Sochacki, A., Hasty, S., Li Calzi, S., Kim, S., Duclas, S. K., Segal, M. S., Guberski, D. L., Esselman, W. J., Boulton, M.E., Grant, M. B., 2009. *Diabetic retinopathy is associated with bone marrow neuropathy and a depressed peripheral clock. J. Exp. Med.* 206, 2897–2906. https://doi.org/10.1084/jem.20090889.

Cahill GM, Besharse JC. *Circadian rhythmicity in vertebrate retinas: regulation by a photoreceptor oscillator. Progress in Retinal and Eye Research.* 1995; 14:267–291. https://doi.org/10.1016/1350-9462(94)00001-Y.

Cahill, G. M., & Besharse, J. C. (1991). Resetting the circadian clock in cultured Xenopus eyecups: regulation of retinal melatonin rhythms by light and D2 dopamine receptors. *The Journal of neuroscience: the official journal of the Society for Neuroscience*, *11*(10), 2959–2971. https://doi.org/10.1523/JNEUROSCI.11-10-02959.1991.

Chakraborty, R., Ostrin, L. A., Nickla, D. L., Iuvone, P. M., Pardue, M. T., & Stone, R. A. (2018). Circadian rhythms, refractive development, and myopia. *Ophthalmic & physiological optics: the journal of the British College of Ophthalmic Opticians (Optometrists)*, *38*(3), 217–245. https://doi.org/10.1111/opo.12453.

Chakraborty, R., Read, S. A., & Collins, M. J. (2012). Monocular myopic defocus and daily changes in axial length and choroidal thickness of human eyes. *Experimental eye research*, *103*, 47–54. https://doi.org/10.1016/j.exer.2012.08.002.

Chakraborty, R., Read, S. A., & Collins, M. J. (2012). Monocular myopic defocus and daily changes in axial length and choroidal thickness of human eyes. *Experimental eye research*, *103*, 47–54. https://doi.org/10.1016/j.exer.2012.08.002.

Chew, K. S., Renna, J. M., McNeill, D. S., Fernandez, D. C., Keenan, W. T., Thomsen, M. B., Ecker, J. L., Loevinsohn, G. S., VanDunk, C., Vicarel, D. C., Tufford, A., Weng, S., Gray, P. A., Cayouette, M., Herzog, E. D., Zhao, H., Berson, D. M., & Hattar, S. (2017). A subset of ipRGCs regulates both maturation of the circadian clock and segregation of retinogeniculate projections in mice. *eLife*, *6*, e22861. https://doi.org/10.7554/eLife.22861.

Chhunchha, B., Kubo, E., & Singh, D. P. (2020). Clock Protein Bmal1 and Nrf2 Cooperatively Control Aging or Oxidative Response and Redox Homeostasis by Regulating Rhythmic Expression of Prdx6. *Cells*, *9*(8), 1861. https://doi.org/10.3390/cells9081861.

Ciulla, L., Moorthy, M., Mathew, S., Siesky, B., Verticchio Vercellin, A. C., Price, D., Januleviciene, I., & Harris, A. (2020). Circadian Rhythm and Glaucoma: What do We Know?. *Journal of glaucoma*, *29*(2), 127–132. https://doi.org/10.1097/IJG.0000000000001402.

Cox, K. H., & Takahashi, J. S. (2019). Circadian clock genes and the transcriptional architecture of the clock mechanism. *Journal of molecular endocrinology*, *63*(4), R93–R102. https://doi.org/10.1530/JME-19-0153.

Dalvin, L. A., Fautsch, M. P., (2015). Analysis of circadian rhythm gene expression with reference to diurnal pattern of intraocular pressure in mice. *Invest. Ophthalmol. Vis. Sci.* 56, 2657–2663. https://doi.org/10.1167/iovs.15-16449.

Dinet, V., Ansari, N., Torres-Farfan, C., & Korf, H. W. (2007). Clock gene expression in the retina of melatonin-proficient (C3H) and melatonin-deficient (C57BL) mice. *Journal of pineal research*, *42*(1), 83–91. https://doi.org/10.1111/j.1600-079X.2006.00387.x.

Doyle, S. E., Grace, M. S., McIvor, W., & Menaker, M. (2002). Circadian rhythms of dopamine in mouse retina: the role of melatonin. *Visual neuroscience*, *19*(5), 593–601. https://doi.org/10.1017/s0952523802195058.

Dubrovsky, Y. V., Samsa, W. E., & Kondratov, R. V. (2010). Deficiency of circadian protein CLOCK reduces lifespan and increases age-related cataract development in mice. *Aging*, *2*(12), 936–944. https://doi.org/10.18632/aging.100241.

Fanjul-Moles, M. L., & López-Riquelme, G. O. (2016). Relationship between Oxidative Stress, Circadian Rhythms, and AMD. *Oxidative medicine and cellular longevity*, *2016*, 7420637. https://doi.org/10.1155/2016/7420637.

French, A. N., Ashby, R. S., Morgan, I. G., & Rose, K. A. (2013). Time outdoors and the prevention of myopia. *Experimental eye research*, *114*, 58–68. https://doi.org/10.1016/j.exer.2013.04.018.

Hastings, M. H., Reddy, A. B., McMahon, D. G., & Maywood, E. S. (2005). Analysis of circadian mechanisms in the suprachiasmatic nucleus by transgenesis and biolistic transfection. *Methods in enzymology*, *393*, 579–592. https://doi.org/10.1016/S0076-6879(05)93030-9.

Hobday R. (2016). Myopia and daylight in schools: a neglected aspect of public health?. *Perspectives in public health*, *136*(1), 50–55. https://doi.org/10.1177/1757913915576679.

Hysi, PG, Choquet, H, Khawaja, AP, Wojciechowski, R, Tedja, MS, Yin, J, Simcoe, MJ, Patasova, K, Mahroo, OA, Thai, KK, Cumberland, PM, Melles, RB, Verhoeven, VJM, Vitart, V, Segre, A, Stone, RA, Wareham, N, Hewitt, AW, Mackey, DA, Klaver, CCW, MacGregor, S, Khaw, PT, Foster, PJ, Guggenheim, JA, Rahi, JS, Jorgenson, E, Hammond, CJ, 2020. Meta-analysis of 542,934 subjects of European ancestry identifies new genes and mechanisms predisposing to refractive error and myopia. *Nat. Genet.* 52, 401–407. https://doi.org/10.1038/s41588-020-0599-0.

Ikegami, K., Shigeyoshi, Y., & Masubuchi, S. (2020). Circadian Regulation of IOP Rhythm by Dual Pathways of Glucocorticoids and the Sympathetic Nervous System. *Investigative ophthalmology & visual science*, *61*(3), 26. https://doi.org/10.1167/iovs.61.3.26.

Jadhav, V., Luo, Q., M Dominguez, J., 2nd, Al-Sabah, J., Chaqour, B., Grant, M. B., & Bhatwadekar, A. D. (2016). Per2-Mediated Vascular Dysfunction Is Caused by the Upregulation of the Connective Tissue Growth Factor (CTGF). *PloS one*, *11*(9), e0163367. https://doi.org/10.1371/journal.pone.0163367.

Jaliffa, C. O., Saenz, D., Resnik, E., Keller Sarmiento, M. I., & Rosenstein, R. E. (2001). Circadian activity of the GABAergic system in the golden hamster retina. *Brain research*, *912*(2), 195–202. https://doi.org/10.1016/s0006-8993(01)02736-6.

Janssen, S. F., Gorgels, T. G., Ramdas, W. D., Klaver, C. C., van Duijn, C. M., Jansonius, N. M., & Bergen, A. A. (2013). The vast complexity of primary open angle glaucoma: disease genes, risks, molecular mechanisms and pathobiology. *Progress in retinal and eye research*, *37*, 31–67. https://doi.org/10.1016/j.preteyeres.2013.09.001.

Jun, G., Nicolaou, M., Morrison, M. A., Buros, J., Morgan, D. J., Radeke, M. J., Yonekawa, Y., Tsironi, E. E., Kotoula, M. G., Zacharaki, F., Mollema, N., Yuan, Y., Miller, J. W., Haider, N. B., Hageman, G. S., Kim, I. K., Schaumberg, D. A., Farrer, L. A., & DeAngelis, M. M. (2011). Influence of ROBO1 and RORA on risk of age-related macular degeneration reveals genetically distinct phenotypes in disease pathophysiology. *PloS one*, *6*(10), e25775. https://doi.org/10.1371/journal.pone.0025775.

Kamphuis, W., Cailotto, C., Dijk, F., Bergen, A., & Buijs, R. M. (2005). Circadian expression of clock genes and clock-controlled genes in the rat retina. *Biochemical and biophysical research communications*, *330*(1), 18–26. https://doi.org/10.1016/j.bbrc.2005.02.118.

Kondratov, R. V., Kondratova, A. A., Gorbacheva, V. Y., Vykhovanets, O. V., & Antoch, M. P. (2006). Early aging and age-related pathologies in mice deficient in BMAL1, the core component of the circadian clock. *Genes & development*, *20*(14), 1868–1873. https://doi.org/10.1101/gad.1432206.

Lee, H. S., Nelms, J. L., Nguyen, M., Silver, R., & Lehman, M. N. (2003). The eye is necessary for a circadian rhythm in the suprachiasmatic nucleus. *Nature neuroscience*, *6*(2), 111–112. https://doi.org/10.1038/nn1006.

Liu, A. C., Welsh, D. K., Ko, C. H., Tran, H. G., Zhang, E. E., Priest, A. A., Buhr, E. D., Singer, O., Meeker, K., Verma, I. M., Doyle, F. J., 3rd, Takahashi, J. S., & Kay, S. A. (2007). Intercellular coupling confers robustness against mutations in the SCN circadian clock network. *Cell*, *129*(3), 605–616. https://doi.org/10.1016/j.cell.2007.02.047.

Liu, J. H., Kripke, D. F., Hoffman, R. E., Twa, M. D., Loving, R. T., Rex, K. M., Gupta, N., & Weinreb, R. N. (1998). Nocturnal elevation of intraocular pressure in young adults. *Investigative ophthalmology & visual science*, *39*(13), 2707–2712.

Liu, W. J., Chen, J. Y., Niu, S. R., Zheng, Y. S., Lin, S., & Hong, Y. (2023). Recent advances in the study of circadian rhythm disorders that induce diabetic retinopathy. *Biomedicine & pharmacotherapy = Biomedecine & pharmacotherapie*, *166*, 115368. https://doi.org/10.1016/j.biopha.2023.115368.

Lozano, D. C., Hartwick, A. T., & Twa, M. D. (2015). Circadian rhythm of intraocular pressure in the adult rat. *Chronobiology international*, *32*(4), 513–523. https://doi.org/10.3109/07420528.2015.1008135.

Maeda, A., Tsujiya, S., Higashide, T., Toida, K., Todo, T., Ueyama, T., Okamura, H., & Sugiyama, K. (2006). Circadian intraocular pressure rhythm is generated by clock genes. *Investigative ophthalmology & visual science*, *47*(9), 4050–4052. https://doi.org/10.1167/iovs.06-0183.

Maywood, E. S., Reddy, A. B., Wong, G. K., O'Neill, J. S., O'Brien, J. A., McMahon, D. G., Harmar, A. J., Okamura, H., & Hastings, M. H. (2006). Synchronization and maintenance of timekeeping in suprachiasmatic circadian clock cells by neuropeptidergic signaling. *Current biology: CB*, *16*(6), 599–605. https://doi.org/10.1016/j.cub.2006.02.0232006; 16:599–605. [PubMed: 16546085] doi: 10.1016/j.cub.2006.02.023.

McMahon, D. G., Iuvone, P. M., & Tosini, G. (2014). Circadian organization of the mammalian retina: from gene regulation to physiology and diseases. *Progress in retinal and eye research*, *39*, 58–76. https://doi.org/10.1016/j.preteyeres.2013.12.001.

Myung, J., Schmal, C., Hong, S., Tsukizawa, Y., Rose, P., Zhang, Y., Holtzman, M. J., De Schutter, E., Herzel, H., Bordyugov, G., & Takumi, T. (2018). The choroid plexus is an important circadian clock component. *Nature communications*, *9*(1), 1062. https://doi.org/10.1038/s41467-018-03507-2.

Nickla D. L. (2013). Ocular diurnal rhythms and eye growth regulation: where we are 50 years after Lauber. *Experimental eye research*, *114*, 25–34. https://doi.org/10.1016/j.exer.2012.12.013.

Nickla, D. L., Wildsoet, C., & Wallman, J. (1998). The circadian rhythm in intraocular pressure and its relation to diurnal ocular growth changes in chicks. *Experimental eye research*, *66*(2), 183–193. https://doi.org/10.1006/exer.1997.0425.

Nir, I., Haque, R., & Iuvone, P. M. (2000). Diurnal metabolism of dopamine in the mouse retina. *Brain research*, *870*(1-2), 118–125. https://doi.org/10.1016/s0006-8993(00)02409-4.

Ogilvie, J. M., & Speck, J. D. (2002). Dopamine has a critical role in photoreceptor degeneration in the rd mouse. *Neurobiology of disease*, *10*(1), 33–40. https://doi.org/10.1006/nbdi.2002.0489.

Peirson, S. N., Butler, J. N., Duffield, G. E., Takher, S., Sharma, P., & Foster, R. G. (2006). Comparison of clock gene expression in SCN, retina, heart, and liver of mice. *Biochemical and biophysical research communications*, *351*(4), 800–807. https://doi.org/10.1016/j.bbrc.2006.10.118.

Pendergast, J. S., Friday, R. C., & Yamazaki, S. (2010). Distinct functions of Period2 and Period3 in the mouse circadian system revealed by in vitro analysis. *PloS one*, *5*(1), e8552. https://doi.org/10.1371/journal.pone.0008552.

Read, S. A., Collins, M. J., & Iskander, D. R. (2008). Diurnal variation of axial length, intraocular pressure, and anterior eye biometrics. *Investigative ophthalmology & visual science*, *49*(7), 2911–2918. https://doi.org/10.1167/iovs.08-1833.

Reppert, S., Weaver, D. Coordination of circadian timing in mammals. *Nature* 418, 935–941 (2002). https://doi.org/10.1038/nature00965.

Ruan, Y., Jiang, S., & Gericke, A. (2021). Age-Related Macular Degeneration: Role of Oxidative Stress and Blood Vessels. *International journal of molecular sciences*, *22*(3), 1296. https://doi.org/10.3390/ijms22031296.

Sandu, C., Hicks, D., & Felder-Schmittbuhl, M. P. (2011). Rat photoreceptor circadian oscillator strongly relies on lighting conditions. *The European journal of neuroscience*, *34*(3), 507–516. https://doi.org/10.1111/j.1460-9568.2011.07772.x.

Sarfare, S., Yang, J., & Nickla, D. L. (2020). The effects of brief high intensity light on ocular growth in chicks developing myopia vary with time of day. *Experimental eye research*, *195*, 108039. https://doi.org/10.1016/j.exer.2020.108039.

Schneider, K., Tippmann, S., Spiwoks-Becker, I., Holthues, H., Wolloscheck, T., Spatkowski, G., Engel, L., Frederiksen, U., & Spessert, R. (2010). Unique clockwork in photoreceptor of rat. *Journal of neurochemistry*, *115*(3), 585–594. https://doi.org/10.1111/j.1471-4159.2010.06953.x.

Sekaran, S., Lupi, D., Jones, S. L., Sheely, C. J., Hattar, S., Yau, K. W., Lucas, R. J., Foster, R. G., & Hankins, M. W. (2005). Melanopsin-dependent photoreception provides earliest light detection in the mammalian retina. *Current biology: CB*, *15*(12), 1099–1107. https://doi.org/10.1016/j.cub.2005.05.053.

Silveira, A .C., Morrison, M. A., Ji, F., Xu, H., Reinecke, J. B., Adams, S. M., Arneberg, T. M., Janssian, M., Lee, J. E., Yuan, Y., Schaumberg, D. A., Kotoula, M. G., Tsironi, E. E., Tsiloulis, A. N., Chatzoulis, D. Z., Miller, J. W., Kim, I. K., Hageman, G. S., Farrer, L. A., Haider, N. B., DeAngelis, M. M., 2010. Convergence of linkage, gene expression and association data demonstrates the influence of the RAR-related orphan receptor alpha (RORA) gene on neovascular AMD: a systems biology based approach. *Vis. Res. 50*, 698–715. https://doi.org/10.1016/j.visres.2009.09.016.

Stone, R. A., Lin, T., Desai, D., & Capehart, C. (1995). Photoperiod, early post-natal eye growth, and visual deprivation. *Vision research*, *35*(9), 1195–1202. https://doi.org/10.1016/0042-6989(94)00232-b.

Stone, R. A., McGlinn, A. M., Chakraborty, R., Lee, D. C., Yang, V., Elmasri, A., Landis, E., Shaffer, J., Iuvone, P. M., Zheng, X., Sehgal, A., & Pardue, M. T. (2019). Altered ocular parameters from circadian clock gene disruptions. *PloS one*, *14*(6), e0217111. https://doi.org/10.1371/journal.pone.0217111.

Stone, R. A., Pardue, M. T., Iuvone, P. M., & Khurana, T. S. (2013). Pharmacology of myopia and potential role for intrinsic retinal circadian rhythms. *Experimental eye research*, *114*, 35–47. https://doi.org/10.1016/j.exer.2013.01.001.

Stone, R. A., Wei, W., Sarfare, S., McGeehan, B., Engelhart, K. C., Khurana, T. S., Maguire, M. G., Iuvone, P. M., & Nickla, D. L. (2020). Visual Image Quality Impacts Circadian Rhythm-Related Gene Expression in Retina and in Choroid: A Potential Mechanism for Ametropias. *Investigative ophthalmology & visual science*, *61*(5), 13. https://doi.org/10.1167/iovs.61.5.13.

Storch, K. F., Paz, C., Signorovitch, J., Raviola, E., Pawlyk, B., Li, T., & Weitz, C. J. (2007). Intrinsic circadian clock of the mammalian retina: importance for retinal processing of visual information. *Cell*, *130*(4), 730–741. https://doi.org/10.1016/j.cell.2007.06.045.

Sugawara, T., Sieving, P. A., Iuvone, P. M., & Bush, R. A. (1998). The melatonin antagonist luzindole protects retinal photoreceptors from light damage in the rat. *Investigative ophthalmology & visual science*, *39*(12), 2458–2465.

Takahashi, J. S., Hong, H. K., Ko, C. H., & McDearmon, E. L. (2008). The genetics of mammalian circadian order and disorder: implications for physiology and disease. *Nature reviews. Genetics*, *9*(10), 764–775. https://doi.org/10.1038/nrg2430.

Teirstein, P. S., Goldman, A. I., & O'Brien, P. J. (1980). Evidence for both local and central regulation of rat rod outer segment disc shedding. *Investigative ophthalmology & visual science*, *19*(11), 1268–1273.

Tosini, G., & Menaker, M. (1996). Circadian rhythms in cultured mammalian retina. *Science (New York, N.Y.)*, *272*(5260), 419–421. https://doi.org/10.1126/science.272.5260.419.

Tosini, G., & Menaker, M. (1998). The clock in the mouse retina: melatonin synthesis and photoreceptor degeneration. *Brain research*, *789*(2), 221–228. https://doi.org/10.1016/s0006-8993(97)01446-7.

Tsuchiya, S., Buhr, E. D., Higashide, T., Sugiyama, K., & Van Gelder, R. N. (2017). Light entrainment of the murine intraocular pressure circadian rhythm utilizes non-local mechanisms. *PloS one*, *12*(9), e0184790. https://doi.org/10.1371/journal.pone.0184790.

Van Hook, M. J., Wong, K. Y., & Berson, D. M. (2012). Dopaminergic modulation of ganglion-cell photoreceptors in rat. *The European journal of neuroscience*, *35*(4), 507–518. https://doi.org/10.1111/j.1460-9568.2011.07975.x.

Vancura, P., Wolloscheck, T., Baba, K., Tosini, G., Iuvone, P. M., & Spessert, R. (2016). Circadian and Dopaminergic Regulation of Fatty Acid Oxidation Pathway Genes in Retina and Photoreceptor Cells. *PloS one*, *11*(10), e0164665. https://doi.org/10.1371/journal.pone.0164665.

von Schantz, M., Lucas, R. J., & Foster, R. G. (1999). Circadian oscillation of photopigment transcript levels in the mouse retina. *Brain research. Molecular brain research*, *72*(1), 108–114. https://doi.org/10.1016/s0169-328x(99)00209-0.

Wallman, J., & Winawer, J. (2004). Homeostasis of eye growth and the question of myopia. *Neuron*, *43*(4), 447–468. https://doi.org/10.1016/j.neuron.2004.08.008.

Weng, S., Wong, K. Y., & Berson, D. M. (2009). Circadian modulation of melanopsin-driven light response in rat ganglion-cell photoreceptors. *Journal of biological rhythms*, *24*(5), 391–402. https://doi.org/10.1177/0748730409343767.

Witkovsky P. (2004). Dopamine and retinal function. *Documenta ophthalmologica. Advances in ophthalmology*, *108*(1), 17–40. https://doi.org/10.1023/b:doop.0000019487.88486.0a.

Xue, Y., Liu, P., Wang, H., Xiao, C., Lin, C., Liu, J., Dong, D., Fu, T., Yang, Y., Wang, Z., Pan, H., Chen, J., Li, Y., Cai, D., Li, Z., 2017. Modulation of circadian rhythms affects corneal epithelium renewal and repair in mice. *Invest. Ophthalmol. Vis. Sci.* 58, 1865–1874. https://doi.org/10.1167/iovs.16-21154.

Yamaguchi, S., Isejima, H., Matsuo, T., Okura, R., Yagita, K., Kobayashi, M., & Okamura, H. (2003). Synchronization of cellular clocks in the suprachiasmatic nucleus. *Science (New York, N.Y.)*, *302*(5649), 1408–1412. https://doi.org/10.1126/science.1089287.

Yang, G., Chen, L., Grant, G. R., Paschos, G., Song, W. L., Musiek, E. S., Lee, V., McLoughlin, S. C., Grosser, T., Cotsarelis, G., & FitzGerald, G. A. (2016). Timing of expression of the core clock gene Bmal1 influences its effects on aging and survival. *Science translational medicine*, *8*(324), 324ra16. https://doi.org/10.1126/scitranslmed.aad3305.

Zhang, D. Q., Belenky, M. A., Sollars, P. J., Pickard, G. E., & McMahon, D. G. (2012). Melanopsin mediates retrograde visual signaling in the retina. *PloS one*, *7*(8), e42647. https://doi.org/10.1371/journal.pone.0042647.

Zhang, D. Q., Wong, K. Y., Sollars, P. J., Berson, D. M., Pickard, G. E., & McMahon, D. G. (2008). Intraretinal signaling by ganglion cell photoreceptors to dopaminergic amacrine neurons. *Proceedings of the National Academy of Sciences of the United States of America*, *105*(37), 14181–14186. https://doi.org/10.1073/pnas.0803893105.

Zhou, X., Pardue, M. T., Iuvone, P. M., & Qu, J. (2017). Dopamine signaling and myopia development: What are the key challenges. *Progress in retinal and eye research*, *61*, 60–71. https://doi.org/10.1016/j.preteyeres.2017.06.003.

Chapter 17

Physiopathology of Allergic Diseases and Their Relation to Circadian Rhythm

Gül Şahika Gökdemir*, PhD
Department of Physiology, Faculty of Medicine Mardin Artuklu University Mardin, Turkiye

Abstract

Allergic diseases have become a major health problem in modern society. These diseases are caused by an overreaction of the immune system and are often triggered by exposure to environmental allergens. Allergic diseases include asthma, allergicrhinitis, eczema, food allergies, and anaphylaxis. In recent years, research on the effectof circadian rhythm on the immune system has shown that there is an important relationship between the pathophysiology of allergic diseases and circadian rhythm. The pathophysiology of allergic diseases begins with responses to the immune system and the effect of allergens. The immune system is a complex network that regulates the response of immune cells. Immunoglobulin E (IgE) antibodies play an important role inreactions of hypersensitivity to allergens. Exposure to allergens triggers the activation of mast cells and basophils, resulting in the release of inflammatory mediators. The circadian rhythm is an internal clock system that regulates the 24-hour cycle of biological processes. The human body adapts various physiological and metabolic processes to this rhythm. The relationship of allergic diseases with the circadian rhythmis related to their effects on both the immune system and tissue and organ function. The circulation and activity of immune cells can change depending on the circadian rhythm. These changes can influence the immune system's

* Corresponding Author's Email: gulsahikagokdemir@gmail.com.

In: Human Health is a Matter of Timing
Editors: Sumeyya Deniz Aybek, Gonca Gulbay and Mucahit Secme
ISBN: 979-8-89113-467-6

response to exposure to allergens. In addition, the symptoms and severity of allergic diseases are also related to the circadian rhythm. Some studies have shown that allergic symptoms increase at night or in the morning. This suggests that the circadian rhythm may influence the severity of allergic reactions by affecting the release of immunoglobulins, the inflammatory response, and bronchial hyperreactivity. This chapter aims to provide researchers, clinicians, and healthcare professionals with an important resource on recent research findings that advance our understanding of the relationship between the pathophysiology of allergic diseases and the relationship between circadian rhythm.

Keywords: allergic diseases, pathophysiology, circadian rhythm, immune system

Introduction

Worldwide, the prevalence of allergic diseases is increasing (Wangetal., 2023). Comparison of the prevalence of allergic diseases using international systematic methods is necessary to understand the global epidemiology of these diseases, to formulate new hypotheses, and to evaluate the possible causes of existing hypotheses. In the early 2000s, about 20% of adults and about one-third of schoolchildren were reported to suffer from allergies (Behrendt and Becker, 2001; González -Buitrago et al., 2007). Allergic diseases such as asthma, allergic rhinitis, atopic dermatitis, and food allergy significantly affect the quality of life and constitute a significant burden on health (Schoenwetteret al., 2004; Rothe et al., 2018; Bachertetal., 2002).

Some symptoms that can be attributed to allergic diseases date back to ancient times (Epöztürk and Görkey, 2018). The concep of "allergy" was firstused by Austrian pediatrician Clemens Pirquetin 1906 after he noticed that patients who received injections of horse serum or smallpox vaccine usually reacted more severely to the second injection (Ring, 1985). Today, it is still used as a concept that includes hypersensitivity reactions of theimmune system to any substance. Allergic diseases are among the major health problems ofmodern societies and adversely affect approximately 25% of the population (Behrendt and Becker, 2001; González-Buitragoetal., 2007). Allergy can be defined as an abnormal response of the body to normally harmless substances. Some of the most common allergens are dust, insects, various foods, and pollen. While there is no problem when healthy people encounter these substances, called allergens, in people with allergic diseases, the body assumes these substances as "threats" to itself and reacts. As a result, allergic reactions may occur in people with allergic diseases. Allergic reactions can be very mild or life-threatening (Thomsen, 2015).

Diseases occur depending on the organs in which the allergic reaction develops. In the respiratory system, allergic rhinitis occurs when allergic reactions occur in the nose and asthma occurs when allergic reactions occur in the airways of the lungs. Since both organs are components of the respiratory system, both diseases often occur together. Allergens are not only taken in through the respiratory tract. Proteins in food can also cause allergic reactions. Today, food allergies are the most common cause of anaphylaxis in children, while drug allergies are the most common cause of anaphylaxis in adults. However, food allergens may also cause other diseases other than anaphylaxis. They may also play a role in the development of diseases such as eosinophilic oesophagitis, proctocolitis, or atopic dermatitis (eczema). On the other hand, allergic reactions, such as severe anaphylaxis, can develop due to bee stings. These reactions can be fatal.

The pathophysiology of allergic diseases is associated with the immune system developing hypersensitivity to allergens and an excessive immune response. In this process, T cells, B cells, mast cells, and other immune cells play an important role. Upon contact with allergens, allergen-specific antibodies are produced via receptors on immune cells and immune system activation begins. Activated immune cells trigger inflammatory responses by increasing the release of various cytokines (Galli et al., 2008). In recent years, the relationship between the pathophysiology of allergic diseases and the circadian rhythm has been increasingly investigated.

The circadian rhythm is the body's internal clock system that regulates various biological processes in a 24-hour cycle. Many physiological processes, such as the sleep-wake cycle, hormonal release, metabolic activity, and immune functions, vary depending on the circadian rhythm. Recent studies show that circadian rhythm has a significant effect on the immune system and plays a role in the development and course of allergic diseases (Labrecque and Cermakian, 2015; Nakao, 2020; Silveretal., 2012).

The effect of circadian rhythm on the immune system is mediated through many mechanisms. For example, gene expression in immune cells is regulated depending on the circadian rhythm. This regulation can affect the circulation, activity, and cytokine release ofimmune cells. Furthermore, circadian rhythm is thought to modulate the immune response by influencing hormonal and metabolic processes (Silver et al., 2012; Durrington et al., 2014; Labrecque and Cermakian, 2015).

Although the relationship between the pathophysiology of allergic diseases and circadian rhythm is not yet fully understood, some findings support this relationship. For example, it has been observed that symptoms in asthma patients follow a certain pattern during the day and intensify at night. In addition, some studies have shown that allergic diseases change in accordance with the circadian rhythm due to seasonal changes.

Pathophysiology of Allergic Diseases

The pathophysiology of allergic diseases is characterized by the interaction of complex immunological mechanisms, inflammatory processes, and genetic factors. Allergic diseases are the result of a complex interaction of genetic and environmental factors. Allergic reactionsare usually mediated by immunoglobulin E (IgE) and lead to inflammatory responses. The pathophysiology of allergic diseases is associated with changes in immune system cells, immunoglobulins, inflammatory mediators, and target organs (Akdisand Akdis, 2014).

Immune System and Overreaction: Allergens and Immune Response

A hypersensitivity reaction initiated by specific immunological mechanisms can be defined as an allergy. Allergens are proteinaceous substances that are generally recognized as harmless but cause allergic reactions in sensitive individuals. They stimulate the formation ofspecific IgE. In allergic diseases, people have allergen-specific IgE antibodies and symptoms occur when they encounter the allergen (Johansson et al., 2004). Exposure to an allergen at a dose tolerated by normal individuals can cause hypersensitivity in allergic individuals. Hypersensitivity reactions are examined in four groups according to the pathophysiology of the immunological mechanism (Dispenza, 2019; Knol and Gilles, 2022).

Type 1 Hypersensitivity: Type 1 or immediate hypersensitivity reactions are mediated by allergen-specific IgE antibodies. It is an allergic reaction triggered by repeated exposure to aspecific antigen, called an allergen. IgE antibodies bind to mast cells and basophils, which contain histamine granules. Subsequent exposure to the same allergen causes degranulation of bound IgE and release of mediators such as histamine, leukotrienes, and prostaglandins. Allergen exposure occurs by ingestion, inhalation, injection, or direct contact. There action may be local or systemic. The main effects are vasodilatation and smooth muscle contraction. Symptoms can range from a mild reaction to anaphylactic shock to sudden death (Agnihotriand McGrath, 2019; Son et al.,2018; Justiz Vaillant and Zito, 2019; Simon, 2018; Knol and Gilles, 2022).

Type 2 Hypersensitivity: It is a hypersensitivity reaction that is effective in organs or cells to which the antibody binds and in which the antibody to cell membrane antigens activates the complement system. Immunoglobulin G (IgG) and Immunoglobulin M (IgM) antibodies are involved in the type II hypersensitivity reaction and the immunoglobulin A (IgA) antibody is involved to a lesser extent. IgG and IgM antibodies are the main components of host defense that bind to microbiological agents and help them to be killed directly through multiple mechanisms. However, when these antibodies bind to the host's own antigens, they can direct this cytotoxic response to the host itself and cause damage. These antigens arefound in circulating blood cells such as erythrocytes, platelets, neutrophils, or epithelial cellson mucosal surfaces and basement membranes. The antigen can be formed by the patient's own cells (autoimmunity), or a foreign protein can attack the cell membrane.

Type 3 Hypersensitivity: When the organism is exposed to a foreign protein, antibodies are formed against this antigenic substance after 7-10 days. In type III responses, IgG, and IgM antibodies bind to antigens to form immune complexes. These complexes accumulate in tissues and cause organ damage by activating complement. Common sites of complex deposition include small arteries, renal glomeruli, and synovial capsules of joints. Complement deposition causes vasculitis, glomerulonephritis, and arthritis (Knol and Gilles, 2022).

Type 4 Hypersensitivity: Type IV hypersensitivity reactions are so-called delayed reactions and involve T cells as the main effector cells. Stimulated T cells can directly cause damage, as in the case of cytotoxic T cells, or Th cells can activate other leukocytes such a macrophages, neutrophils, and eosinophils that can cause tissue damage through the production and release of reactive oxygen radicals and lysosomal enzymes and inflammatory cytokines (Uzzamanand Cho, 2012; Dispenza, 2019; Knol and Gilles, 2022).

T Cells, B Cells, and Antibody Production

T cells, B cells, and antibodies are important components of the immune system that come together. T cells recognize antigens, while B cells produce antibodies that bind to antigens and initiate the immune response.

From birth, our organism is constantly exposed to self-antigens and foreign pathogens. The immune system has developed strategies against foreign antigens. Among these strategies, effector T cells are the main players regulating immune responses. T cells have a regulatory role in many pathways of the immune system with the soluble mediators they produce and receptor-ligand inter actions on their surface. T cell activation is activated by antigen binding to the T cell receptor (TCR) and signal transduction. Unlike B cells that react to soluble antigens, T cells are stimulated by small peptides presented on the surface of other cells. Antigen presentation can occur when these peptides bind to the protein groove of the major histocompatibility complex (MHC). The ligand required for TCR consists of aminoacids of the antigenic peptide and residues of the MHC molecule. Binding of the peptide-MHC complex to the TCR triggers a series of biochemical events leading to T cell activation (Delves and Roitt, 2000; Abbas and Lichtman, 2005; Bonilla and Oettgen, 2010; Mesquita Júnior et al., 2010).

The development and maturation of B cells take place in the bone marrow independently of antigen. These cells express surface antigen receptors during the complex maturation process in the bone marrow and gain functional and phenotypic maturation. The surface antigen receptors of mature naive B cells are IgM and IgD molecules. Mature naive B cells that have completed their development and maturation in the bone marrow migrate to peripheral lymphoid tissues and wait to encounter the antigen. The humoral immune response begins with the encounter of antigen-specific B cells with antigen in these peripheral lymphoid tissues. Antigen receptors of maturenaive B cells can recognize various antigens such as polysaccharides, lipids, glycolipids, nucleic acids, and small soluble molecules that are not recognized by T cells, and B cells can be directly activated by these types of antigens. However, $CD4^+$ T cell assistance is required for B cell activation with protein antigens. B cell activation is a process consisting of successive complex steps. The sequential steps of the humoral immune response for protein antigens can be listed as follows:

1. Antigen recognition and intra cellular signaling by B cells.
2. Antigen presentation of B cells to Th cells.

3. B cell activation by Th cells.
4. B cell differentiation (formation of antibody-releasing effector B cells, heavy chain isotype/class change, affinity maturation, formation of memory B cells).
5. Elimination of antigen by released antibodies.
6. Haemostasis (termination of the humoral imune response).

Furthermore, B cells produce specialized cells called memory cells so that they can mount a faster and more effective immune response to subsequent infections (Abbas et al., 2012; Delves and Roitt, 2000; Bonilla and Oettgen, 2010; Mesquita Júnior et al., 2010).

Antibodies are a fundamental part of the defense mechanism of the immune system. They are protein molecules produced by B cells. Antibodies with antigen-specific binding sites bind to antigens on the surface of pathogens or foreign substances. This binding process leads to aseries of immunological responses to inactivate pathogens. Antibodies neutralize pathogens such as viruses, bacteria, and other infectious agents while activating other cells of the immune system in the process.

Antibody production usually occurs as the primary response of the immune system. After the initial exposure, memory B cells develop to provide a faster and more effective response to the same antigen. In this way, the body can mount a more effective immune response to pathogens it has previously encountered (Delves and Roitt, 2000; Bonilla and Oettgen, 2010; Mesquita Júnioretal., 2010).

Allergic Inflammation

T cell activation is the key event in allergic inflammation. The basis of this reaction is a pathological event resulting in the secretion of mediators (LTC4, PGD2, Histamine) in the early phase and the arrival of T-lymphocytes and eosinophils in the late phase. The cell group that plays a key role in the development of the immune response, which is effective in the development of allergic diseases, is Th2-type lymphocytes; the basic mediators directing the response are IgE and lipid metabolism intermediates; and the effector cell group is basophils, mastcells, and eosinophils.

The cornerstone of inflammation is the formation of specific IgE against any allergen. There are 2 stages in the development of allergic inflammation. The first phase is the sensitization phase. Allergic inflammation begins with the uptake of allergens through the skin, upper and lower airways. In general, protein allergens require an intermediary cell in order to stimulate the immune system to create a response. Cells called 'antigen presenting cells' present antigens to T lymphocytes. Cytokines released after allergen presentation stimulate IgE synthesis from B lymphocytes. IgE provides the migration of inflammatory cells that will be important in the allergic response phase. Thus, allergen-specific IgE is synthesized in theperson who comesinto contact with the allergen, and a sensitized individual is now in question. After this phase, the allergic response phase begins. After allergen-specific IgE is synthesized, it binds to high-affinity IgE receptors on the surface of mast cells and basophils. When the allergen is contacted again, mast cells in the target tissue bind to the IgE molecule on the surface, and mediator release occurs. This event is defined as the "early stage" of allergic inflammation. Mediators such as histamine, prostaglandins, cysteinyl leukotrienes, platelet activating factor, and bradykinin are released from mast cells. Some of the mediators secreted from mast cells are pre-synthesized and readily stored in the granules, while some are synthesized as a result of allergen IgE in corporation.

The early phase of allergic inflammation is characterized by the onset of symptoms within minutes after inhalation of the allergen. In this phase, mediators are released from mast cells. A few hours after the early phase, symptoms may reappear in people exposed to the allergen; this event is called the "late phase" of allergic inflammation. The late phase reactionis caused by the migration of inflammatory cells into the environment; mediators released from monocytes, dendritic cells, neutrophils, T lymphocytes, basophils, and eosinophils in the environment in the late phase cause symptoms to reappear hours after the allergen exposure (Vignolaetal., 2001; Barners, 2003; Sohetal., 2023).

Genetic Predisposition and Role of Environmental Factors

The development of allergic diseases is often associated with the influence of genetic predisposition. Genetic predisposition refers to the presence of genetic factors that increase an individual's susceptibility to allergic diseases. Current estimates suggest that a child with one allergic parent has a 30-50% risk of developing allergies, increasing to 60-80% if both parents are allergic. Research has shown that multiple genes play a role in the development of allergic diseases. Genes related to the immune system, such as cytokines, immunoglobulins, and HLA (human leukocyte antigen) genes, play an important role in the development of allergic diseases. However, genetic predisposition alone does not guarantee the development of allergic diseases; it is also important that it interacts with environmental factors. Genetic predisposition is an important focus of research to understand the mechanisms and causes of allergic diseases and guides individuals for early diagnosis and treatment (Dold et al., 1992; Oberand Yao, 2010).

The development of allergic diseases is associated with environmental factors, as well as genetic predisposition. Studies on identical twins reveal a strong role of non-genetic factors. A person who has a high level of exposure to a certain allergen over a certain period of time has a higher chance of becoming sensitized to that allergen than a person with less exposure (Portelli et al., 2015). Environmental factors are the factors to which people are exposed in their environment and play an important role in the development of allergic diseases. The effect of environmental factors exposed, especially during childhood, is more pronounced. Exposure to allergens such as cigarette smoke, house dust mites, pollen, animal hair, mold fungi, and some foods may contribute to the development of allergic diseases. In addition, environmental factors such as air pollution, industrial chemicals, indoor humidity, and hygiene levels can also influence the risk of allergic diseases. Furthermore, the use of antibiotics at anearly age may affect the development of the immune system and trigger the emergence ofallergic diseases. The influence of environmental factors on allergic diseases interacts in a complex way and may vary depending on the type of disease, the genetic predisposition of the individual, and the duration of exposure to environmental factors. Therefore, measures to be taken at the individual and societal levels, taking into account environmental factors, are important in the prevention and management of allergic diseases (Xing and Wong, 2022; Murrisonetal, 2019).

Relationship of Allergic Diseases with Circadian Rhythm

Allergic reactions occur as a result of an over reaction of the immune system when a person is exposed to allergens. These reactions can be triggered by inhalation, contact, or consumption of allergens and can manifest themselves as symptoms such as nasal congestion, sneezing, watery eyes, itching, skin rashes, and even breathing difficulties. Although allergic diseases (allergic rhinitis, asthma, atopic dermatitis, food allergy, etc.) are an important public health problem, their causes are not fully understood (Reynolds and Finlay, 2017).

Circadian clocks are internal clocks that drive behavior and physiological processes such as sleep-wake cycles, body temperature, and hormonal secretions, which have approximately 24-hour rhythms. These rhythms enable organisms to anticipate environmental changes and respond accordingly (Dibneretal., 2010; Takahashietal., 2008).

The circadian clock system in mammals consists of molecular oscillators controlled by several clock genes within cells. The circadian clock mechanism causes periodic expression in thousands of genes, regulating the timing of cellular activities and ensuring rhythmic physiology in various organs. This system also plays an important role in the regulation of many basic physiological processes such as metabolism, immune system, development, and reproduction by influencing nuclear hormone receptors (Turek, 2016; Scheiermann et al., 2018). In mammals, the circadian clock system consists of a central oscillator called the supra chiasmatic nucleus (SCN) in the hypothalamus and peripheral oscillators found in almost all cell types. The SCN functions as a central clock that is influenced by the activation of specific photoreceptors in the retina that respond to light. The molecular mechanisms of rhythm generation are cell-specificand are regulated and maintained by transcriptional and translational feedback networks consisting of clock genes such as Clock, Bmal1, Period (Per), and Cryptochrome (Cry). This circadian rhythm mechanism affects genes containing transcription factors, enzymes, and molecules involved in various physiological processes. For example, in mice, the CLOCK/BMAL1 complex regulates various processes, such as immune functions. Peripheral clocks can also be influenced by non-fotic environmental cues and metabolic signals. Factors such as the timing of feeding can influence the phase angle in gene expression in organs such as the liver. Studies in mice have shown that gene expression in the liver of mice fed only at night or during the day has different phases (Patke et al., 2020; Panda, 2016; Stokkan et al., 2001; Takahashi, 2017; Dibneretal., 2010; Takahashietal., 2008).

The clock system regulates various processes in the body in synchronization with environmental signals and is important for maintaining healthy rhythmic physiology. Circadian disruption is the result of a mismatch between the internal circadian clock and environmental cycles. The mismatch between the circadian clock and environmental cycles results in reduced circadian rhythms and the occurrence of circadian disruption. Conditions such as night shiftwork, time zone changes (jet lag), or constant exposure to artificial light can lead to rapid or severe disruption of circadian rhythms. Disruption of the circadian rhythm can affect the balance in the immune system and increase susceptibility to allergic reactions (Roenneberg and Merrow 2016; Walker et al., 2020).

Recent studies have shown that allergic reactions are related to circadian rhythms. The circadian clock is an intrinsic time-keeping mechanism that enables organisms to adapt to 24-hour daily rhythmic changes. In allergic diseases, symptoms and laboratory parameters change in 24-hour cycles, indicating that allergic diseases are related to circadian rhythms. Allergic diseases show marked day-night variations in symptoms, laboratory parameters, and response to treatment. In diseases such as allergic rhinitis, asthma, and chronic urticaria, symptoms often worsen during the night or early morning. This suggests that an allergic reaction is related to circadian rhythms (Smolensky et al., 2007).

Allergen exposure and allergic reactions can affect the circadian rhythm. Allergic diseases are characterized by impaired epithelial barrier function and dysregulated immune response. In atopic dermatitis, defects in various components of the skin barrier allow allergens to pass through the skin, leading to the release of cytokines that trigger allergic reactions. Inflammatory responses in the immune system after allergen exposure may affect the circadian rhythm (Figure 1). Because immune functions and inflammation processes are associated with circadian rhythms (Golevaetal., 2019).

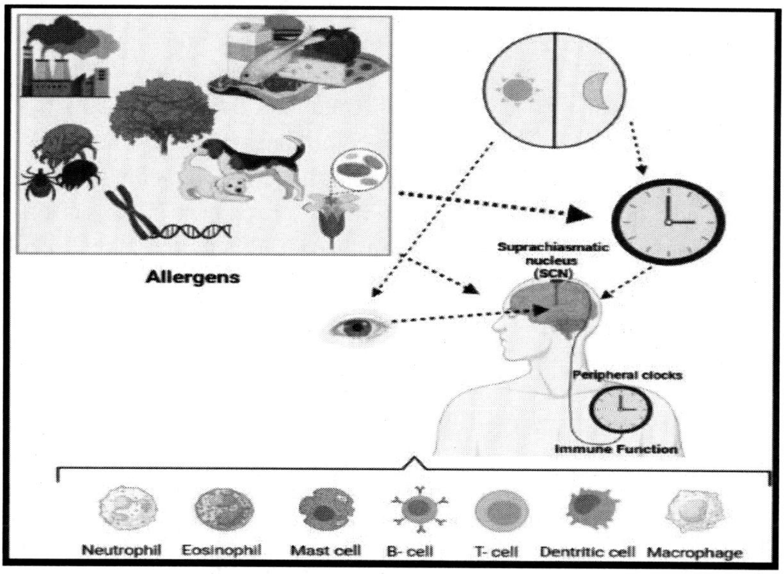

Figure 1. Allergens cause the release of cytokines that trigger allergic reactions.

In allergic rhinitis, symptoms such as sneezing, runny nose, stuffy nose, and itchy nose increase during the night or early morning. These symptoms are accompanied by nasal reactivity to methacholine in the nasal mucosa and circadian differences in eosinophil and basophil activity. Therefore, circadian rhythms play an important role in allergic rhinitis (Smolenskyetal., 2007).

Aurelianus Caelius' observations of asthma attacks have been associated with rhythmic changes in bronchial hyper-reactivity. However, the mechanisms underlying these observations are still unclear (Caelius, 1709). Asthmatic patients experience nocturnal exacerbations similar to those of allergic rhinitis. Asthma symptoms and bronchial reactivity peak at midnight or early in the morning. Alveolar eosinophil activity follows the same cycle, supporting the circadian nature of asthma (Kellyetal., 2004).

In patients with chronic urticaria, symptoms are usually more pronounced in the evening. This suggests that skin reactions to histamine or other triggering factors increase in the evening. Therefore, the effect of circadian rhythms is important in chronic urticaria (Maureretal., 2009).

Epithelial cells in the skin, intestines, and airwaysactasa barrier against external pathogens, chemicals, and allergens. Disruption of this epithelial barrier function plays an important role in the development of allergic diseases (Golevaetal, 2019). Impairment of epithelial barrier function facilitates the entry of allergens into the body and causes the triggering of an allergic immune response. Genetic factors (filaggrin deficiency) and non-genetic factors (protease activity of allergens, chemical agents, and injury/itching) may contribute to this barrier disruption (Schleimer and Berdnikovs, 2017).

The skin barrier is provided by many components such as filaggrin, lipid, skin pH level, tight junctions (TJs), antimicrobial peptides, commensal bacteria, and Aquaporin-3, most of which show circadian rhythms (Goleva et al.,2019; Vaughnetal., 2018). Aquaporin-3 (AQP3) is a protein that regulates the entry of water and glycerol into the skin and is controlled by CLOCK. Clock disruption can reduce stratum corneum hydration. Disruption of circadian rhythm may affect the normal function of proteins such as AQP3 and disrupt the moisture balance of the skin barrier (Matsunaga et al., 2014).

Intestinal epithelial cells form a barrier with components such as TJs, mucus, and anti-microbial peptides. Intestinal barrier function is regulated by clock genes. The clock gene CLOCK regulates the expression of TJ molecules such as Occludin and Claudin-1, which affect intestinal permeability. Clock disruption can lead to intestinal barrier dysfunction and exacerbate food allergy symptoms (Kyokoetal, 2014).

The airway epithelial barrier consists of components such as TJs, mucus-producing cells, ciliated cells, and epithelium-derived cytokines/chemokines. Defects in airway barrier function may be associated with allergic diseases, such as asthma. Disruptions in TJs and increased inflammation may be observed in allergic diseases such as asthma. Clock genes can regulate the responses to infection and inflammation in the lung. Disruption of the clock mechanism may affect the development and severity of allergic diseases by affecting responses in the lung (Ehlers et al., 2018).

Mast cells and basophils are innate immune cells that play an important role in allergic diseases. In IgE-mediated allergic diseases such as allergic rhinitis, asthma, and food allergy, mast cells, and basophils are activated by an IgE-dependent mechanism.

IgE/mast cell-mediated allergic reactions vary depending on circadian rhythms. Studies in both mice and humans have shown that the IgE/mast cell-mediated allergic reaction is subject to 24-hour cycles. In experiments in mice, it has been observed that anaphylactic sensitizationin the auricle changes daily and that skin hypersensitivity reactions in patients with nocturnal asthma exhibit a circadian rhythm. Symptoms, nasal or bronchial reactivity, and inflammatory activity become more pronounced in the early morning and at midnight. Skin hypersensitivity to allergens may also vary according to the time of day.

Mast cells are cells with a functional molecular clock. In studies on mast cells, it has been found that core clock genes are expressed rhythmically and that some genes show circadian oscillations. After IgE-mediated activation, circadian variations occur in histamine release, cysteinyl leukotriene production, and the expression of some cytokines in mast cells (Nakao et al., 2015).

In animal studies, a day-dependent variation in IgE/mast cell-mediated allergic reactions were observed in mice, but not in mice with impaired circadian clock activity or in adrenalectomized mice. These findings suggest that humoral factors released from the adrenal gland, such as corticosterone, may play an important role in synchronizing the circadian clock mechanism in mast cells. In aged mice, no time-dependent variation in the passive cutaneous anaphylactic reaction was observed in the presence of abnormal circadian clock activity. These findings suggest that the circadian clock plays an important role in the establishment of daily rhythms inIgE/mastcell-mediated allergic reactions (Nakaoetal, 2015).

It is not fully understood why the IgE/mast cell-mediated allergic reaction exhibits circadian rhythms. It is thought that the IgE/mast cell-mediated allergic reaction may be one of the body's defense mechanisms against macroparasites. Parasites and biting arthropods may be carriers of microorganisms that are potentially harmful to humans. These parasites and biting arthropods are known to have circadian rhythms in their behavior. Circadian control of the IgE/mast cell-mediated allergic reaction may have evolved to provide an evolutionary advantage. In this way, the immune system can anticipate the risk of attack by parasites and biting arthropods and prepare by increasing the IgE/mast cell reaction (Nakaoetal, 2015).

In addition to playing an important role in the control of parasitic infections, there is evidence that eosinophils have regulatory roles in tissue homeostasis and repair. In allergic diseases, eosinophils contribute to effect or functions through mechanisms such as degranulation, extracellular traps, andcytolysis (Chusid, 2018).

Human eosinophils show circadian oscillations in basal ECP (eosinophil cationic protein) expression and release of IL-8 (CXCL8) and CCL2 (chemokine [CC motif] ligand 2) in response to stimulation with fMLP (N-formyl-methionyl-leucyl-phenylalanine) (Baumann et al., 2014). Blood and sputum eosinophils and serum IL-5 levels may vary depending on the time of day in asthma patients and control subjects. Moreover, the circadian variation of blood eosinophils has been associated with neuroendocrine and metabolic cycles (Nussbaum et al., 2013). These findings suggest that circadian control of eosinophil homeostasis is consistent with activation and migration in stable states and allergic disease.

Macrophages are versatile innate immune cells that function in many aspects of physiology and disease. Their role in allergic disease is generally unclear, but in allergic asthma, macrophages can trigger inflammatory responses such as lung injury, fibrosis, and hyperplasia of goblet cells (Shapouri-Moghaddam et al., 2018).

Circadian clock components regulate various functions in macrophages, such as lipopolysaccharide (LPS) loading. In peritoneal macrophages, approximately 8% of genes containing key elements of LPS/TLR4 signaling are rhythmically expressed. These findings emphasize the importance of circadian clock disruption, which may affect asthma by altering the responses of macrophages and bronchial epithelial cells to LPS (Kitchenetal, 2020).

Innate lymphoid cells (ILCs) are the most recently discovered family of immune cells. ILCs are divided into three different groups: ILC1s, ILC2s, and ILC3s. ILC2s are master regulators of allergic immune responses and are activated by epithelium-derived cytokines. Activated ILC2s initiate and increase allergic inflammation by secreting substances such as IL-5 and IL-13, affecting eosinophils and epithelial cells (Bartemesetal, 2014).

The role of ILC2s in the circadian clock is still unclear, but RORa, a circadian clock component, is thought to be involved in ILC2 differentiation and IL-5 production. In addition, circadian rhythms associated with blood eosinophil counts have been shown to be effective in the development and function of ILC2s (Nakao, 2020).

ILC3s provide mucosal defense via IL-22 and IL-17 and are thought to be under strong control of the circadian clock. Since ILC3s are associated with obesity-induced asthma, clock disruption through metabolic disorders in obese patients may increase ILC3 responses and predispose patients to asthma (Everaere et al., 2016).

Dendritic cells (DCs), known as professional antigen-presenting cells (APCs), the activation and function of DCs influence various responses of the immune system. The ability of DCs to trigger immunity or tolerance through co-stimulatory or inhibitory molecules may play a role in the development of allergic disease. The roles of the circadian clock in DCs are still unclear.

The clock genes are genes that are expressed rhythmically in T and B cells. These genes temporally control lymphocyte trafficking, development, and immune responses to various pathogens. However, there are limited studies investigating the roles of circadian clock components in T and B cell responses associated with allergic disease (Silver et al., 2012; Scheiermann et al., 2018).

The Th1 and Th2 are two different response pathways of the immune system. The Th1 response is effective against infections by increasing cellular immunity, while the Th2 response can be effective against parasites by increasing antibody production. In one study, the effects of deletion of Bmal1, a gene in dendritic cells, on Th1 and Th2 responses in mice were examined. It showed that deletion of the Bmal1 gene in dendritic cells suppressed the Th1 response in mice and at the same time enhanced the Th2 response against the intestinal parasite Trichuris muris. Thus, the disruption of the clock in dendritic cells may influence allergic diseases by affecting the Th1/Th2 balance. However, since this study was conducted only on a mouse model, further research is needed on whether the same effects are seen in humans and its direct relationship with allergic diseases (Nakao, 2020).

In mouse models of skin hypersensitivity reactions, Th2 cells play an important role. Mice with clock mutations exhibit severe inflammation, IL-4/IL-13 expression, mast cell counts, and elevated serum IgE levels. These findings suggest that circadian clock components may play an important role in the development and function of different subsets of T cells, Th2, and Th17 cells.

Th17 cells provide protection against bacterial and fungal infections on mucosal surfaces. Circadian proteins regulate Th17 cell differentiation. Since Th17 cells are associated with neutrophilic asthma, clock disruption may affect specific phenotypes of asthma.

Regulatory Tcells (Tregs) contribute to the prevention of allergic disease. Genetic deficiency of Tregs is observed in people with allergic symptoms. Clock disruption can reduce the number of Tregs and thus accelerate the allergic disease. Studies suggest that irregular light/dark cycles or rotation of working hours may increase the risk of allergic disease due to reduced Treg numbers and the development of food allergies (Nakao, 2020).

The relationship between the clock and B cells has not yet been well studied, and its relationship with allergy is not yet fully understood.

Animal Models and Clinical Studies

Animal Models

Animal models are an important tool to understand the effect of allergic diseases on circadian rhythm and to develop potential treatment methods. Laboratory animals are the most widely used animal models to study the circadian rhythm and the interaction of immune system cells. The main components of the circadian rhythm are the molecular clock genes and their products, proteins. Genetic modification techniques have enabled the creation of mouse models that mimic changes in clock genes in mice and rats. Due to these animal models, great progress has been made in the study of the circadian rhythm.

The effects of clock genes on the autonomic cell patterns that constitute the circadian rhythm have been studied in detail. These studies have shown that the circadian rhythm can influence allergic responses by regulating the function of immune system cells.

The effectof allergic diseases on circadian rhythm has been established by clinical observations and studies on animal models. Experiments in laboratory animals have shown that allergen exposure can affect circadian rhythm and regulate allergic responses. Forexample, exposure to the allergen at night can increase the severity of allergic reactions whereas mice exposed during the day may show fewer responses. These findings suggest that the circadian rhythm should be considered in the treatment of allergic diseases.

Studies on the effect of allergic diseases on the circadian rhythm have led to the developmentof new therapeutic strategies. Correction or targeting of the circadian rhythm may be a potential approach to reduce or prevent symptoms of allergic diseases. Animal models are the tools used to evaluate the efficacy of these treatment strategies.

There are many studies investigating the relationship between circadian rhythm disruption and allergic diseases in mouse and rat models. In mice and rats, methods have been used to change the light-dark cycle or completely eliminate the cycle. At the same time, studies have been carried out on mice with mutations such as clock mutations and mast cell deficiency.

In these models, the exacerbation of inflammatory responses, changes in immune responses, and activation of immune cells have been investigated (Cheng et al., 2022; Curtis et al., 2015; Silveretal, 2012; Herichováetal., 2013).

For example, PER2 LUC knock-in mice are a model used in research to study circadian rhythms at the molecular level and to understand the circadian clock mechanism. These mice can be a valuable tool for investigating how circadian rhythms are regulated, how external factors (light, hormones, etc.) affect circadian rhythms, and the effects of diseases on circadian rhythms (Nakaoetal, 2015).

BMMCs are mast cells obtained from the bone marrow. These cells are grown in the laboratory and used in research. In particular, studying the mechanisms and functions of mast cells can contribute to the understanding of diseases such as allergies, asthma, and other immune disorders. They can also be used to test the effects of drugs on mast cells and develop new treatment approaches (Christetal, 2018).

Hamster Models: Other animal models such as hamsters and primates have also been used to study the relationship between allergic diseases and circadian rhythm. In these models, an increase in allergic diseases and changes in inflammatory responses can be observed as a result of circadian rhythm disruption (Prendergast and Freeman, 1999).

There have been many clinical studies on allergic asthma and allergic rhinitis. In clinical studies in patients with allergic asthma, it has been observed that pulmonary function changes during the day, and symptoms increase at certain times of the day. In addition, circadian rhythm-related changes have been found between bronchial hyperreactivity, inflammation, and pulmonary function. In patients with allergic rhinitis, it has been observed that symptoms and nasal mucosa change with circadian rhythm. Itis known that symptoms are exacerbatedin the morning hours and the nasal mucosa is more reactive (Smolensky et al., 2007; Comas et al., 2017; Manetal, 2016).

Advanced Research and Clinical Applications

Circadian variations support the use of chronotherapy in the treatment of allergic diseases. Chronotherapy aims to improve the efficacy of treatment and minimize side effects by using the optimal timing of the medications. For example, dosing allergy medications at night may provide better efficacy in allergic rhinitis. In the treatment of nocturnal asthma, the use of steroids in the evening is also advantageous in terms of efficacy. Similarly, evening doses of long-acting bronchodilators may be effective in controlling asthma symptoms.

Other classes of drugs are also being investigated for the chronotherapy of allergic diseases. Treatment strategies based on circadian rhythms may help patients optimally control symptoms and improve the response to treatment (Paudel et al., 2021; Nakamura et al., 2016; Smolenskyetal, 2016).

Conclusion

Although the relationship between the pathophysiology of allergic diseases and circadian rhythm is still not fully understood, research supports this relationship. The effects of the circadian rhythm on the immune system appear to play an important role in the severity and symptoms of allergic diseases. The observation of significant day-night variations in the symptoms, laboratory findings, and treatment responsesof allergic diseases shows the effect of the circadian rhythm on allergic diseases. In this context, the regulation of circadian rhythms and clock proteins is important for understanding the pathophysiology of allergic diseases and developing new treatment strategies. The effect of allergic diseases on the circadian rhythm; studies on animal models show that circadian rhythm plays an important role in the pathophysiology of allergic diseases. Understanding the potential of the circadian rhythm in thetreatment and prevention of allergic diseases may help the development of new approaches and treatment methods.

References

Abbas, A. K., Lichtman, A. H., & Pillai, S. (2012). B cell activation and antibody production. In Abbas A. K., Lichtman A. H., Pillai S. (Eds.), *Cellular and molecular immunology* (7th ed., pp. 243-268). Philadelphia, PA: ElsevierSaunders.

Abbas, A. K., & Lichtman, A. H. (2005). *Cellular and molecular immunology* (5th ed., pp. 163-188). Philadelphia, PA: ElsevierSaunders.

Agnihotri, N. T., & McGrath, K. G. (2019). Allergic and nonallergic rhinitis. *Allergy Asthma Proc.,* 40(6):376-9. https://doi.org/10.2500/aap.2019.40.4251.

Akdis, M., & Akdis, C. A. (2014). Mechanisms of allergen-specific immunotherapy: multiple suppress or factors at work in immune tolerance to allergens. *J Allergy Clin Immunol.* 133(3):621-31. https://doi.org/10.1016/j.jaci.2013.12.1088.

Bachert, C., van Cauwenberge, P., Khaltaev, N., & World Health O. (2002). Allergic rhinitis and its impact on asthma. In collaboration with the World Health Organization. Executive summary of the workshop report.7-10 December 1999, Geneva, Switzerland. *Allergy.* 57(9):841-55. https://doi.org/10.1034/j.1398-9995.2002.23625.x.

Barners, P. (2003). Pathophysiology of allergic inflammation. In Middleton, E., Reed, C. E., Ellis, E. F., Adkinson, N. F., Yunginger, J. W., & Buse, W. W. (Eds.), *Allergy. Volume I* (6th ed., pp. 483-499). St. Louis, MO: Mosby-YearBookInc.

Bartemes, K. R., Kephart, G. M., Fox, S. J., & Kita, H. (2014). Enhanced innate type 2 immune response in peripheral blood from patients with asthma. *J Allergy Clin Immunol.* 134:671–8.e4. https://doi.org/10.1016/j.jaci.2014.06.024.

Baumann, A., Feilhauer, K., Bischoff, S. C., Froy, O., & Lorentz, A. (2015). IgE-dependent activation of human mastcells and fMLP-mediatedactivation of humaneosinophils is controlled by the circadian clock. *MolImmunol.* 64:76–81. https://doi.org/10.1016/j.molimm.2014.10.026/

Behrendt, H., & Becker, W. M., (2001). Localization, release and bioavailability of pollen allergens: the influence of environmentalfactors, *Currentopinion in immunology,* 13(6), 709–715. https://doi.org/10.1016/s0952-7915(01)00283-7.

Bonilla, F. A., & Oettgen, H. C. (2010). Adaptive immunity. *J Allergy Clin Immunol* 125:33-40. https://doi.org/10.1016/j.jaci.2009.09.017.

Caelius, A. (1709). *De Morbis Acuitis et Chronicis.* Amsterdam: Wetsteniand.

Cheng, F. L., An, Y. F., Xue, J. M., Wang, Y. J., Ding, X. W., Zhang, Y. T., & Zhao, C. Q. (2022). Circadian rhythm disruption exacerbates Th2-like immune response in murine allergic airway inflammation. *Int Forum Allergy Rhinol.* 12(5), 757-770. https://doi.org/10.1002/alr.22914.

Christ, P., Sowa, A. S., Froy, O., & Lorentz, A. (2018). The Circadian Clock Drives Mast Cell Functions in Allergic Reactions. *Front Immunol.,* 9, 1526. https://doi.org/10.3389/fimmu.2018.01526.

Chusid, M. J. (2018). Eosinophils: Friends or foes? *J Allergy Clin Immunol Pract.*, 6, 1439–44. https://doi.org/10.1016/j.jaip.2018.04.031/

Comas, M., Gordon, C. J., Oliver, B. G., Stow, N. W., King, G., Sharma, P., Ammit, A. J., Grunstein, R. R., & Phillips, C. L. (2017). A circadian based inflammatory response–

implications for respiratory disease and treatment. *Sleep Science and Practice*, *1*, 1-19. https://doi.org/10.1186/s41606-017-0019-2.

Curtis, A. M., Fagundes, C. T., Yang, G., Palsson-McDermott, E. M., Wochal, P., McGettrick, A. F., Foley, N. H., Early, J. O., Chen, L., Zhang, H., Xue, C., Geiger, S. S., Hokamp, K., Reilly, M. P., Coogan, A. N., Vigorito, E., FitzGerald, G. A., &O'Neill, L. A. (2015). Circadian control of innate immunity in macrophages by miR-155 targeting Bmal1. *Proc Natl Acad Sci USA.*, 112(23):7231-6. https://doi.org/10.1073/pnas.1501327112.

Delves, P. J., & Roitt, I. M. (2000). The immune system. First of two parts. *N Engl J Med*, 343:37-49. https://doi.org/10.1056/NEJM200007063430107.

Dibner, C., Schibler, U., & Albrecht, U. (2010). The mammalian circadian timing system: organization and coordination of central and peripheral clocks. *Annu Rev Physiol*, 517– 549. https://doi.org/10.1146/annurev-physiol-021909-135821.

Dispenza, M. C. (2019). Classification of hyper sensitivity reactions. *AllergyAsthmaProc.*, 40(6):470. https://doi.org/10.2500/aap.2019.40.4274.

Dold, S., Wjst, M., Von Mutıus, E., Reıtmeır, P., & Stıepel, E. (1992). Genetic risk for asthma, allergic rhinitis, and atopic dermatitis. *ArchDis Child*, 67, 1018-1022. https://doi.org/10.1136/adc.67.8.1018.

Durrington, H. J., Farrow, S. N., Loudon, A. S., & Ray, D. W. (2014). The circadian clock and asthma. *Thorax*. 69(1), 90-2. https://doi.org/10.1136/thoraxjnl-2013-203482.

Ehlers, A., Xie, W., Agapov, E., Brown, S., Steinberg, D., Tidwell, R., Sajol G, Schutz R, Weaver R, Yu H, Castro, M., Bacharier, L. B., Wang, X., Holtzman, M. J., & Haspel, J. A. (2018). BMAL1 links the circadian clock to viral airway pathology and asthma phenotypes. *Mucosal Immunol.*, 11, 97-111. https://doi.org/10.1038/mi.2017.24.

Epöztürk, K., & Görkey, Ş. (2018). Were Allergic Diseases Prevalent in Antiquity. *Asthma Allergy Immunol*, 17, 1-6. https://doi.org/10.21911/aai.406.

Everaere, L., Ait-Yahia, S., Molendi-Coste, O., Vorng, H., Quemener, S., LeVu, P., Fleury, S., Bouchaert, E., Fan, Y., Duez, C., de Nadai, P., Staels, B., Dombrowicz, D., Tsicopoulos, A.(2016). In nate lymphoid cells contribute to allergic airway disease exacerbation by obesity. *Journal of Allergy and Clinical Immunology*, 138(5), 1309-1318.e11. https://doi.org/10.1016/j.jaci.2016.03.019.

Galli, S. J., Tsai, M., & Piliponsky, A. M. (2008). Thedevelopment of allergicinflammation. *Nature*, 454(7203), 445-454. https://doi.org/10.1038/nature07204.

Goleva, E., Berdyshev, E., & Leung, D. Y. (2019). Epithelial barrier repair and prevention of allergy. *Journal of Clinical Investigation*, 129, 1463-1474. https://doi.org /10.1172/JCI124608.

González-Buitrago, J. M., Ferreira, L., Isidoro-García, M., Sanz, C., Lorente, F., &Dávila, I. (2007). Proteomic approaches for identifying new allergens and diagnosing allergic diseases. *Clinica Chimica Acta*, 385(1-2), 21-27. https://doi.org/10.1016/j.cca. 2007.07.010.

Herichová, I., Šoltésová, D., Szántóová, K., Mravec, B., Neupauerová, D., Veselá, A., &Zeman, M. (2013). Effect of angiotensin II on rhythmic per2 expression in the suprachiasmatic nucleus and heart and daily rhythm of activity in Wistarrats. *Regulatory Peptides*, 186, 49-56. https://doi.org/10.1016/j.regpep.2013.06.016.

Johansson, S. G., Bieber, T., Dahl, R., Friedmann, P. S., Lanier, B. Q., Lockey, R. F., Motala, C., Ortega Martell, J. A., Platts-Mills, T. A., Ring, J., Thien, F., Van Cauwenberge, P., & Williams, H. C. (2004). Revised nomenclature for allergy for global use: Report of the Nomenclature Review Committee of the World Allergy Organization, October 2003. *Journal of Allergy and Clinical Immunology*, 113(5), 832-836. https://doi.org/10.1016/j.jaci.2003.12.591.

Justiz Vaillant, A. A., & Zito, P. M. (2019). *Immediate Hypersensitivity Reactions*. StatPearls. https://www.ncbi.nlm.nih.gov/books/NBK534870.

Kelly, E. A., Houtman, J. J., & Jarjour, N. N. (2004). Inflammatory changes associated with circadian variation in pulmonary function in subjects with mild asthma. *Clinical and Experimental Allergy*, 34, 227-233. https://doi.org/10.1111/j.1365-2222.2004.01866.x.

Kitchen, G. B., Cunningham, P. S., Poolman, T. M., Iqbal, M., Maidstone, R., Baxter, M., Bagnall, J., Begley, N., Saer, B., Hussell, T., Matthews, L. C., Dockrell, D. H., Durrington, H. J., Gibbs, J. E., Blaikley, J. F., Andrew S. Loudon, A. S., & David W. Ray, D. W. (2020). The clock gene Bmal1 inhibits macrophagemotility, phagocytosis, and impairs defense against pneumonia. *Proceedings of the National Academy of Sciences USA*, 117, 1543-1551. https://doi.org/10.1073/pnas.1915932117.

Knol, E. F., & Gilles, S. (2022). Allergy: Type I, II, III, and IV. *Handbook of Experimental Pharmacology*, 268, 31-41. https://doi.org/10.1007/164_2021_510.

Kyoko, O. O., Kono, H., Ishimaru, K., Miyake, K., Kubota, T., Ogawa, H., Okumura, K., Shibata, S., & Nakao, A. (2014). Expressions of tight junction proteins occludin and claudin-1 are under the circadian control in the mouselargeintestine: Implications in in testinal permeability and susceptibility to colitis. *PLo SONE*, 9, e98016. https://doi.org/10.1371/journal.pone.0098016.

Labrecque, N., & Cermakian, N. (2015). Circadian Clocks in the Immune System. *Journal of Biological Rhythms*, 30(4), 277-290. https://doi.org/10.1177/0748730415577723.

Man, K., Loudon, A., & Chawla, A. (2016). Immunity around the clock. *Science*, 354, 999-1003. https://doi.org/10.1126/science.aah4966.

Matsunaga, N., Itcho, K., Hamamura, K., Ikeda, E., Ikeyama, H., Furuichi, Y., Watanabe, M., Koyanagi, S., & Ohdo, S.(2014). 24-hour rhythm of aquaporin-3 function in theepidermis is regulated by molecular clocks. *Journal of Investigative Dermatology*, 134, 1636-1644. https://doi.org/10.1038/jid.2014.13.

Maurer, M., Ortonne, J. P., & Zuberbier, T. (2009). Chronic urticaria: An internet survey of health behaviors, symptom patterns and treatment needs in Europeanadultpatients. *British Journal of Dermatology*, 160, 633-641. https://doi.org/10.1111/j.1365-2133.2008.08920.x.

Mesquita Júnior, D., Araújo, J. A., Catelan, T. T., Souza, A. W., Cruvinel, W. M., Andradc, L. E., & Silva, N. P. (2010). Immune system - Part II: Basis of the immunological response mediated by T and B lymphocytes. *Revista Brasileira de Reumatologia*, 50, 552-580.

Murrison, L. B., Brandt, E. B., Myers, J. B., & Hershey, G. K. K. (2019). Environmental exposures and mechanisms in allergy and asthma development. *Journal of Clinical Investigation*, 129(4), 1504-1515. https://doi.org/10.1172/JCI124612.

Nakao, A. (2020). Circadian Regulation of the Biology of Allergic Disease: Clock Disruption Can Promote Allergy. *Frontiers in Immunology*, 11, 1237. https://doi.org/10.3389/fimmu.2020.01237.

Nakao, A., Nakamura, Y., & Shibata, S. (2015). The circadian clock functions as a potent regulator of allergic reaction. *Allergy*, 70, 467-473. https://doi.org/10.1111/all.12596.

Nakamura, Y., Nakano, N., Ishimaru, K., Ando, N., Katoh, R., Suzuki-Inoue, K., Koyanagki, S., Ogawa, H., Okumura, K., Shibata, S., & Nakao, A. (2016). Inhibition of IgE-mediated allergic reactions by pharmacologically targeting the circadian clock. *Journal of Allergy and Clinical Immunology*, 137, 1226-1235. https://doi.org/10.1016/j.jaci.2015.08.052.

Nussbaum, J. C., van Dyken, S. J., von Moltke, J., Cheng, L. E., Mohapatra, A., Molofsky, A. B., Thornton, E. E., Krummel, M. F., Chawla, A., Liang, H. E., & Locksley, R. M. (2013). Type 2 innate lymphoid cells control eosinophil homeostasis. *Nature*, 502, 245-248. https://doi.org/10.1038/nature12526.

Ober, C., & Yao, T. C. (2011). The genetics of asthma and allergic disease: A 21st-century perspective. *Immunological Reviews*, 242(1), 10-30. https://doi.org/10.1111/j.1600-065X.2011.01029.x.

Panda, S. (2016). Circadian physiology of metabolism. *Science*, 354, 1008-1015. https://doi.org/10.1126/science.aah4967.

Patke, A., Young, M. W., & Axelrod, S. (2020). Molecular mechanisms and physiological importance of circadian rhythms. *Nature Reviews Molecular Cell Biology*, 21, 67-84. https://doi.org/10.1038/s41580-019-0179-2.

Paudel, K. R., Jha, S. K., Allam, V. S. R. R., Prasher, P., Gupta, P. K., Bhattacharjee, R., Jha, N. K.,Vishwas, S., Singh, S. K., Shrestha, J., Imran, M., Panth, N., Chellappan, D. K., Ebrahimi Warkiani, M., Hansbro, P. M., & Dua, K. (2021). Recent Advances in Chronotherapy Targeting Respiratory Diseases. *Pharmaceutics*, 13(12), 2008. https://doi.org/10.3390/pharmaceutics13122008.

Prendergast, B. J., &Freeman, D. A. (1999). Pineal-independent regulation of photo-nonresponsiveness in the Siberian hamster (Phodopussungorus). *Journal of Biological Rhythms*, 14(1), 62-71. https://doi.org/10.1177/074873099129000452.

Portelli, M. A., Hodge, E., & Sayers, I. (2015). Genetic risk factors for the development of allergic disease identified by genome-wide association. *Clinical and Experimental Allergy*, 45(1), 21-31. https://doi.org/10.1111/cea.12327.

Reynolds, L. A., & Finlay, B. B. (2017). Early life factors that affect allergy development. *Nature Reviews Immunology*, 17, 518-528. https://doi.org/10.1038/nri.2017.39.

Ring, J. (1985). Erstbeschreibungeiner "atopischenFamilienanamnese" im Julisch-ClaudischenKaiserhaus: Augustus, Claudius, Britannicus [1st description of an "atopicfamilyanamnesis" in the Julio-Claudianimperialhouse: Augustus, Claudius, Britannicus]. *Der Hautarzt; Zeitschriftfur Dermatologie, Venerologie, und verwandte Gebiete*, 36(8), 470-471.

Roenneberg, T., & Merrow, M. (2020). The circadian clock and human health. *Current Biology,* 26, R432-R443. https://doi.org/10.1016/j.cub.2016.04.011 28.

Rothe, T., Spagnolo, P., Bridevaux, P. O., Clarenbach, C., Eich-Wanger, C., Meyer, F., Miedinger, D., Möller, A., Nicod, L. P., Nicolet-Chatelain, G., Sauty, A., Steurer-Stey, C., & Leuppi, J. D. (2018). Diagnosis and management of asthma- The Swiss guidelines. *Respiration; International Review of Thoracic Diseases,* 95(5), 364-380. https://doi.org/10.1159/000486797.

Scheiermann, C., Gibbs, J., Ince, L., & Loudon, A. (2018). Clocking in toimmunity. *Nature Reviews Immunology,* 18, 423-437.10.1038/s41577-018-0008-4.

Schleimer, R. P., & Berdnikovs, S. (2017). Etiology of epithelial barrier dysfunction in patients with type 2 inflammatory diseases. *Journal of Allergy and Clinical Immunology,* 139, 1752-1761. https://doi.org/10.1016/j.jaci.2017.04.010.

Schoenwetter, W. F., Dupclay, L., Appajosyula, S., Botteman, M. F., & Pashos, C. L. (2004). Economic impact and quality-of-life burden of allergicrhinitis. *Current Medical Research and Opinion,* 20(3), 305-317. https://doi.org/10.1185/030079903125003053.

Shapouri-Moghaddam, A., Mohammadian, S., Vazini, H., Taghadosi, M., Esmaeili, S. A., Mardani, F., Seifi, B., Mohammadi, A., Afshari, J. T., Sahebkar, A. (2018). Macrophageplasticity, polarization, and function in healthanddisease. *Journal of Cellular Physiology,* 233, 6425-6440. https://doi.org/10.1002/jcp.26429.

Silver, A. C., Arjona, A., Hughes, M. E., Nitabach, M. N., & Fikrig, E. (2012). Circadian expression of clock genes in mouse macrophages, dendritic cells, and B cells. *Brain, Behavior, and Immunity,* 26(3), 407-413. https://doi.org/10.1016/j.bbi.2011.10.001.

Simon, D. (2018). Recent Advances in Clinical Allergy and Immunology. *International Archives of Allergy and Immunology,* 177, 324-333. https://doi.org/10.1159/000494931.

Smolensky, M. H., Hermida, R. C., Reinberg, A., Sackett-Lundeen, L., & Portaluppi, F. (2016). Circadian disruption: New clinical perspective of disease pathology and basis for chronotherapeutic intervention. *Chronobiology International,* 33, 1101-1119. https://doi.org/10.1080/07420528.2016.1184678.

Smolensky, M. H., Lemmer, B., & Reinberg, A. E. (2007). Chronobiology and chronotherapy of allergic rhinitis and bronchial asthma. *Advanced Drug Delivery Reviews,* 59(9-10), 852-882. https://doi.org/10.1016/j.addr.2007.08.016.

Soh, W. T., Zhang, J., Hollenberg, M. D., Vliagoftis, H., Rothenberg, M. E., Sokol, C. L., Robinson, C. & Jacquet, A. (2023). Protease allergens as initiators-regulators of allergic inflammation. *European Journal of Allergy and Clinical Immunology,* 78, 1148-1168. https://doi.org/10.1111/all.15678.

Son, J. H., Park, S. Y., Cho, Y. S., Chung, B. Y., Kim, H. O., & Park, C. W. (2018). Immediate hypersensitivity reactions induced by triamcinolone in a patient with atopic dermatitis. *Journal of Korean Medical Science,* 33(12), e87. https://doi.org/10.3346/jkms.2018.33.e87.

Stokkan, K. A., Yamazaki, S., Tei, H., Sakaki, Y., & Menaker, M. (2001). Entrainment of the circadian clock in the liver by feeding. *Science,* 291, 490-493. https://doi.org/10.1126/science.291.5503.490.

Takahashi, J. S. (2017). Transcriptional architecture of the mammalian circadian clock. *Nature Reviews Genetics,* 18, 164-179. https://doi.org/10.1038/nrg.2016.150.

Takahashi, J. S., Hong, H. K., Ko, C. H., &McDearmon, E. L. (2008). The genetics of mammalian circadian order and disorder: Implications for physiology and disease. *Nature Reviews Genetics,* 9, 764-775. https://doi.org/10.1038/nrg2430.

Thomsen, S. F. (2015). Epidemiology and natural history of atopic diseases. *European Clinical Respiratory Journal,* 2(1), .https://doi.org/10.3402/ecrj.v2.24642.

Turek, F. W. (2016). Circadian clocks: Not your grandfather'sclock. *Science,* 354, 992-993. https://doi.org/10.1126/science.aal2613.

Uzzaman, A., & Cho, S. H. (2012). Chapter 28: Classification of hypersensitivity reactions. *Allergy and Asthma Proceedings,* 33(Suppl 1), 96-99. https://doi.org/10.2500/aap.2012.33.3561.

Vaughn, A. R., Clark, A. K., Sivamani, R. K., & Shi, V. Y. (2018). Circadian rhythm in atopic dermatitis: Pathophysiology and implications for chronotherapy. *Pediatric Dermatology,* 35, 152-157. https://doi.org/10.1111/pde.13364.

Vignola, A. M., Chiappare, G., Siena, L., Ganglierdo, P. C., & Bousqet, J. (2001). Fibro proliferative response in matrix deposition. *Clinical and ExperimentalAllergyReviews,* 1, 111-115. https://doi.org/10.1046/j.1472-9725.2001.00019.x.

Xing, Y., & Wong, G. W. (2022). Environmental influences and allergic diseases in the Asia-Pacific region: What will happen in the next 30 years? *Allergy, Asthma & Immunology Research,* 14(1), 21-39. https://doi.org/10.4168/aair.2022.14.1.21.

Walker, W. H., Walton, J. C., De Vries, A. C., & Nelson, R. J. (2020). Circadian rhythm disruption and mental health. *Translational psychiatry, 10*(1), 28. https://doi.org/10.1038/s41398-020-0694-0.

Wang, S., Liu, H., Yang, P., Wang, Z., Hu, P., Ye, P., & Chen, J. X. S. (2023). Exploring genetic association of allergic disease with cardiovascular disease: A bidirectional Mendelianr and omization study. Preprint (Version 1), Retrieved Research Square from https://doi.org/10.21203/rs.3.rs-2463442/v1.

Chapter 18

Roles of Light and the Circadian Rhythm in Response to Viral, Bacterial, and Parasitic Infections

Aydan Çevik Varol*, MD

Department of Department of Family Medicine, Namık Kemal University, Tekirdag, Turkiye

Abstract

This chapter examines the roles of light and the circadian rhythm in the response to viral, bacterial, and parasitic infections. Light serves as an environmental cue that synchronizes the circadian rhythm, which regulates immune function. Disruptions in the circadian rhythm, caused by altered light exposure patterns, can significantly impact the immune response of the body. The section explores the influence of light on viral, bacterial, and parasitic infections separately. It discusses how light affects viral replication, the host immune response, and antiviral therapies. It also explores the impact of light on bacterial toxin production, biofilm formation, and antibiotic effectiveness. Additionally, it investigates the influence of light on the life cycles, transmission, and immune evasion mechanisms of parasites. Furthermore, the section highlights the relationship between the circadian rhythm and the immune system. It examines how the circadian clock regulates immune cell function, cytokine production, and susceptibility to infections. It also explores the consequences of disrupted circadian rhythms on immune responses. By exploring these topics, this section contributes to future

---

* Corresponding Author's Email: dracevik@gmail.com

In: Human Health is a Matter of Timing
Editors: Sumeyya Deniz Aybek, Gonca Gulbay and Mucahit Secme
ISBN: 979-8-89113-467-6

research and therapeutic interventions targeting a wide range of infections.

Keywords: role of light, circadian rhythm, immune response, infection

Introduction

In recent years, research has shed light on the intricate interplay between light, the circadian rhythm, and the immune system. The circadian rhythm, often referred to as our body's internal clock, regulates a wide array of physiological processes, including sleep-wake cycles, hormone production, metabolism, and immune function. Light serves as a crucial environmental cue that synchronizes the circadian rhythm, helping to maintain its optimal functioning (Pearson et al., 2021; Bellet et al., 2020; Costantini et al., 2020; Scheiermann et al., 2013).

The influence of light and the circadian rhythm on infection response has emerged as a fascinating area of investigation. It is now recognized that disruptions to the circadian rhythm, such as those caused by shift work, jet lag, or irregular sleep patterns, can significantly impact the immune system's ability to mount an effective defense against pathogens. Similarly, exposure to light, particularly at specific times of the day, has been found to modulate immune responses and affect susceptibility to infections functioning (Pearson et al., 2021; Bellet et al., 2020; Costantini et al., 2020; Scheiermann et al., 2013).

The circadian regulation of the immune system is a complex and finely orchestrated process. Immune cells, such as lymphocytes, monocytes, and macrophages, exhibit circadian variations in their activation, migration, and cytokine production. These rhythmic immune processes ensure that the body is prepared to defend against potential pathogens at optimal times, aligning with the recurring environmental challenges it faces functioning (Scheiermann et al., 2013; Cox et al., 2022; Chang & Qiu, 2022; Al-Abri et al., 2023).

Moreover, emerging evidence suggests that the circadian rhythm influences the production and release of immune-related molecules, including cytokines, chemokines, and antimicrobial peptides. These molecules play crucial roles in the coordination of immune responses and in the regulation of the recruitment and activation of immune cells at the site of infection. Disruptions in circadian rhythm can dysregulate these immune signaling pathways, compromising the body's ability to effectively combat infections functioning (Pearson et al., 2021; Scheiermann et al., 2013; Cox et al., 2022; Chang & Qiu, 2022; Al-Abri et al., 2023; Scheiermann et al., 2018).

Light, as an external stimulus, plays a vital role in the entrainment of the circadian rhythm. The master circadian clock, located in the suprachiasmatic nucleus of the brain, receives input from specialized retinal cells known as intrinsically photosensitive retinal ganglion cells (ipRGCs). These cells are particularly sensitive to blue light and transmit signals to synchronize the internal clock with the external light-dark cycle. By influencing the circadian rhythm, light exposure can regulate immune processes and impact infection outcomes functioning (Cox et al., 2022; Chang & Qiu, 2022; Al-Abri et al., 2023; Scheiermann et al., 2018; Palomino-Segura & Hidalgo, 2021; Besedovsky et al., 2012; Haspel et al., 2020).

Furthermore, recent studies have unveiled direct interactions between light and immune cells. Photoreceptors present in immune cells, such as T cells and macrophages, can respond to light by altering cellular functions and immune signaling pathways. Light exposure can affect immune cell activation, proliferation, cytokine production, and phagocytic activity, thereby influencing the overall immune response to infections functioning (Scheiermann et al., 2013; Cox et al., 2022; Chang & Qiu, 2022; Al-Abri et al., 2023; Scheiermann et al., 2018; Palomino-Segura & Hidalgo, 2021; Besedovsky et al., 2012).

Understanding the roles of light and the circadian rhythm in infection response has significant implications for various fields, including infectious diseases, immunology, and chronobiology. By deciphering the mechanisms underlying these interactions, researchers aim to develop novel therapeutic strategies that leverage the circadian-immune axis to improve infection control. Manipulating light exposure and circadian timing may offer promising approaches to enhance immune defense, optimize vaccine efficacy, and minimize the impact of infectious diseases functioning (Besedovsky et al., 2012; Haspel et al., 2020; Fagiani et al., 2022; Duan et al., 2021; Olejniczak et al., 2022; Holtkamp et al., 2021; Ramsey et al., 2020; Brooks 2nd Behrendt et al., 2021; Gray et al., 2022).

Circadian Rhythm and Its Importance in the Immune System

The circadian rhythm is an intrinsic biological system that governs the timing and coordination of various physiological processes in the body, including the immune system. The term "circadian" originates from the Latin words "circa" (meaning "around") and "diem" (meaning "day"), reflecting the approximately 24-hour cycle that characterizes the circadian rhythm functioning. At the core of the circadian system is the master clock located in the suprachiasmatic nucleus of the hypothalamus. The SCN serves as the central pacemaker, orchestrating and synchronizing circadian rhythms throughout the body. It receives information about environmental light and darkness through the retinal pathway, allowing the circadian system to align with the external day-night cycle functioning (Besedovsky et al., 2012; Haspel et al., 2020; Fagiani et al., 2022; Duan et al., 2021; Olejniczak et al., 2022).

The circadian rhythm is regulated by a complex network of genes and proteins that interact in a feedback loop. The primary transcriptional activators, known as clock genes (e.g., CLOCK and BMAL1), promote the expression of other clock genes and proteins. These proteins, in turn, repress the activity of clock genes, forming a self-sustaining oscillation with a period of approximately 24 hours of functioning (Fagiani et al., 2022; Duan et al., 2021; Olejniczak et al., 2022; Holtkamp et al., 2021; Ramsey et al., 2020).

In addition to its role in the regulation of sleep-wake cycles and metabolism, the circadian rhythm exerts significant control over immune system functions. The immune system displays robust circadian variations in its activity, with numerous immune cells and molecular processes exhibiting rhythmic patterns functioning (Haspel et al., 2020; Fagiani et al., 2022; Duan et al., 2021; Olejniczak et al., 2022; Holtkamp et al., 2021; Ramsey et al., 2020; Brooks 2nd Behrendt et al., 2021; Gray et al., 2022; Logan & Sarkar, 2012; Liu et al., 2022; Shivshankar et al., 2020; Labrecque & Cermakian, 2015; Godinho-Silva et al., 2019).

One key aspect of circadian regulation in the immune system is the trafficking and migration of immune cells. Lymphocytes, for instance, exhibit circadian variations in their movement between lymphoid organs, blood circulation, and peripheral tissues. The timing of immune cell migration is thought to be crucial for effective immune surveillance and response to infections functioning (Cox et al., 2022; Chang & Qiu, 2022; Al-Abri et al., 2023).

Moreover, various immune functions, such as the production of cytokines, chemokines, and immune signaling molecules, are under circadian control. These molecules serve as important mediators of immune cell communication and coordination. Their rhythmic release ensures that immune responses are finely tuned to the time of day, optimizing defense mechanisms against pathogens functioning (Palomino-Segura & Hidalgo, 2021; Besedovsky et al., 2012; Haspel et al., 2020; Fagiani et al., 2022).

Circadian regulation also extends to the functioning of immune cells themselves. Different immune cell populations, including monocytes, macrophages, dendritic cells, and natural killer cells, display circadian variations in their activation, phagocytic activity, and antigen presentation capabilities. These rhythmic changes in immune cell function contribute to the overall robustness and efficiency of immune responses functioning (Pearson et al., 2021; Bellet et al., 2020; Fagiani et al., 2022; Duan et al., 2021; Olejniczak et al., 2022).

The significance of the circadian rhythm in the immune system is further highlighted by observations of immune dysregulation in circadian disruption conditions. Shift work, jet lag, and sleep disorders are examples of situations that can disturb the circadian rhythm. These disruptions have been associated with altered immune cell functionality, increased susceptibility to infections, and heightened inflammatory responses functioning (Holtkamp et al., 2021; Ramsey et al., 2020; Brooks 2nd Behrendt et al., 2021).

The molecular mechanisms underlying the circadian-immune interaction are complex and multifaceted. Clock genes, in addition to their role in maintaining the circadian rhythm, can directly modulate immune processes. They can influence the expression of immune-related genes, regulate immune cell differentiation and function, and affect the production of cytokines and other immune mediators functioning (Olejniczak et al., 2022; Holtkamp et al., 2021; Ramsey et al., 2020; Brooks 2nd Behrendt et al., 2021; Gray et al., 2022; Logan & Sarkar, 2012).

Furthermore, the circadian rhythm intersects with other signaling pathways and molecular processes that impact immune responses. For instance, the circadian system interacts with the hypothalamic-pituitary-adrenal (HPA) axis and the sympathetic nervous system, both of which play critical roles in immune regulation. These interactions contribute to the circadian modulation of immune functions and responses to infectious challenges functioning (Gray et al., 2022; Logan & Sarkar, 2012; Liu et al., 2022; Shivshankar et al., 2020).

Understanding the importance circadian rhythm in the immune system has broad implications for human health and disease. Disruptions to the circadian rhythm, such as those experienced during shift work or international travel, can compromise immune function, leading to increased susceptibility to infections and inflammatory disorders. Conversely, optimizing circadian alignment and promoting healthy sleep-wake cycles may enhance immune defense mechanisms and overall well-being functioning (Duan et al., 2021; Olejniczak et al., 2022; Holtkamp et al., 2021; Ramsey et al., 2020).

The Impact of Light on the Immune Response to Infections

Light, as an environmental cue, plays a vital role in modulating various physiological processes in the human body, including the immune response to infections. The effects of light on the immune system have gained significant attention in recent years, highlighting its potential as a powerful regulator of immune function and infection outcomes. One of the primary ways light influences the immune response is through its impact on the circadian rhythm. Light exposure, particularly in the blue spectrum, is a crucial entrainment signal for the master circadian clock in the suprachiasmatic nucleus of the brain. By aligning the circadian rhythm with the external light-dark cycle, light helps synchronize the timing of immune processes, ensuring optimal immune defense against pathogens functioning (Pearson et al., 2021; Bellet et al., 2020; Logan & Sarkar, 2012; Liu et al., 2022).

Studies have shown that disruptions of the natural light-dark cycle, such as those experienced during shift work or frequent travel across time zones, can impair immune function. These disruptions can lead to dysregulation of the circadian rhythm and compromise the timing of immune cell activities and the release of immune mediators. Consequently, this misalignment may result in decreased immune surveillance, reduced pathogen clearance, and an increased susceptibility to infections functioning (Logan & Sarkar, 2012; Liu et al., 2022; Shivshankar et al., 2020; Labrecque & Cermakian, 2015; Godinho-Silva et al., 2019).

Moreover, exposure to light can directly influence immune cells and immune responses. Photoreceptors present in immune cells, such as T cells, B cells, and macrophages, allow them to respond to light stimuli. These photoreceptors, including opsins and cryptochromes, can sense and transduce light signals into intracellular biochemical pathways, affecting immune cell activation, proliferation, and cytokine production functioning (Brooks 2nd Behrendt et al., 2021; Gray et al., 2022; Logan & Sarkar, 2012).

Research has demonstrated that exposure to specific wavelengths and intensities of light can have distinct effects on immune cell behavior. Blue light, for example, has been shown to enhance the phagocytic activity of macrophages and stimulate the production of antimicrobial peptides. On the other hand, red and infrared light has been found to promote tissue healing and reduce inflammation, thereby modulating the immune response to the functioning of infections (Palomino-Segura & Hidalgo, 2021; Besedovsky et al., 2012; Mavroudis et al., 2013; Bellet et al., 2013; Borrmann et al., 2020; Lee et al., 2021).

Furthermore, light exposure can impact the production and release of cytokines and chemokines, which are crucial for coordinating immune responses. Different wavelengths of light have been shown to affect the expression of pro-inflammatory and anti-inflammatory cytokines, influencing the balance between immune activation and resolution. This modulation of cytokine profiles can influence the magnitude and duration of immune responses to infections functioning (Palomino-Segura & Hidalgo, 2021; Besedovsky et al., 2012; Haspel et al., 2020; Fagiani et al., 2022).

The timing of light exposure also appears to be important to determine its effects on the immune response. Studies have shown that the timing of light exposure can influence the expression of clock genes in immune cells and regulate their immune functions. Light exposure during specific phases of the circadian rhythm can enhance immune cell activity and promote a robust immune response, while exposure at inappropriate times may disrupt immune processes and impair infection defense functioning (Gray et al., 2022; Logan & Sarkar, 2012; Liu et al., 2022; Shivshankar et al., 2020; Labrecque & Cermakian, 2015; Godinho-Silva et al., 2019; Mavroudis et al., 2013).

Collectively, these findings highlight the significant impact of light on the immune response to infections. The ability of light to modulate the circadian rhythm, directly influence immune cell behavior, and regulate cytokine production underscores its potential as a therapeutic tool to enhance immune defense. Light-based interventions, such as bright light therapy, have shown promise in boosting immune responses and improving outcomes in various infectious diseases functioning (Mavroudis et al., 2013; Bellet et al., 2013; Borrmann et al., 2020; Lee et al., 2021; Zandi et al., 2023).

However, it is important to note that the effects of light on the immune system are complex and context-dependent. Factors such as the duration and intensity of light exposure, the specific pathogen involved, and individual variations in circadian biology can all influence the outcomes. Further research is needed to elucidate the underlying mechanisms and optimize the use of light as a modulator of immune response functioning (Pearson et al., 2021; Bellet et al., 2020; Ramsey et al., 2020; Brooks 2nd Behrendt et al., 2021; Gray et al., 2022).

Viral Infections

In recent years, research has revealed intriguing interactions between viral infections, the circadian rhythm, and light exposure, shedding light on the mechanisms that underlie the timing and effectiveness of immune responses functioning (Gray et al., 2022; Logan & Sarkar, 2012; Liu et al., 2022; Shivshankar et al., 2020; Bellet et al., 2013; Blanco et al., 2022; Skrlec & Talapko, 2022; Borrmann et al., 2021; Pearson et al., 2021).

The circadian rhythm has been found to play a critical role in the defense of the host against viral infections. Studies have shown that the timing of viral exposure can influence infection outcomes, with variations observed in viral replication, disease severity, and immune responses depending on the time of day. The circadian regulation of immune cell functions, such as the activity of natural killer (NK) cells and T cells, appears to contribute to this time-of-day-dependent susceptibility to viral infection functioning (Duan et al., 2021; Olejniczak et al., 2022; Holtkamp et al., 2021; Ramsey et al., 2020; Brooks 2nd Behrendt et al., 2021; Gray et al., 2022; Logan & Sarkar, 2012; Liu et al., 2022; Shivshankar et al., 2020; Labrecque & Cermakian, 2015; Bellet et al., 2013; Blanco et al., 2022; Skrlec & Talapko, 2022; Borrmann et al., 2021; Pearson et al., 2021).

Viral infections can also impact the circadian rhythm. Viruses have been shown to disrupt the molecular clock machinery within host cells, altering the rhythmic expression of clock genes, and affecting circadian oscillations. This disruption can have profound effects on immune cell functions and the timing of antiviral immune responses. For instance, the dysregulation of clock genes in response to viral infection may lead to impaired immune cell activation, compromised cytokine production, and suboptimal immune defense functioning (Zandi et al., 2023; Blanco et al., 2022; Skrlec & Talapko, 2022; Borrmann et al., 2021).

Moreover, light exposure has been found to modulate the immune response to viral infections. In the context of viral diseases, light exposure can influence the production of antiviral cytokines, such as interferons, which are critical for controlling viral replication and spreading. It has been observed that blue light exposure can enhance the expression of interferons and stimulate the antiviral activity of immune cells, potentially leading to improved viral clearance functioning (Chang & Qiu, 2022; Al-Abri et al., 2023; Scheiermann et al., 2018; Palomino-Segura & Hidalgo, 2021; Borrmann et al., 2021; Pearson et al., 2021).

Exposure to light can also impact the molecular mechanisms involved in viral replication and host-virus interactions. For instance, certain viruses possess light-sensitive proteins known as photoreceptors that enable them to sense and respond to specific wavelengths of light. Light-induced activation or suppression of these viral photoreceptors can modulate viral replication, gene expression, and host immune response functioning (Mavroudis et al., 2013; Bellet et al., 2013; Borrmann et al., 2020; Lee et al., 2021; Zandi et al., 2023).

Recent studies have suggested that light-based interventions may hold promise in the management of viral infections. For instance, the use of ultraviolet (UV) light in certain wavelengths has been investigated as a potential antiviral therapy. UV light can directly inactivate viral particles and disrupt their genetic material, limiting viral replication and spread. Additionally, bright light therapy has shown promise in enhancing immune responses and reducing the severity of viral infection functioning (Pearson et al., 2021; Zhuang et al., 2022; Chacón et al., 2022; Downton et al., 2020).

Understanding the intricate interactions between viral infections, the circadian rhythm, and light exposure is crucial for developing targeted strategies to combat viral diseases. By optimizing the timing of interventions, such as antiviral treatments or light-based therapies, it may be possible to enhance the effectiveness of immune responses against specific viral pathogens. Furthermore, the integration of light management strategies, such as maintaining appropriate light-dark cycles and minimizing light exposure during vulnerable periods, may contribute to improved outcomes in viral infection control functioning (Zhuang et al., 2022; Chacón et al., 2022; Downton et al., 2020; Carvalho Cabral et al., 2019; Borges-Pereira et al., 2020).

Bacterial Infections

Studies have shown that some bacteria such as *Enterobacter aerogenes, Streptococcus pneumoniae*, *Escherichia coli, Pseudomonas aeruginosa, Legionella pneumophilia, Helicbacter pylori, Bacillus subtilis*, and cyanobacteria such as *Synechococcus elongatus* have circadian rhythms. Some of their actions including cell division, amino acid uptake, photosynthesis, or swarming/motility may vary according to exposure to light. Besides this, recent research provides information about interactions between bacterial infections and the circadian rhythm, revealing the importance of circadian regulation in mounting an effective immune defense against bacterial invaders functioning (Pearson et al., 2021; Bellet et al., 2020; Ramsey et al., 2020; Brooks 2nd Behrendt et al., 2021; Borrmann et al., 2020; Zhuang et al., 2022; Carvalho Cabral et al., 2019; Borges-Pereira et al., 2020).

The circadian rhythm exerts a profound influence on immune cell functions, including those involved in the response to bacterial infections. Various immune cell populations, such as monocytes, macrophages, and neutrophils, exhibit circadian variations in their activation, migration, and cytokine production. These rhythmic immune processes help optimize the timing and coordination of immune responses, ensuring effective defense against bacterial pathogens functioning (Duan et al., 2021; Olejniczak et al., 2022; Holtkamp et al., 2021; Ramsey et al., 2020; Lee et al., 2021; Zandi et al., 2023).

Studies have demonstrated that the time of day at which a bacterial infection occurs can impact infection outcomes. The circadian regulation of immune cells and immune signaling molecules plays a critical role in determining the timing and magnitude of the immune response to bacterial invaders. For example, the activity of phagocytes, key immune cells responsible for engulfing and eliminating bacteria, is subject to circadian control. The phagocytic activity of these cells, along with the production of antimicrobial peptides and pro-inflammatory cytokines, exhibits rhythmic variations that can influence bacterial clearance and infection resolution functioning (Holtkamp et al., 2021; Ramsey et al., 2020; Brooks 2nd Behrendt et al., 2021; Gray et al., 2022; Zhuang et al., 2022; Carvalho Cabral et al., 2019; Borges-Pereira et al., 2020).

The circadian rhythm also influences the expression and activity of pattern recognition receptors (PRRs) involved in the recognition of bacterial components. Toll-like receptors (TLRs), a class of PRRs, exhibit circadian variations in their expression, affecting the recognition and response to bacterial pathogens. The timing of bacterial infection can influence the accessibility and functionality of TLRs, thereby impacting the initiation and coordination of the immune response functioning (Pearson et al., 2021; Al-Abri et al., 2023; Fagiani et al., 2022; Duan et al., 2021; Olejniczak et al., 2022; Borges-Pereira et al., 2020).

The circadian regulation of the gut microbiota, which consists of a diverse community of bacteria residing in the gastrointestinal tract, has implications for host defense against bacterial infections. The circadian rhythm influences various aspects of the gut environment, such as nutrient availability and epithelial integrity, which in turn impact the composition and function of the gut microbiota. Dysregulation of the circadian rhythm can disrupt the delicate balance of the gut microbiota and compromise its protective effects against bacterial pathogens functioning (Haspel et al., 2020; Fagiani et al., 2022; Duan et al., 2021; Mavroudis et al., 2013; Bellet et al., 2013; Borrmann et al., 2020;

Lee et al., 2021; Zandi et al., 2023; Blanco et al., 2022; Skrlec & Talapko, 2022; Borrmann et al., 2021).

Bacteria themselves possess circadian-like mechanisms that can modulate their virulence and interactions with the host's immune system. For instance, certain bacteria exhibit rhythmic expression of virulence factors, such as toxins or adhesive molecules, which may enhance their ability to establish infection or evade immune surveillance during specific times of the day. These temporal variations in bacterial virulence can influence the outcome of bacterial infections and the effectiveness of immune responses functioning (Zhuang et al., 2022; Chacón et al., 2022; Downton et al., 2020; Carvalho Cabral et al., 2019; Borges-Pereira et al., 2020).

The importance of circadian regulation in the immune response to bacterial infections is further underscored by observations of immune dysregulation in circadian disruption conditions. Shift work, for instance, is associated with altered immune cell functions, impaired phagocytosis, and increased susceptibility to bacterial infections. Disruptions in the natural light-dark cycle, such as exposure to artificial light at night or irregular sleep patterns, can disrupt circadian rhythms and compromise the timing and effectiveness of immune defense against bacterial pathogens functioning.

Timing therapeutic interventions to align with the peak immune activity may enhance the effectiveness of antimicrobial treatments. Additionally, strategies aimed at maintaining a healthy circadian rhythm, such as optimizing sleep patterns and promoting regular light-dark cycles, may strengthen the immune system's ability to mount a robust defense against bacterial invaders (Haspel et al., 2020; Fagiani et al., 2022; Duan et al., 2021; Skrlec & Talapko, 2022; Borrmann et al., 2021; Pearson et al., 2021; Zhuang et al., 2022).

Parasitic Infections

Recent research has shed light on the complex interactions between parasitic infections, the circadian rhythm, and light exposure, revealing the importance of circadian regulation in the maintenance of an effective immune defense against parasitic invaders functioning. The circadian rhythm has emerged as a critical regulator of immune responses to parasitic infections. Various immune cell populations, including lymphocytes, macrophages, and dendritic cells, exhibit circadian variations in their activation, migration, and cytokine production. These rhythmic immune processes help optimize the timing and coordination of immune responses, ensuring effective defense against parasitic pathogens functioning (Zhuang et al., 2022; Chacón et al., 2022; Downton et al., 2020; Carvalho Cabral et al., 2019; Borges-Pereira et al., 2020).

The parasites have developed sophisticated strategies to manipulate and exploit the host's circadian rhythm. For example, certain parasitic organisms exhibit rhythmic patterns of activity and reproduction that are synchronized with the host's circadian rhythm. By aligning their life cycles with the host's biological rhythms, parasites can maximize their chances of survival and transmission functioning (Besedovsky et al., 2012; Haspel et al., 2020; Mavroudis et al., 2013; Bellet et al., 2013; Borrmann et al., 2020; Zhuang et al., 2022; Chacón et al., 2022; Downton et al., 2020; Carvalho Cabral et al., 2019; Borges-Pereira et al., 2020).

The circadian rhythm also influences the functioning of immune cells involved in the response to parasitic infections. For instance, studies have shown that natural killer (NK) cells, important effectors of the innate immune response, display circadian variations in their cytotoxic activity against parasitic targets. Additionally, the timing of antigen presentation by dendritic cells to T cells can be influenced by the circadian rhythm, affecting the subsequent adaptive immune response against parasitic pathogens functioning (Blanco et al., 2022; Skrlec & Talapko, 2022; Borrmann et al., 2021; Pearson et al., 2021; Zhuang et al., 2022; Chacón et al., 2022; Downton et al., 2020; Carvalho Cabral et al., 2019; Borges-Pereira et al., 2020).

Light exposure, as a crucial environmental cue, can influence immune responses to parasitic infections. Light information received through specialized retinal cells, called intrinsically photosensitive retinal ganglion cells, helps entrain the master circadian clock in the brain to the external light-dark cycle. Disruptions in the natural light-dark cycle, such as those experienced during shift work or exposure to artificial light at night, can impact the circadian rhythm and compromise immune defense against parasitic invaders functioning (Borrmann et al., 2020; Lee et al., 2021; Zandi et al., 2023; Blanco et al., 2022; Zhuang et al., 2022; Chacón et al., 2022; Downton et al., 2020; Carvalho Cabral et al., 2019; Borges-Pereira et al., 2020).

Interestingly, parasitic infections themselves can be influenced by exposure to light. Certain parasites, such as those causing malaria or sleeping sickness, exhibit phototactic behaviors, meaning they can sense and respond to light stimuli. Light-induced activation or suppression of specific parasite molecules can influence their development, reproduction, and infectivity. Furthermore, light exposure has been shown to affect the activity and growth of some parasitic organisms, potentially impacting the course of infection functioning (Zhuang et al., 2022; Chacón et al., 2022; Downton et al., 2020; Carvalho Cabral et al., 2019; Borges-Pereira et al., 2020).

The timing of light exposure can also modulate immune responses to parasitic infections. The circadian rhythm regulates the expression and activity of immune molecules involved in parasite recognition and defense. For instance, the production of cytokines, chemokines, and antimicrobial peptides that contribute to the immune response against parasitic pathogens can be influenced by the timing of light exposure. Optimizing light exposure to align with the peak immune activity may enhance the immune response and improve outcomes in parasitic infections functioning (Zhuang et al., 2022; Chacón et al., 2022; Downton et al., 2020; Carvalho Cabral et al., 2019; Borges-Pereira et al., 2020).

Some parasites such as Plasmodium falciparum, Leishmania spp., and Schistosoma mansoni have their own circadian rhythm. Additioanlly, Tripanosoma brucei parasitic infection is one of the important parasitic infections that disrupts the patient's circadian rhythm resulting in "sleeping sickness". However, the pathogenesis of this disease is not directly related to light, it's caused because of involvement of the brain and neuroinflammation functioning (Gray et al., 2022; Logan & Sarkar, 2012; Zhuang et al., 2022; Chacón et al., 2022; Downton et al., 2020; Carvalho Cabral et al., 2019; Borges-Pereira et al., 2020).

Understanding the role of light and the circadian rhythm in the immune response to parasitic infections has important implications for infection control and treatment strategies. Chronotherapy approaches that consider the timing of anti-parasitic treatments and interventions may enhance their effectiveness. Additionally, maintaining a healthy circadian rhythm, promoting regular light exposure patterns, and optimizing sleep-wake cycles may strengthen the immune system's ability to combat parasitic invaders functioning (Zhuang et al., 2022; Chacón et al., 2022; Downton et al., 2020; Carvalho Cabral et al., 2019; Borges-Pereira et al., 2020).

Disruptions to Circadian Rhythm and Light Exposure: Implications for Infection Susceptibility

The circadian rhythm and light exposure play crucial roles in maintaining optimal immune function and the body's ability to mount an effective defense against infections. Disruptions in the natural circadian rhythm and alterations in light exposure patterns have been found to have significant implications for infection susceptibility, compromising the immune response and increasing vulnerability to pathogens functioning (Pearson et al., 2021; Gray et al., 2022; Borrmann et al., 2020; Lee et al., 2021; Zandi et al., 2023; Blanco et al., 2022; Skrlec & Talapko, 2022; Borrmann et al., 2021).

Exposure to artificial light at night has become increasingly prevalent with the widespread use of electronic devices and artificial lighting. Exposure to artificial light during the nighttime hours can suppress the release of melatonin, a hormone involved in the regulation of sleep-wake cycles and immune function. The suppression of melatonin and the disruption of the natural light-dark cycle can disrupt the circadian rhythm and compromise immune defense mechanisms functioning (Pearson et al., 2021; Bellet et al., 2020; Holtkamp et al., 2021; Ramsey et al., 2020; Brooks 2nd Behrendt et al., 2021; Gray et al., 2022).

Disruptions to the circadian rhythm and alterations in light exposure have been associated with increased susceptibility to various infections. Studies have shown that individuals with disrupted circadian rhythms, such as shift workers or individuals with sleep disorders, are more prone to respiratory tract infections, gastrointestinal infections, and viral infections. This increased susceptibility is attributed to compromised immune function, impaired antiviral responses, and altered cytokine production functioning (Cox et al., 2022; Chang & Qiu, 2022; Al-Abri et al., 2023; Scheiermann et al., 2018; Palomino-Segura & Hidalgo, 2021; Chacón et al., 2022; Downton et al., 2020).

The ability of the immune system to mount an effective defense against pathogens relies on the precise timing and coordination of immune processes. Disruptions to the circadian rhythm and alterations in light exposure can disrupt the timing of immune cell activities, cytokine release, and immune cell trafficking, leading to suboptimal immune responses functioning (Ramsey et al., 2020; Brooks 2nd Behrendt et al., 2021; Gray et al., 2022; Pearson et al., 2021; Zhuang et al., 2022; Chacón et al., 2022).

One of the mechanisms through which circadian disruption impacts immune function is the dysregulation of clock genes and clock-controlled genes. Clock genes, including CLOCK, BMAL1, PER, and CRY play key roles in maintaining the circadian rhythm and regulating immune cell functions. Disruptions to the circadian rhythm can lead to dysregulated expression and activity of these clock genes, resulting in compromised immune cell responses and impaired infection control functioning (Scheiermann et al., 2013; Cox et al., 2022; Chang & Qiu, 2022; Al-Abri et al., 2023; Brooks 2nd Behrendt et al., 2021; Labrecque & Cermakian, 2015; Zhuang et al., 2022).

Moreover, the suppression of melatonin secretion due to exposure to artificial light at night can impact immune function. Melatonin has immunomodulatory properties and is involved in regulation the activity of immune cells, including T cells, B cells, and natural killer cells. Reduced levels of melatonin can result in diminished immune cell function, decreased antibody production, and impaired immune surveillance against infections functioning (Mavroudis et al., 2013; Bellet et al., 2013; Borrmann et al., 2020; Lee et al., 2021; Zandi et al., 2023; Blanco et al., 2022; Zhuang et al., 2022; Chacón et al., 2022; Borges-Pereira et al., 2020).

The implications of disruptions in the circadian rhythm and light exposure patterns extend beyond the individual level. For example, shift workers in healthcare settings, such as hospitals, face increased risks of infections and impaired immune responses. Additionally, the disturbance of the circadian rhythm in frequent travelers, such as those experiencing jet lag, can have consequences for their susceptibility to infections during and after travel functioning (Godinho-Silva et al., 2019; Mavroudis et al., 2013; Bellet et al., 2013; Zhuang et al., 2022; Chacón et al., 2022).

Understanding the implications of circadian disruption and altered light exposure patterns for infection susceptibility is essential to develop strategies to mitigate these risks. Promoting healthy sleep-wake cycles, minimizing exposure to artificial light at night, and optimizing the timing of light exposure can help restore and maintain circadian alignment. These measures may enhance immune function, reduce infection susceptibility, and improve overall health outcomes functioning (Cox et al., 2022; Chang & Qiu, 2022; Al-Abri et al., 2023; Scheiermann et al., 2018; Palomino-Segura & Hidalgo, 2021; Besedovsky et al., 2012; Haspel et al., 2020; Fagiani et al., 2022; Duan et al., 2021; Labrecque & Cermakian, 2015; Godinho-Silva et al., 2019; Mavroudis et al., 2013).

Therapeutic Approaches: Modulation of Circadian Rhythm and Light to Enhance Immune Defense

The circadian rhythm and light exposure are emerging as promising therapeutic targets for enhancing immune defense against infections. The intricate interplay between the circadian rhythm, light, and the immune system presents opportunities for developing innovative interventions aimed at optimizing immune responses and improving infection control functioning. Chronotherapy, the strategic timing of therapeutic interventions based on the circadian rhythm, has great potential in enhancing immune defense against infections. By aligning the timing of treatments with the circadian phase of optimal immune activity, chronotherapy aims to maximize treatment efficacy while minimizing side effects functioning (Labrecque & Cermakian, 2015; Godinho-Silva et al., 2019; Blanco et al., 2022; Skrlec & Talapko, 2022; Borrmann et al., 2021; Pearson et al., 2021).

Studies have demonstrated that the timing of administration of antiviral medications can impact their effectiveness. Antiviral drugs, such as those used in the treatment of influenza or HIV, may exhibit enhanced efficacy when administered at specific times of the day that align with the highest immune response against viral pathogens. By considering the circadian regulation of immune processes, chronotherapy approaches can optimize treatment outcomes and reduce the risk of drug resistance functioning. Light-based therapies offer another avenue to modulate the immune response and enhance immune defense against infections. Light therapy, also known as phototherapy, involves controlled exposure to specific wavelengths of light to stimulate biological processes. Light therapy has been successfully used in various medical fields, such as dermatology and psychiatry, and is now being explored for its potential in enhancing immune function functioning (Palomino-Segura & Hidalgo, 2021; Besedovsky et al., 2012; Haspel et al., 2020; Fagiani et al., 2022; Duan et al., 2021; Olejniczak et al., 2022; Holtkamp et al., 2021; Zhuang et al., 2022; Chacón et al., 2022; Downton et al., 2020).

Research has shown that exposure to specific wavelengths of light, such as blue or near-infrared light, can modulate immune responses and improve infection control. Blue light has been found to enhance antimicrobial activity in immune cells, stimulate cytokine production, and promote wound healing. Near-infrared light, on the other hand, has shown the potential to reduce inflammation, enhance tissue repair, and improve the functioning of immune function. Light therapy can be delivered through various methods, including light-emitting diodes (LEDs), lasers, or specialized devices. The timing, duration, and intensity of light exposure are important factors to consider when designing light-based therapies to enhance immune defense. Optimizing light exposure parameters to align with the circadian rhythm and specific immune processes can maximize the functioning of therapeutic benefits (Pearson et al., 2021; Bellet et al., 2020; Costantini et al., 2020; Scheiermann et al., 2013; Borrmann et al., 2020; Lee et al., 2021; Zandi et al., 2023; Blanco et al., 2022;

Skrlec & Talapko, 2022; Borrmann et al., 2021; Pearson et al., 2021; Zhuang et al., 2022).

In addition to external light exposure, optimizing the natural light-dark cycle is crucial for maintaining a healthy circadian rhythm and enhancing immune defense. Minimizing exposure to artificial light at night, particularly from electronic devices and indoor lighting, can help promote the secretion of melatonin, which has immunomodulatory effects. Creating a sleep environment that mimics natural darkness and ensuring adequate exposure to natural daylight during the day can help reinforce the circadian rhythm and support optimal immune function. Lifestyle modifications that promote healthy sleep-wake patterns and prioritize regular exposure to light can also contribute to enhancing immune defense. Consistent sleep routines, with sufficient sleep duration and quality, help maintain the circadian rhythm and support robust immune responses. Establishing habits that align with the natural light-dark cycle, such as spending time outdoors during daylight hours, can reinforce the entrainment of the circadian rhythm and optimize the functioning of the immune function (Duan et al., 2021; Olejniczak et al., 2022; Holtkamp et al., 2021; Ramsey et al., 2020; Labrecque & Cermakian, 2015; Godinho-Silva et al., 2019; Mavroudis et al., 2013; Bellet et al., 2013; Carvalho Cabral et al., 2019; Borges-Pereira et al., 2020).

Furthermore, personalized approaches that consider an individual's chronotype, or their propensity to be a morning person or an evening person, can optimize therapeutic strategies. Chronotypes influence an individual's circadian preferences and their response to light exposure at different times of the day. By tailoring interventions based on an individual's chronotype, therapeutic effectiveness may be enhanced, leading to better immune defense and infection control outcomes functioning (Borrmann et al., 2020; Lee et al., 2021; Zandi et al., 2023; Blanco et al., 2022; Skrlec & Talapko, 2022; Borrmann et al., 2021; Pearson et al., 2021; Zhuang et al., 2022; Chacón et al., 2022).

In conclusion, therapeutic approaches that modulate the circadian rhythm and light exposure hold promise for enhancing immune defense against infections. Chronotherapy, through the strategic timing of treatments, can optimize therapeutic outcomes by aligning with the circadian regulation of immune processes. Light-based therapies, such as light therapy and optimized light exposure, offer additional avenues to stimulate immune responses and improve infection control. By leveraging the interplay between the circadian rhythm, light, and the immune system, these innovative approaches may contribute to more effective and personalized strategies for enhancing immune defense and combating infectious diseases functioning (Gray et al., 2022; Logan & Sarkar, 2012; Liu et al., 2022; Shivshankar et al., 2020; Labrecque & Cermakian, 2015).

Conclusion

Light exposure, as a crucial environmental cue, plays a pivotal role in entraining the circadian rhythm and modulating immune responses. Specific wavelengths of light, such as blue or red light, have been found to stimulate immune cell activity, influence cytokine production, and promote wound healing. Conversely, disruptions to the natural light-dark cycle, such as exposure to artificial light at night, can disrupt circadian entrainment and compromise immune defense. Understanding the effects of light exposure on immune function enables the development of interventions that harness its potential to enhance immune responses and improve infection control functioning. Therapeutic approaches that modulate the circadian rhythm and light exposure hold promise for enhancing immune defense against infections. Chronotherapy, with its strategic timing of treatments to align with the circadian rhythm, can optimize the efficacy of treatment and minimize side effects. Light-based therapies, such as phototherapy, offer innovative avenues for stimulating immune responses and improving infection outcomes. By leveraging the interplay between light, the circadian rhythm, and the immune system, these therapeutic approaches may contribute to more effective strategies for infection control functioning (Pearson et al., 2021; Bellet et al., 2020; Gray et al., 2022, 2020; Lee et al., 2021; Zandi et al., 2023; Blanco et al., 2022).

While significant progress has been made, there are still many exciting avenues for future research in this field. Unraveling the underlying molecular mechanisms connecting light exposure, the circadian rhythm, and immune responses will provide deeper insights into the complex interplay between these factors. Further exploration of individual variations, the long-term effects of circadian disruption, and the impact on different types of infections will help tailor interventions and therapies to individuals and specific infectious diseases functioning. Interdisciplinary collaborations will be essential for advancing research and translating findings into practical applications. Collaborations between researchers in immunology, chronobiology, lighting engineering, and healthcare fields can bridge the gap between fundamental research and real-world implementation. Integrating light and circadian management strategies into healthcare settings may contribute to infection control measures and improve patient outcomes functioning (Duan et al., 2021; Olejniczak et al., 2022; Holtkamp et al., 2021; Ramsey et al., 2020; Logan & Sarkar, 2012; Liu et al., 2022; Shivshankar et al., 2020; Labrecque & Cermakian, 2015; Borrmann et al., 2020; Lee et al., 2021; Zandi et al., 2023; Blanco et al., 2022).

In conclusion, the study of light, the circadian rhythm, and the immune response to infections has shed light on the intricate relationship between our environment and our immune system. By understanding and harnessing these interactions, we can develop innovative strategies to improve infection control, enhance immune defense, and optimize treatment outcomes. The path towards improved infection control is illuminated by the growing body of knowledge in this field. It is an exciting journey that will continue to unveil new insights and pave the way for advancements in the prevention, treatment, and management of infectious diseases.

References

Al-Abri, M. A., Al-Yaarubi, S., & Said, E. A. (2023). Circadian Rhythm, Sleep, and Immune Response and the Fight against COVID-19. *Oman medical journal, 38*(2), e477. https://doi.org/10.5001/omj.2023.38.

Bellet, M. M., Deriu, E., Liu, J. Z., Grimaldi, B., Blaschitz, C., Zeller, M., Edwards, R. A., Sahar, S., Dandekar, S., Baldi, P., George, M. D., Raffatellu, M., & Sassone-Corsi, P. (2013). Circadian clock regulates the host response to Salmonella. *Proceedings of the National Academy of Sciences of the United States of America, 110*(24), 9897–9902. https://doi.org/10.1073/pnas.1120636110.

Bellet, M. M., Eckel-Mahan, K., & Romani, L. (2020). Editorial: Circadian Rhythm: From Microbes to Hosts. *Frontiers in cellular and infection microbiology, 10*, 613181. https://doi.org/10.3389/fcimb.2020.613181.

Besedovsky, L., Lange, T., & Born, J. (2012). Sleep and immune function. Pflugers Archiv: *European journal of physiology, 463*(1), 121–137. https://doi.org/10.1007/s00424-011-1044-0.

Blanco, J. R., Verdugo-Sivianes, E. M., Amiama, A., & Muñoz-Galván, S. (2022). The circadian rhythm of viruses and its implications on susceptibility to infection. *Expert review of anti-infective therapy, 20*(8), 1109–1117. https://doi.org/10.1080/14787210.2022.2072296.

Borges-Pereira, L., Dias, B. K. M., Singh, M. K., & Garcia, C. R. S. (2020). Malaria parasites and circadian rhythm: New insights into an old puzzle. Current research in microbial sciences, 2, 100017. https://doi.org/10.1016/j.crmicr.2020.100017.

Borrmann, H., Davies, R., Dickinson, M., Pedroza-Pacheco, I., Schilling, M., Vaughan-Jackson, A., Magri, A., James, W., Balfe, P., Borrow, P., McKeating, J. A., & Zhuang,

X. (2020). Pharmacological activation of the circadian component REV-ERB inhibits HIV-1 replication. *Scientific reports, 10*(1), 13271. https://doi.org/10.1038/s41598-020-70170-3.

Borrmann, H., McKeating, J. A., & Zhuang, X. (2021). The Circadian Clock and Viral Infections. *Journal of biological rhythms, 36*(1), 9–22. https://doi.org/10.1177/0748730420967768.

Brooks, J. F., 2nd, Behrendt, C. L., Ruhn, K. A., Lee, S., Raj, P., Takahashi, J. S., & Hooper, L. V. (2021). The microbiota coordinates diurnal rhythms in innate immunity with the circadian clock. *Cell, 184*(16), 4154–4167.e12. https://doi.org/10.1016/j.cell.2021.07.001.

Carvalho Cabral, P., Olivier, M., & Cermakian, N. (2019). The Complex Interplay of Parasites, Their Hosts, and Circadian Clocks. Frontiers in cellular and infection microbiology, 9, 425. https://doi.org/10.3389/fcimb.2019.00425.

Chacón, F., Muñoz-San Martín, C., Bacigalupo, A., Álvarez-Duhart, B., Solís, R., & Cattan, P. E. (2022). Trypanosoma cruzi Parasite Load Modulates the Circadian Activity Pattern of Triatoma infestans. Insects, 13(1), 76. https://doi.org/10.3390/insects13010076.

Chang, J. L., & Qiu, J. (2022). *Sichuan da xue xue bao. Yi xue ban = Journal of Sichuan University. Medical science edition*, *53*(1), 15–19. https://doi.org/10.12182/20220160502.

Costantini, C., Renga, G., Sellitto, F., Borghi, M., Stincardini, C., Pariano, M., Zelante, T., Chiarotti, F., Bartoli, A., Mosci, P., Romani, L., Brancorsini, S., & Bellet, M. M. (2020). Microbes in the Era of Circadian Medicine. *Frontiers in cellular and infection microbiology*, *10*, 30. https://doi.org/10.3389/fcimb.2020.00030.

Cox, S. L., O'Siorain, J. R., Fagan, L. E., Curtis, A. M., & Carroll, R. G. (2022). Intertwining roles of circadian and metabolic regulation of the innate immune response. *Seminars in immunopathology*, *44*(2), 225–237. https://doi.org/10.1007/s00281-021-00905-5.

Downton, P., Early, J. O., & Gibbs, J. E. (2020). Circadian rhythms in adaptive immunity. Immunology, 161(4), 268–277. https://doi.org/10.1111/imm.13167.

Duan, J., Greenberg, E. N., Karri, S. S., & Andersen, B. (2021). The circadian clock and diseases of the skin. *FEBS letters, 595*(19), 2413–2436. https://doi.org/10.1002/1873-3468.14192.

Fagiani, F., Di Marino, D., Romagnoli, A., Travelli, C., Voltan, D., Di Cesare Mannelli, L., Racchi, M., Govoni, S., & Lanni, C. (2022). Molecular regulations of circadian rhythm and implications for physiology and diseases. *Signal transduction and targeted therapy, 7*(1), 41. https://doi.org/10.1038/s41392-022-00899-y.

Godinho-Silva, C., Domingues, R. G., Rendas, M., Raposo, B., Ribeiro, H., da Silva, J. A., Vieira, A., Costa, R. M., Barbosa-Morais, N. L., Carvalho, T., & Veiga-Fernandes, H. (2019). Light-entrained and brain-tuned circadian circuits regulate ILC3s and gut homeostasis. *Nature, 574*(7777), 254–258. https://doi.org/10.1038/s41586-019-1579-3.

Gray, K. J., & Gibbs, J. E. (2022). Adaptive immunity, chronic inflammation and the clock. *Seminars in immunopathology, 44*(2), 209–224. https://doi.org/10.1007/s00281-022-00919-7.

Haspel, J. A., Anafi, R., Brown, M. K., Cermakian, N., Depner, C., Desplats, P., Gelman, A. E., Haack, M., Jelic, S., Kim, B. S., Laposky, A. D., Lee, Y. C., Mongodin, E., Prather, A. A., Prendergast, B. J., Reardon, C., Shaw, A. C., Sengupta, S., Szentirmai, É., Thakkar, M., Walker, W. E., Solt, L. A. (2020). Perfect timing: circadian rhythms, sleep, and immunity - an NIH workshop summary. *JCI insight, 5*(1), e131487. https://doi.org/10.1172/jci.insight.131487.

Holtkamp, S. J., Ince, L. M., Barnoud, C., Schmitt, M. T., Sinturel, F., Pilorz, V., Pick, R., Jemelin, S., Mühlstädt, M., Boehncke, W. H., Weber, J., Laubender, D., Philippou-Massier, J., Chen, C. S., Holtermann, L., Vestweber, D., Sperandio, M., Schraml, B. U., Halin, C., Dibner, C., Scheiermann, C. (2021). Circadian clocks guide dendritic cells into skin lymphatics. *Nature immunology, 22*(11), 1375–1381. https://doi.org/10.1038/s41590-021-01040-x.

Labrecque, N., & Cermakian, N. (2015). Circadian Clocks in the Immune System. *Journal of biological rhythms, 30*(4), 277–290. https://doi.org/10.1177/0748730415577723.

Lee, Y., Field, J. M., & Sehgal, A. (2021). Circadian Rhythms, Disease and Chronotherapy. *Journal of biological rhythms, 36*(6), 503–531. https://doi.org/10.1177/07487304211044301.

Liu, Y., Zhang, H., Yuan, G., Yao, M., Li, B., Chen, J., Fan, Y., Mo, R., Lai, F., Chen, X., Li, M., Chen, B., Lord, J. M., Peng, S., Cheng, K., & Xiao, H. (2022). The impact of circadian rhythms on the immune response to influenza vaccination in middle-aged and older adults (IMPROVE): a randomised controlled trial. *Immunity & ageing : I & A, 19*(1), 46. https://doi.org/10.1186/s12979-022-00304-w.

Logan, R. W., & Sarkar, D. K. (2012). Circadian nature of immune function. *Molecular and cellular endocrinology, 349*(1), 82–90. https://doi.org/10.1016/j.mce.2011.06.039.

Mavroudis, P. D., Scheff, J. D., Calvano, S. E., & Androulakis, I. P. (2013). Systems biology of circadian-immune interactions. *Journal of innate immunity, 5*(2), 153–162. https://doi.org/10.1159/000342427.

Olejniczak, I., Oster, H., & Ray, D. W. (2022). Glucocorticoid circadian rhythms in immune function. *Seminars in immunopathology, 44*(2), 153–163. https://doi.org/10.1007/s00281-021-00889-2.

Palomino-Segura, M., & Hidalgo, A. (2021). Circadian immune circuits. *The Journal of experimental medicine, 218*(2), e20200798. https://doi.org/10.1084/jem.20200798.

Pearson, J. A., Voisey, A. C., Boest-Bjerg, K., Wong, F. S., & Wen, L. (2021). Circadian Rhythm Modulation of Microbes During Health and Infection. *Frontiers in microbiology, 12*, 721004. https://doi.org/10.3389/fmicb.2021.721004.

Ramsey, A. M., Stowie, A., Castanon-Cervantes, O., & Davidson, A. J. (2020). Environmental Circadian Disruption Increases Stroke Severity and Dysregulates Immune Response. *Journal of biological rhythms, 35*(4), 368–376. https://doi.org/10.1177/0748730420929450.

Scheiermann, C., Gibbs, J., Ince, L., & Loudon, A. (2018). Clocking in to immunity. *Nature reviews. Immunology, 18*(7), 423–437. https://doi.org/10.1038/s41577-018-0008-4.

Scheiermann, C., Kunisaki, Y., & Frenette, P. S. (2013). Circadian control of the immune system. *Nature reviews. Immunology, 13*(3), 190–198. https://doi.org/10.1038/nri3386.

Shivshankar, P., Fekry, B., Eckel-Mahan, K., & Wetsel, R. A. (2020). Circadian Clock and Complement Immune System-Complementary Control of Physiology and Pathology?. *Frontiers in cellular and infection microbiology, 10*, 418. https://doi.org/10.3389/fcimb.2020.00418.

Skrlec, I., & Talapko, J. (2022). Hepatitis B and circadian rhythm of the liver. *World journal of gastroenterology, 28*(27), 3282–3296. https://doi.org/10.3748/wjg.v28.i27.3282.

Zandi, M., Shafaati, M., Shapshak, P., & Hashemnia, S. M. R. (2023). Monkeypox virus replication underlying circadian rhythm networks. *Journal of neurovirology, 29*(1), 1–7. https://doi.org/10.1007/s13365-023-01118-2.

Zhuang, X., Edgar, R. S., & McKeating, J. A. (2022). The role of circadian clock pathways in viral replication. *Seminars in immunopathology, 44*(2), 175–182. https://doi.org/10.1007/s00281-021-00908-2.

Chapter 19

Roles of Light and the Circadian Rhythm in Cancer Pathogenesis

Ayse Kocak*, **PhD**
Department of Biochemistry, Faculty of Medicine, Kutahya Health Sciences University, Kutahya, Turkiye

Abstract

All living creatures have circadian clock processes that regulate physiological, biochemical, and metabolic activities. The circadian clock can be defined as completely natural hemostasis. There are many studies describing the relationship between cancer and the circadian clock, and it is known that clock molecules have a role in the pathogenesis of cancer. This chapter summarizes circadian clock mechanisms and their role in cancer.

Keywords: circadian clock, cancer, cancer pathogenesis

Introduction

The circadian clock is the well-preserved molecular clock valid in all organisms evolutionarily. In fact, the circadian clock is exactly a timing mechanism (especially daily), and this mechanism includes the regulation of all behaviour and biological processes in an organism (Delaunay and Laudet, 2002; Panda et al., 2002; Fu and Kettner, 2013; Sancar and Brunner, 2014).

---

* Corresponding Author's Email: kocak.ayse@gmail.com

In: Human Health is a Matter of Timing
Editors: Sumeyya Deniz Aybek, Gonca Gulbay and Mucahit Secme
ISBN: 979-8-89113-467-6

This circadian clock is governed mainly in the suprachiasmatic nucleus (SCN) of the hypothalamus section and it is completely well maintained; however, secondary clocks, which are cell-autonomous regulators, are found in metabolic organs such as the liver, heart, pancreas, ovary, lung, kidney, intestine, skin and five sense organs. They are synchronized with each other by the suprachiasmatic nucleus clock via neural and humoral inputs. The suprachiasmatic nucleus governs molecular and physiological functions on a 24-hour cycle; these synchronize with ambient light and environmental factors to coordinate the circadian clock (Stevens et al., 2007; Welsh et al., 2010). Although the basic molecular working mechanism of the suprachiasmatic nucleus and peripheral clocks seems to be the same; It synchronizes all peripheral clocks including the active autonomic nervous system and neuroendocrine system in metabolism, and it is considered as the main mechanism or main clock. The circadian clock is very important and has a vital role in biochemical and physiological balance and especially for cellular homeostasis in all living creatures.

Daily changes in cortisol are very important for the circadian clock. The indoleamine hormone melatonin (N-acetyl-5-methoxetamine) is mainly produced by the pineal gland. Cortisol production is very low during the day but increases in the evening and peaks between 02:00 and 04:00 at night. Then, with the sunrise, its amount in metabolism gradually decreases.

The circadian clock is disrupted by exposure to direct light at night; this exposure to light also suppresses melatonin production, and in this process, the irregularity of circadian genes that play a role in the development of many cancers occurs (Stevens et al., 2007). The role of the circadian clock in the initiation and pathogenesis of cancer is now better known and is still being studied more intensively.

Recently, several studies have explored the idea of using circadian clocks for the treatment of cancer, with ameliorative modulation of circadian clock activity (Sulli et al., 2019). In this section, the author discusses the role of circadian rhythm in cancer pathogenesis and potential therapeutic strategies targeting the circadian clock.

Circadian Clock Mechanism

In mammals, cryptochromes are molecularly specifically circadian photoreceptors and form different regional expression patterns in the retina-neuroanatomical system. The main task of these molecules is to absorb light and transmit the electromagnetic signal to the circadian molecular clock using a pterin and flavin adenine dinucleotide as chromophore-cofactors. At the core of these molecules is the DNA repair enzyme photolyase (A. Sancar, 2000). In the retina, cryptochromes-1 (Cry-1) and cryptochromes-2 (Cry-2) are differentially expressed relative to opsin-based visual photoreceptors. In the retina of the eye, the axons of some ganglion cells enter the retinohypothalamic pathway, which leaves the dorsal surface of the optic chiasm and synapses with the suprachiasmatic nucleus. As mentioned above, the main regulator of the circadian clock is actually the SCN. Its neurons are tightly interconnected and synchronized as an organ by cross-talk coupling mediated by vasoactive intestinal polypeptide and other neurotransmitters (Aton et al., 2005; Liu et al., 2007; Welsh et al., 2010) . In the suprachiasmatic nucleus, it is the Cry1 molecule that conforms to the circadian periodic table and has a high expression. In a study of pancreatic adenocarcinomas or osteosarcomas, when the SCN was excised, it had a very rapid tumor growth rate compared to control mice (Filipski, 2002). In a daylight cycle of 24 hours, visual inputs lead to synchronization of the circadian neuronal firing rhythm of suprachiasmatic neurons with the environment, and with daylight, the suprachiasmatic nuclei in turn synchronize the peripheral molecular clock in each cell metabolism (Reppert & Weaver, 2002; Stephan & Zucker, 1972). This process is dependent on the anatomically altered ambient light levels on gonadotropin secretion from the gland of pituitary and on the effect of melatonin on pineal secretion.

The main mechanism of the circadian clock is basically completely self-controlled, automatic regulators consisting of negative and also positive transcription and feedback of translation (Ko & Takahashi, 2006; Miller et al., 2007; Young & Kay, 2001). The circadian clock in cell metabolism is completely molecularly regulated. Autoregulators are present in this molecular regulation and are translationally and transcriptionally regulated. This molecular regulation of the circadian clock includes core helix-loop-helix heterodimeric transcription factors (CLOCK & BMAL-1 or BMAL-1-NPAS-2) and negative regulator cryptochromes (Cry-1 and Cry-2) and Period (Per-1, Per-2, Per-3) genes, and most regulation is by these genes. is managed. Cryptochromes and period form a transcriptional repressor complex that enters the nucleus to suppress genes of CLOCK and BMAL-1 activity, thereby creating a negative feedback loop to control the clock. BMAL-1 is also rhythmically controlled by its transcriptional target. Briefly, Rev-erba, RORa, and Rev-erbb. RORa stimulates Bmal-1 expression while Rev-erba suppresses Bmal-1 expression. The importance of these master clock regulators is highlighted by the observation that CLOCK & BMAL-1 controls the expression of clock-controlled genes that regulate molecular, biochemical, and physiological processes (Delaunay & Laudet, 2002; Fu & Kettner, 2013; Panda et al., 2002; G. Sancar & Brunner, 2014). In circadian clock regulation, post-translational modifications of cryptochromes and period genes regulate protein stability, control the nuclear entry of cryptochromes and period repressors, and affect autoregulatory clock feedback loops (Becker-Weimann et al., 2004; Ko & Takahashi, 2006; Ye et al., 2011).

Circadian Clock and Cancer

Circadian Clock and Cancer Pathogenesis

Genes of the circadian clock are very common in human metabolism and are often affected by environmental factors such as light and nutrition. They are widely expressed and affected by environmental factors (light and food). The circadian rhythm is disturbed by many external factors, and thus the biological functions and properties of organs and cells change. These changes cause the pathogenesis of many diseases, especially cancer, psychological disorders, and endocrine disorders (Cederroth et al., 2019; Cox & Takahashi, 2019; Finger et al., 2020; Kinouchi & Sassone-Corsi, 2020; Leng et al., 2019; Patke et al., 2020; Schibler et al., 2015; Xie et al., 2019).

There are some mechanisms directly affected by the circadian clock in cancer pathogenesis. These mechanisms can be summarized as follows:

- In the formation of tumour, cell proliferation, and growth, cell experience, DNA damage repair mechanisms, and apoptosis mechanisms are effective and the circadian clock can directly affect all these processes (P. Chen et al., 2021; Kinouchi & Sassone-Corsi, 2020; Koritala et al., 2021; Pavlova & Thompson, 2016; A. Sancar & van Gelder, 2021; Shafi & Knudsen, 2019; Sulli et al., 2019; Yang et al., 2019; Zhou et al., 2020)
- In some types of cancer, especially in cancer cells such as acute myeloid leukemia (AML) and pleomorphic glioblastoma, which can be renewed, may have effects of the circadian clock on the stem cells (P. Chen et al., 2021; Dong et al., 2019; Puram et al., 2016),

- The circadian clock regulates the expression of angogenic factors in the cell such as nuclear translocator (ARNT), hypoxia, in durable factor 1α (HIF-1α), vascular endothelial growth factor (VEGF). Especially in the formation of tumor, the change of these angogenic factors is important and can promote metastasis (Hanahan, 2022; Hu et al., 2015; X. Jiang et al., 2020; Y. Wang et al., 2017).
- The circadian clock regulates inflammation in myeloid cells (Hanahan, 2022; Shalapour & Karin, 2019).

The circadian clock is known to play an important role in cancer stem cell heterogeneity and plasticity (De et al., 2020; Diamantopoulou et al., 2022; Matsunaga et al., 2018). Jatlag models mimicking circadian perturbations induce an immunosuppressive shift in tumor cells, accelerating and promoting tumor aggressiveness (Hadadi et al., 2020). Molecular and cellular levels of the clock from the circadian in cellular events and especially in the functioning of the molecular level, there is a close mixing of DNA between the circadian clock mechanism and the cell cycle repair, apoptosis, senescence, autophagy, and other oncogenic and immune pathways (Sulli et al., 2019). The circadian clock has an impact on DNA repair mechanisms, autophagy, apoptosis, aging, and other oncogenic processes, and in an impaired circadian rhythm this causes angiogenesis, escape from apoptosis, uncontrolled cell growth, escape from immune cells, and metastasis, all of which are important mechanisms of cancerization processes (Hanahan, 2022). For this reason, cell culture and experimental animal studies have shown that circadian clock genes play a direct role in cancer formation and development. Epigenetic or genetic inactivation of BMAL-1 and/or CLOCK has been shown to increase tumour growth in various cancer cells such as glioblastoma, breast, colon, and lung (Fekry et al., 2018a, 2018b; Gwon et al., 2020; W. Jiang et al., 2016; Korkmaz et al., 2018a, 2018b; Papagiannakopoulos et al., 2016; Peng et al., 2019; Tang et al., 2017; Taniguchi et al., 2009; Zhang et al., 2020). It has been shown to increase proliferation or growth rates. Furthermore, epigenetic or genetic inactivation of BMAL-1 and/or CLOCK has been shown to increase tumour growth in various cancer cells such as glioblastoma, breast, colon, and lung. In another study, it was shown that Cry1, the target gene of CLOCK & BMAL-1, Per-1, and Per-2, promotes or suppresses tumour incidence and proliferation in various cancer types(Gong et al., 2021; Hanoun et al., 2012; Nirvani et al., 2017; Papagiannakopoulos et al., 2016; Sun et al., 2010; Z. Wang et al., 2020; Zhanfeng et al., 2016).

Circadian Clock and Cancer Metabolism

In healthy non-cancerous cells, maintaining homeostasis is physiologically very important. A coordinated interaction between the molecular circadian clock and the complex network of metabolic pathways is necessary to maintain this homeostasis. The metabolic circadian clock identified in mammalian red blood cells (O'Neill, 2011) is independent of transcriptional activity and is maintained by the redox cycle of peroxiredoxin/thioredoxin/NADPH enzymes (Ray, 2016). This important structure metabolizes H2O2 in cells and tissues, and this process continues for 24 hours.

Thiols (glutathione-GSH/GSSG) and coenzymes (FADH2/FAD+, NADH/NAD+ and NADPH/NADP+) multiple redox pairs regulate electron flow and cellular homeostasis (Rey er al. 2016). In tissues and cells, NADPH in particular can prolong or shorten the 24-hour circadian rhythm. Therefore, NADPH is an important cofactor in cancer and functions as a circadian-regulated and cancer-promoting metabolite.

In cancer, there is a strong relationship between tumorigenesis, nutritional metabolism, and the circadian clock. BMAL1, CRY1, and CRY2 can lengthen and shorten metabolite rhythms in the circadian rhythm cycle. Another sensor, AMPK, is an important nutrient sensor that can disturb the balance. In addition, CRY1 and PER2 can alter the circadian rhythm through phosphorylation (Lamia et al., 2009). MYC directly activates the negative regulators of CLOCK/BMAL1, leading to the disruption of circadian metabolic oscillation. The insulin-FOXO3-CLOCK signaling cascade mediates function in hepatic metabolism and oxidative sensitivity. Finally, a recent study showed that a high-fat diet affects the circadian transcriptome and metabolome due to impaired BMAL1 and PPARγ uptake. Thus, through transcriptional remodeling and posttranslational modifications, the circadian clock regulates metabolism and integrates nutrient signals critical to sustain tumorigenesis.

Single amino acid substitutions of PER2S662G and PER2S662D in transgenic mice can shorten or lengthen the circadian clock. In humans, the PER2S662G mutation causes familial advanced sleep phase syndrome, characterized by sleep onset in the early evening between 18:00-20:00 hours; these humans have wakefulness in the early morning like that between 13:00-15:00hours (Jones et al., 1999; Toh et al., 2001; Xu et al., 2005, 2007). PER2S662 mutations also increase resistance to x-ray-induced apoptosis and enhance RAS and E1A-mediated oncogenic transformation. Tumorigenesis in p53R172H+/- mice (a cancer susceptible genetic background) is affected by

PER2S662 mutations and the risk of developing cancer conferred by the specific PER2S662 mutation is increased (Gu et al., 2012) . Another study showed that the PER2S662G mutation increased cancer risk and alterations in PER2 are often found in human breast cancer in humans (S.-T. Chen et al., 2005; Winter et al., 2007). Per2m/m mice develop colon polyps and have increased levels of small intestinal mucosal cyclin D and β-catenin protein compared to control mice. This is consistent with findings from human colonic cell lines where down-regulation of PER2 increases β-catenin and cyclin D as well as the rate of proliferation of cells (Wood et al., 2008). Interestingly, APC is another component of the WNT signaling pathway involved in the β-catenin degradation complex. In the results, the number of small intestine and colon polyps was increased 2-fold in ApcMin/+Per2m/m mice compared to ApcMin/+ mice. It is concluded that the Per2 gene product suppresses tumor formation in the colon and small intestine through the down-regulation of β-catenin.

A study showed that ın hepatocyte cells, the c-myc gene is expressed with full circadian expression. However, there is a change in c-myc expression in Per2 mutant mice, and this level is significantly increased. There is also the circadian expression of Gadd45 and cyclin D1, two genes that regulate c-myc in Per2 wild-type mice, and their circadian expression is altered in mutant mice. Per2-deficient mice also have abnormal temporal expression of MDM-2 and cyclin A (Canaple et al., 2003). In summary, it has been shown that there is a very strong link between proliferation and circadian rhythm in liver cells. This relationship is based on molecular pathways.

There are many studies on cancer and circadian rhythm in humans. In terms of breast cancer, the increased risk of breast cancer, especially in women who work night shifts, has been evaluated in murine model systems of xenografted breast cancer (Blask et al., 2005). Moreover, tumors perfused with melatonin-rich blood at night had suppressed proliferative activity and linoleic acid uptake/metabolism compared to melatonin-deprived blood collected during the day. Furthermore, a nested case-control study of urinary melatonin levels and postmenopausal breast cancer risk was conducted in 18,643 participants of the Nurses' Health Study (Schernhammer & Hankinson, 2009). 357 postmenopausal women who developed breast cancer and 533 matched controls had increased concentrations of 6-sulfatoxymelatonin, the main metabolite of melatonin. The increase in 6-sulfatoxymelatonin concentration in urine was significantly associated with a lower risk of breast cancer, with an odds ratio of 0.62 for the highest and lowest quartile of morning urinary 6-sulfatoxymelatonin (C.I. 0.41-0.95; Ptrend = 0.004). This important evidence further confirmed the evidence of an inverse correlation between breast cancer risk and melatonin levels. Suggested reasons for how melatonin exerts a protective effect on breast cancer risk include that it reduces circulating estrogen by down-regulating the hypothalamic-pituitary axis, alters aromatase activity and expression *in vitro* and *in vivo*, or that melatonin may be considered an indirect indicator of environmental circadian effects exerted on components of the molecular clock (Schernhammer & Hankinson, 2009; Stevens, 1987).

Circadian Clock and Cancer Therapy

Chronotherapy is also functional in cancer and is a type of therapy aimed at restoring the appropriate circadian pattern of the sleep-wake cycle through the use of chronobiotic drugs such as melatonin, which affect the output phase of circadian rhythms and thus control the circadian clock.

A phase III study enrolling 186 patients aimed at the benefit of chronotherapy in chemotherapy (Levi et al., 1997). The investigators observed that the proportion of cells in the S phase in the skin, bone marrow, gut, and oral mucosa changed by 50% during each 24-hour period (Smaland, et al., 1991).

The response rate to treatment was 51% for chronotherapy versus 29% for flat-rate administration ($p = 0.003$). The median time to failure of treatment in chronotherapy was 6.4 months for chronotherapy and 4.9 months for fixed-rate infusion ($p = 0.006$). Median survival and 3-year survival were similar in both cohorts at 15.9 and 16.9 months, respectively.

Conclusion

The molecular mechanisms of the circadian clock have an effect on cancer pathogenesis and disease severity in recent studies with cancer and the circadian clock. Disruption of molecular pathways in the circadian clock increases the risk and progression of cancer and directly affects the entire metabolism. At the same time, the circadian clock has a role in cancer and cancer treatment. Although there have been many studies on melatonin in particular, more studies are needed on circadian clock molecular interactions due to the heterogeneity of cancer itself.

References

Aton, S. J., Colwell, C. S., Harmar, A. J., Waschek, J., & Herzog, E. D. (2005). Vasoactive intestinal polypeptide mediates circadian rhythmicity and synchrony in mammalian clock neurons. *Nature Neuroscience*, *8*(4), 476–483. https://doi.org/10.1038/nn1419.

Becker-Weimann, S., Wolf, J., Herzel, H., & Kramer, A. (2004). Modeling Feedback Loops of the Mammalian Circadian Oscillator. *Biophysical Journal*, *87*(5), 3023–3034. https://doi.org/10.1529/biophysj.104.040824.

Blask, D. E., Brainard, G. C., Dauchy, R. T., Hanifin, J. P., Davidson, L. K., Krause, J. A., Sauer, L. A., Rivera-Bermudez, M. A., Dubocovich, M. L., Jasser, S. A., Lynch, D. T., Rollag, M. D., & Zalatan, F. (2005). Melatonin-Depleted Blood from Premenopausal Women Exposed to Light at Night Stimulates Growth of Human Breast Cancer Xenografts in Nude Rats. *Cancer Research*, *65*(23), 11174–11184. https://doi.org/10.1158/0008-5472.CAN-05-1945.

Canaple, L., Kakizawa, T., & Laudet, V. (2003). The days and nights of cancer cells. *Cancer Research*, *63*(22), 7545–7552.

Cederroth, C. R., Albrecht, U., Bass, J., Brown, S. A., Dyhrfjeld-Johnsen, J., Gachon, F., Green, C. B., Hastings, M. H., Helfrich-Förster, C., Hogenesch, J. B., Lévi, F., Loudon, A., Lundkvist, G. B., Meijer, J. H., Rosbash, M., Takahashi, J. S., Young, M., & Canlon, B. (2019). Medicine in the Fourth Dimension. *Cell Metabolism*, *30*(2), 238–250. https://doi.org/10.1016/j.cmet.2019.06.019.

Chen, P., Hsu, W.-H., Han, J., Xia, Y., & DePinho, R. A. (2021). Cancer Stemness Meets Immunity: From Mechanism to Therapy. *Cell Reports*, *34*(1), 108597. https://doi.org/10.1016/j.celrep.2020.108597.

Chen, S. T., Choo, K. B., Hou, M. F., Yeh, K. T., Kuo, S. J., & Chang, J. G. (2005). Deregulated expression of the PER1, PER2 and PER3 genes in breast cancers. *Carcinogenesis*, *26*(7), 1241–1246. https://doi.org/10.1093/carcin/bgi075.

Cox, K. H., & Takahashi, J. S. (2019). Circadian clock genes and the transcriptional architecture of the clock mechanism. *Journal of Molecular Endocrinology*, *63*(4), R93–R102. https://doi.org/10.1530/JME-19-0153.

De, A., Beligala, D. H., Sharma, V. P., Burgos, C. A., Lee, A. M., & Geusz, M. E. (2020). Cancer stem cell generation during epithelial-mesenchymal transition is temporally gated by intrinsic circadian clocks. *Clinical & Experimental Metastasis*, *37*(5), 617–635. https://doi.org/10.1007/s10585-020-10051-1.

Delaunay, F., & Laudet, V. (2002). Circadian clock and microarrays: mammalian genome gets rhythm. *Trends in Genetics*, *18*(12), 595–597. https://doi.org/10.1016/S0168-9525(02)02794-4.

Diamantopoulou, Z., Castro-Giner, F., Schwab, F. D., Foerster, C., Saini, M., Budinjas, S., Strittmatter, K., Krol, I., Seifert, B., Heinzelmann-Schwarz, V., Kurzeder, C., Rochlitz, C., Vetter, M., Weber, W. P., & Aceto, N. (2022). The metastatic spread of breast cancer accelerates during sleep. *Nature*, *607*(7917), 156–162. https://doi.org/10.1038/s41586-022-04875-y.

Dong, Z., Zhang, G., Qu, M., Gimple, R. C., Wu, Q., Qiu, Z., Prager, B. C., Wang, X., Kim, L. J. Y., Morton, A. R., Dixit, D., Zhou, W., Huang, H., Li, B., Zhu, Z., Bao, S., Mack, S. C., Chavez, L., Kay, S. A., & Rich, J. N. (2019). Targeting Glioblastoma Stem Cells through Disruption of the Circadian Clock. *Cancer Discovery*, *9*(11), 1556–1573. https://doi.org/10.1158/2159-8290.CD-19-0215.

Fekry, B., Ribas-Latre, A., Baumgartner, C., Deans, J. R., Kwok, C., Patel, P., Fu, L., Berdeaux, R., Sun, K., Kolonin, M. G., Wang, S. H., Yoo, S. H., Sladek, F. M., & Eckel-Mahan, K. (2018a). Incompatibility of the circadian protein BMAL1 and HNF4α in hepatocellular carcinoma. *Nature Communications*, *9*(1), 4349. https://doi.org/10.1038/s41467-018-06648-6.

Fekry, B., Ribas-Latre, A., Baumgartner, C., Deans, J. R., Kwok, C., Patel, P., Fu, L., Berdeaux, R., Sun, K., Kolonin, M. G., Wang, S. H., Yoo, S. H., Sladek, F. M., & Eckel-Mahan, K. (2018b). Incompatibility of the circadian protein BMAL1 and HNF4α in hepatocellular carcinoma. *Nature Communications*, *9*(1), 4349. https://doi.org/10.1038/s41467-018-06648-6.

Filipski, E. (2002). Host Circadian Clock as a Control Point in Tumor Progression. *CancerSpectrum Knowledge Environment*, *94*(9), 690–697. https://doi.org/10.1093/jnci/94.9.690.

Finger, A., Dibner, C., & Kramer, A. (2020). Coupled network of the circadian clocks: a driving force of rhythmic physiology. *FEBS Letters*, *594*(17), 2734–2769. https://doi.org/10.1002/1873-3468.13898.

Fu, L., & Kettner, N. M. (2013). *The Circadian Clock in Cancer Development and Therapy* (pp. 221–282). https://doi.org/10.1016/B978-0-12-396971-2.00009-9.

Gong, X., Tang, H., & Yang, K. (2021). PER1 suppresses glycolysis and cell proliferation in oral squamous cell carcinoma via the PER1/RACK1/PI3K signaling complex. *Cell Death & Disease*, *12*(3), 276. https://doi.org/10.1038/s41419-021-03563-5.

Gu, X., Xing, L., Shi, G., Liu, Z., Wang, X., Qu, Z., Wu, X., Dong, Z., Gao, X., Liu, G., Yang, L., & Xu, Y. (2012). The circadian mutation PER2S662G is linked to cell cycle progression and tumorigenesis. *Cell Death & Differentiation*, *19*(3), 397–405. https://doi.org/10.1038/cdd.2011.103.

Gwon, D. hyeong, Lee, W. Y., Shin, N., Kim, S. I., Jeong, K., Lee, W., Kim, D. W., Hong, J., & Lee, S. Y. (2020). BMAL1 Suppresses Proliferation, Migration, and Invasion of U87MG Cells by Downregulating Cyclin B1, Phospho-AKT, and Metalloproteinase-9. *International Journal of Molecular Sciences*, *21*(7), 2352. https://doi.org/10.3390/ijms21072352.

Hadadi, E., Taylor, W., Li, X. M., Aslan, Y., Villote, M., Rivière, J., Duvallet, G., Auriau, C., Dulong, S., Raymond-Letron, I., Provot, S., Bennaceur-Griscelli, A., & Acloque, H. (2020). Chronic circadian disruption modulates breast cancer stemness and immune microenvironment to drive metastasis in mice. *Nature Communications*, *11*(1), 3193. https://doi.org/10.1038/s41467-020-16890-6.

Hanahan, D. (2022). Hallmarks of Cancer: New Dimensions. *Cancer Discovery*, *12*(1), 31–46. https://doi.org/10.1158/2159-8290.CD-21-1059.

Hanoun, M., Eisele, L., Suzuki, M., Greally, J. M., Hüttmann, A., Aydin, S., Scholtysik, R., Klein-Hitpass, L., Dührsen, U., & Dürig, J. (2012). Epigenetic Silencing of the Circadian Clock Gene CRY1 is Associated with an Indolent Clinical Course in Chronic Lymphocytic Leukemia. *PLoS ONE*, *7*(3), e34347. https://doi.org/10.1371/journal.pone.0034347.

Hu, Z., Brooks, S. A., Dormoy, V., Hsu, C.-W., Hsu, H. Y., Lin, L. T., Massfelder, T., Rathmell, W. K., Xia, M., Al-Mulla, F., Al-Temaimi, R., Amedei, A., Brown, D. G., Prudhomme, K. R., Colacci, A. M., Hamid, R. A., Mondello, C., Raju, J., Ryan, E. P., Woodrick J, Scovassi AI, Singh N, Vaccari M, Roy R, Forte S, Memeo L, Salem HK, Lowe L, Jensen L, Bisson WH, & Kleinstreuer, N. (2015). Assessing the carcinogenic potential of low-dose exposures to chemical mixtures in the environment: focus on the cancer hallmark of tumor angiogenesis. *Carcinogenesis*, *36*(Suppl 1), S184–S202. https://doi.org/10.1093/carcin/bgv036.

Jiang, W., Zhao, S., Jiang, X., Zhang, E., Hu, G., Hu, B., Zheng, P., Xiao, J., Lu, Z., Lu, Y., Ni, J., Chen, C., Wang, X., Yang, L., & Wan, R. (2016). The circadian clock gene Bmal1 acts as a potential anti-oncogene in pancreatic cancer by activating the p53 tumor suppressor pathway. *Cancer Letters*, *371*(2), 314–325. https://doi.org/10.1016/j.canlet.2015.12.002.

Jiang, X., Wang, J., Deng, X., Xiong, F., Zhang, S., Gong, Z., Li, X., Cao, K., Deng, H., He, Y., Liao, Q., Xiang, B., Zhou, M., Guo, C., Zeng, Z., Li, G., Li, X., & Xiong, W. (2020). The role of microenvironment in tumor angiogenesis. *Journal of Experimental & Clinical Cancer Research*, *39*(1), 204. https://doi.org/10.1186/s13046-020-017 09-5.

Jones, C. R., Campbell, S. S., Zone, S. E., Cooper, F., DeSano, A., Murphy, P. J., Jones, B., Czajkowski, L., & Ptček, L. J. (1999). Familial advanced sleep-phase syndrome: A short-period circadian rhythm variant in humans. *Nature Medicine*, *5*(9), 1062–1065. https://doi.org/10.1038/12502.

Kinouchi, K., & Sassone-Corsi, P. (2020). Metabolic rivalry: circadian homeostasis and tumorigenesis. *Nature Reviews Cancer*, *20*(11), 645–661. https://doi.org/10.1038/s41568-020-0291-9.

Ko, C. H., & Takahashi, J. S. (2006). Molecular components of the mammalian circadian clock. *Human Molecular Genetics*, *15*(suppl_2), R271–R277. https://doi.org/10.1093/hmg/ddl207.

Koritala, B. S. C., Porter, K. I., Arshad, O. A., Gajula, R. P., Mitchell, H. D., Arman, T., Manjanatha, M. G., Teeguarden, J., van Dongen, H. P. A., McDermott, J. E., & Gaddameedhi, S. (2021). Night shift schedule causes circadian dysregulation of DNA repair genes and elevated DNA damage in humans. *Journal of Pineal Research*, *70*(3). https://doi.org/10.1111/jpi.12726.

Korkmaz, T., Aygenli, F., Emisoglu, H., Ozcelik, G., Canturk, A., Yilmaz, S., & Ozturk, N. (2018a). Opposite Carcinogenic Effects of Circadian Clock Gene BMAL1. *Scientific Reports*, *8*(1), 16023. https://doi.org/10.1038/s41598-018-34433-4.

Korkmaz, T., Aygenli, F., Emisoglu, H., Ozcelik, G., Canturk, A., Yilmaz, S., & Ozturk, N. (2018b). Opposite Carcinogenic Effects of Circadian Clock Gene BMAL1. *Scientific Reports*, *8*(1), 16023. https://doi.org/10.1038/s41598-018-34433-4.

Leng, Y., Musiek, E. S., Hu, K., Cappuccio, F. P., & Yaffe, K. (2019). Association between circadian rhythms and neurodegenerative diseases. *The Lancet Neurology*, *18*(3), 307–318. https://doi.org/10.1016/S1474-4422(18)30461-7.

Liu, A. C., Welsh, D. K., Ko, C. H., Tran, H. G., Zhang, E. E., Priest, A. A., Buhr, E. D., Singer, O., Meeker, K., Verma, I. M., Doyle, F. J., Takahashi, J. S., & Kay, S. A. (2007). Intercellular Coupling Confers Robustness against Mutations in the SCN

Circadian Clock Network. *Cell*, *129*(3), 605–616. https://doi.org/10.1016/j.cell.2007.02.047.

Matsunaga, N., Ogino, T., Hara, Y., Tanaka, T., Koyanagi, S., & Ohdo, S. (2018). Optimized Dosing Schedule Based on Circadian Dynamics of Mouse Breast Cancer Stem Cells Improves the Antitumor Effects of Aldehyde Dehydrogenase Inhibitor. *Cancer Research*, *78*(13), 3698–3708. https://doi.org/10.1158/0008-5472.CAN-17-4034.

Miller, B. H., McDearmon, E. L., Panda, S., Hayes, K. R., Zhang, J., Andrews, J. L., Antoch, M. P., Walker, J. R., Esser, K. A., Hogenesch, J. B., & Takahashi, J. S. (2007). Circadian and CLOCK-controlled regulation of the mouse transcriptome and cell proliferation. *Proceedings of the National Academy of Sciences*, *104*(9), 3342–3347. https://doi.org/10.1073/pnas.0611724104.

Nirvani, M., Khuu, C., Utheim, T., Sand, L., & Sehic, A. (2017). Circadian clock and oral cancer (Review). *Molecular and Clinical Oncology*. https://doi.org/10.3892/mco.2017.1518.

Panda, S., Antoch, M. P., Miller, B. H., Su, A. I., Schook, A. B., Straume, M., Schultz, P. G., Kay, S. A., Takahashi, J. S., & Hogenesch, J. B. (2002). Coordinated Transcription of Key Pathways in the Mouse by the Circadian Clock. *Cell*, *109*(3), 307–320. https://doi.org/10.1016/S0092-8674(02)00722-5.

Papagiannakopoulos, T., Bauer, M. R., Davidson, S. M., Heimann, M., Subbaraj, L., Bhutkar, A., Bartlebaugh, J., Vander Heiden, M. G., & Jacks, T. (2016). Circadian Rhythm Disruption Promotes Lung Tumorigenesis. *Cell Metabolism*, *24*(2), 324–331. https://doi.org/10.1016/j.cmet.2016.07.001.

Patke, A., Young, M. W., & Axelrod, S. (2020). Molecular mechanisms and physiological importance of circadian rhythms. *Nature Reviews Molecular Cell Biology*, *21*(2), 67–84. https://doi.org/10.1038/s41580-019-0179-2.

Pavlova, N. N., & Thompson, C. B. (2016). The Emerging Hallmarks of Cancer Metabolism. *Cell Metabolism*, *23*(1), 27–47. https://doi.org/10.1016/j.cmet.2015.12.006.

Peng, H., Zhang, J., Zhang, P. P., Chen, L., Tang, L. L., Yang, X. J., He, Q. M., Wen, X., Sun, Y., Liu, N., Li, Y. Q., & Ma, J. (2019). ARNTL hypermethylation promotes tumorigenesis and inhibits cisplatin sensitivity by activating CDK5 transcription in nasopharyngeal carcinoma. *Journal of Experimental & Clinical Cancer Research*, *38*(1), 11. https://doi.org/10.1186/s13046-018-0997-7.

Puram, R. V., Kowalczyk, M. S., de Boer, C. G., Schneider, R. K., Miller, P. G., McConkey, M., Tothova, Z., Tejero, H., Heckl, D., Järås, M., Chen, M. C., Li, H., Tamayo, A., Cowley, G. S., Rozenblatt-Rosen, O., Al-Shahrour, F., Regev, A., & Ebert, B. L. (2016). Core Circadian Clock Genes Regulate Leukemia Stem Cells in AML. *Cell*, *165*(2), 303–316. https://doi.org/10.1016/j.cell.2016.03.015.

Reppert, S. M., & Weaver, D. R. (2002). Coordination of circadian timing in mammals. *Nature*, *418*(6901), 935–941. https://doi.org/10.1038/nature00965.

Sancar, A. (2000). Cryptochrome: The Second Photoactive Pigment in the Eye and Its Role in Circadian Photoreception. *Annual Review of Biochemistry*, *69*(1), 31–67. https://doi.org/10.1146/annurev.biochem.69.1.31.

Sancar, A., & van Gelder, R. N. (2021). Clocks, cancer, and chronochemotherapy. *Science, 371*(6524). https://doi.org/10.1126/science.abb0738.

Sancar, G., & Brunner, M. (2014). Circadian clocks and energy metabolism. *Cellular and Molecular Life Sciences*, *71*(14), 2667–2680. https://doi.org/10.1007/s00018-014-1574-7.

Schernhammer, E. S., & Hankinson, S. E. (2009). Urinary Melatonin Levels and Postmenopausal Breast Cancer Risk in the Nurses' Health Study Cohort. *Cancer Epidemiology, Biomarkers & Prevention*, *18*(1), 74–79. https://doi.org/10.1158/1055-9965.EPI-08-0637.

Schibler, U., Gotic, I., Saini, C., Gos, P., Curie, T., Emmenegger, Y., Sinturel, F., Gosselin, P., Gerber, A., Fleury-Olela, F., Rando, G., Demarque, M., & Franken, P. (2015). Clock-Talk: Interactions between Central and Peripheral Circadian Oscillators in Mammals. *Cold Spring Harbor Symposia on Quantitative Biology*, *80*, 223–232. https://doi.org/10.1101/sqb.2015.80.027490.

Shafi, A. A., & Knudsen, K. E. (2019). Cancer and the Circadian Clock. *Cancer Research*, *79*(15), 3806–3814. https://doi.org/10.1158/0008-5472.CAN-19-0566.

Shalapour, S., & Karin, M. (2019). Pas de Deux: Control of Anti-tumor Immunity by Cancer-Associated Inflammation. *Immunity*, *51*(1), 15–26. https://doi.org/10.1016/j.immuni.2019.06.021.

Stephan, F. K., & Zucker, I. (1972). Circadian Rhythms in Drinking Behavior and Locomotor Activity of Rats Are Eliminated by Hypothalamic Lesions. *Proceedings of the National Academy of Sciences*, *69*(6), 1583–1586. https://doi.org/10.1073/pnas.69.6.1583.

Stevens, R. G. (1987). Electric Power Use and Breast Cancer: A Hypothesis. *American Journal of Epidemiology*, *125*(4), 556–561. https://doi.org/10.1093/oxfordjournals.aje.a114569.

Stevens, R. G., Blask, D. E., Brainard, G. C., Hansen, J., Lockley, S. W., Provencio, I., Rea, M. S., & Reinlib, L. (2007). Meeting Report: The Role of Environmental Lighting and Circadian Disruption in Cancer and Other Diseases. *Environmental Health Perspectives*, *115*(9), 1357–1362. https://doi.org/10.1289/ehp.10200.

Sulli, G., Lam, M. T. Y., & Panda, S. (2019). Interplay between Circadian Clock and Cancer: New Frontiers for Cancer Treatment. *Trends in Cancer*, *5*(8), 475–494. https://doi.org/10.1016/j.trecan.2019.07.002.

Sun, C., Huang, S., Zeng, J., Liu, D., Xiao, Q., Tian, W., Zhu, X., Huang, Z., & Feng, W. (2010). Per2 Inhibits K562 Leukemia Cell Growth In Vitro and In Vivo Through Cell Cycle Arrest and Apoptosis Induction. *Pathology & Oncology Research*, *16*(3), 403–411. https://doi.org/10.1007/s12253-009-9227-0.

Tang, Q., Cheng, B., Xie, M., Chen, Y., Zhao, J., Zhou, X., & Chen, L. (2017). Circadian Clock Gene *Bmal1* Inhibits Tumorigenesis and Increases Paclitaxel Sensitivity in Tongue Squamous Cell Carcinoma. *Cancer Research*, *77*(2), 532–544. https://doi.org/10.1158/0008-5472.CAN-16-1322.

Taniguchi, H., Fernández, A. F., Setién, F., Ropero, S., Ballestar, E., Villanueva, A., Yamamoto, H., Imai, K., Shinomura, Y., & Esteller, M. (2009). Epigenetic Inactivation of the Circadian Clock Gene *BMAL1* in Hematologic Malignancies.

Cancer Research, *69*(21), 8447–8454. https://doi.org/10.1158/0008-5472.CAN-09-0551.

Toh, K. L., Jones, C. R., He, Y., Eide, E. J., Hinz, W. A., Virshup, D. M., Ptáček, L. J., & Fu, Y. H. (2001). An h *Per2* Phosphorylation Site Mutation in Familial Advanced Sleep Phase Syndrome. *Science*, *291*(5506), 1040–1043. https://doi.org/10.1126/science.1057499.

Wang, Y., Sun, N., Lu, C., Bei, Y., Qian, R., & Hua, L. (2017). Upregulation of circadian gene 'hClock' contribution to metastasis of colorectal cancer. *International Journal of Oncology*, *50*(6), 2191–2199. https://doi.org/10.3892/ijo.2017.3987.

Wang, Z., Li, F., Wei, M., Zhang, S., & Wang, T. (2020). <p>Circadian Clock Protein PERIOD2 Suppresses the PI3K/Akt Pathway and Promotes Cisplatin Sensitivity in Ovarian Cancer</p>. *Cancer Management and Research*, *Volume 12*, 11897–11908. https://doi.org/10.2147/CMAR.S278903.

Welsh, D. K., Takahashi, J. S., & Kay, S. A. (2010). Suprachiasmatic Nucleus: Cell Autonomy and Network Properties. *Annual Review of Physiology*, *72*(1), 551–577. https://doi.org/10.1146/annurev-physiol-021909-135919.

Winter, S. L., Bosnoyan-Collins, L., Pinnaduwage, D., & Andrulis, I. L. (2007). Expression of the Circadian Clock Genes Pert, Per2 in Sporadic, Familial Breast Tumors. *Neoplasia*, *9*(10), 797–800. https://doi.org/10.1593/neo.07595.

Wood, P. A., Yang, X., Taber, A., Oh, E. Y., Ansell, C., Ayers, S. E., Al-Assaad, Z., Carnevale, K., Berger, F. G., Peña, M. M. O., & Hrushesky, W. J. M. (2008). *Period 2* Mutation Accelerates *ApcMin/+* Tumorigenesis. *Molecular Cancer Research*, *6*(11), 1786–1793. https://doi.org/10.1158/1541-7786.MCR-08-0196.

Xie, Y., Tang, Q., Chen, G., Xie, M., Yu, S., Zhao, J., & Chen, L. (2019). New Insights Into the Circadian Rhythm and Its Related Diseases. *Frontiers in Physiology*, *10*. https://doi.org/10.3389/fphys.2019.00682.

Xu, Y., Padiath, Q. S., Shapiro, R. E., Jones, C. R., Wu, S. C., Saigoh, N., Saigoh, K., Ptáček, L. J., & Fu, Y. H. (2005). Functional consequences of a CKIδ mutation causing familial advanced sleep phase syndrome. *Nature*, *434*(7033), 640–644. https://doi.org/10.1038/nature03453.

Xu, Y., Toh, K. L., Jones, C. R., Shin, J.-Y., Fu, Y.-H., & Ptáček, L. J. (2007). Modeling of a Human Circadian Mutation Yields Insights into Clock Regulation by PER2. *Cell*, *128*(1), 59–70. https://doi.org/10.1016/j.cell.2006.11.043.

Yang, Y., Yuan, G., Xie, H., Wei, T., Zhu, D., Cui, J., Liu, X., Shen, R., Zhu, Y., & Yang, X. (2019). Circadian clock associates with tumor microenvironment in thoracic cancers. *Aging*, *11*(24), 11814–11828. https://doi.org/10.18632/aging.102450.

Ye, R., Selby, C. P., Ozturk, N., Annayev, Y., & Sancar, A. (2011). Biochemical Analysis of the Canonical Model for the Mammalian Circadian Clock. *Journal of Biological Chemistry*, *286*(29), 25891–25902. https://doi.org/10.1074/jbc.M111.254680.

Young, M. W., & Kay, S. A. (2001). Time zones: a comparative genetics of circadian clocks. *Nature Reviews Genetics*, *2*(9), 702–715. https://doi.org/10.1038/35088576.

Zhanfeng, N., Chengquan, W., Hechun, X., Jun, W., Lijian, Z., Dede, M., Wenbin, L., & Lei, Y. (2016). Period2 downregulation inhibits glioma cell apoptosis by activating the MDM2-TP53 pathway. *Oncotarget*, *7*(19), 27350–27362. https://doi.org/10.18632/oncotarget.8439.

Zhang, Y., Devocelle, A., Souza, L., Foudi, A., Tenreira Bento, S., Desterke, C., Sherrard, R., Ballesta, A., Adam, R., Giron-Michel, J., & Chang, Y. (2020). BMAL1 knockdown triggers different colon carcinoma cell fates by altering the delicate equilibrium between AKT/mTOR and P53/P21 pathways. *Aging*, *12*(9), 8067–8083. https://doi.org/10.18632/aging.103124.

Zhou, L., Luo, Z., li, Z., & Huang, Q. (2020). Circadian clock is associated with tumor microenvironment in kidney renal clear cell carcinoma. *Aging*, *12*(14), 14620–14632. https://doi.org/10.18632/aging.103509.

Chapter 20

Recent Advances in Chronotherapeutic Applications

Ekrem Dutoğlu*, MD
Department of Internal Medicine, Tokat Medical Park Hospital, Tokat, Türkiye

Abstract

Chronotherapy aims to plan treatment for diseases according to endogenous biological rhythms. Endogenous biological rhythms are controlled by the suprachiasmatic nucleus and hypothalamus. Many diseases and medications are associated with circadian rhythm. In many diseases and drug use, the right timing can produce surprising results in the course of treatment. Especially in cancer, autoimmune diseases, and mood disorders, many studies in favor of chronotherapy have satisfactory results. The frequent variation in response in patients suggests that individualization of chronotherapy will yield better results. By blending statistical methods with clinical experience by using technological developments, creating an individual-specific chronotherapy plan will provide much more efficient results. In this chapter, we will discuss the latest developments in chronotherapy in the light of current data.

Keywords: chronotherapy, circadian rhythm, cancer, autoimmune diseases, mood disorders

* Corresponding Author's Email: dredutoglu@gmail.com

In: Human Health is a Matter of Timing
Editors: Sumeyya Deniz Aybek, Gonca Gulbay and Mucahit Secme
ISBN: 979-8-89113-467-6

Introduction

Chronotherapy is the science of preventing and treating diseases according to biological rhythms (Halberg et al., 1973). Chronotherapy uses pharmacological, non-pharmacological, psychotherapeutic, or physical agents by planning on timing. The goal here is to minimize toxicity and improve response and success of treatment (Selfridge et al., 2016). Chronotherapy aims to make pharmacologically or non-pharmacologically optimal planning in diseases according to the body's circadian rhythm by evaluating various periods by using the biological timing system (Levi & Schibler, 2007). Understanding that circadian rhythms are endogenous has led preclinical studies to investigate the effect of the temporal relationship of biological functions on drug effects. In some experiments, the adrenal cortex inhibitor metapranon, which is used at different times at the same dose each time, has been shown to cause different toxicities (Ertel & Ungar, 1964). Lidocaine hydrochloride (Lutsch & Morris, 1967), morphine (Morris & Lutsch, 1967), methadone (Lenox & Frazier, 1972), arabinocytosine (Haus et al., 1972), lithium (Hawkins et al., 1978), and many other samples given at the same dose and at different times have been found to have different side effects as a result of treatment. In this way, different results were obtained depending on circadian time, including approximately 400 drugs, and 50 of them cancer drugs (Dallmann et al., 2016; Lévi et al., 2010). These studies clearly reveal the importance of circadian rhythm.

Chronotolerance and chronoactivity result from a set of cellular rhythms involving drug transporters as well as drug detoxification and/or bioactivation enzymes. These cellular rhythms can now be investigated in synchronized cell cultures (Le ́vi et al., 2010; Ballesta et al. 2011). They are translated into well-known circadian changes implicated in drug exposure and elimination at the whole organism level. In mice, circadian clocks control Phase I metabolism enzymes such as CYP450 and carboxylesterases, as well as Phase II detoxification enzymes such as glucuronosyltransferases and glutathione S-transferases enzymes (Martin et al. 2003) and ABC transporters including abcb1a/b and abcc2 (Okyar et al., 2011).

Chronotherapy and Clinical Developments

As the awareness of clinicians increases in chronotherapy, beautiful studies emerge. In a meta-analysis study, chronotherapy was shown to have a positive effect on survival in male patients (Giacchetti et al., 2012). However, similar results were obtained in a randomized controlled trial compared in terms of timing (Dallmann et al., 2016). These findings show us that the study should target the optimal timing and that it is necessary to be sensitive in determining the adequate dose range. For example, while some drugs are evaluated among their own groups, chronotherapeutic results can be seen in the groupings of anti-cancer cytotoxic drugs due to different pharmacodynamic and pharmacokinetic differences (Lévi et al., 2010). Experimental and clinical data have shown that there are wide differences in terms of chronotherapy between individuals. Here, we conclude that each individual should be evaluated separately. Because there are a lot of variables that affect this. Genetics, epigenetics, gender, age, and lifestyle are the differences that require individuals to be evaluated separately. However, there are of course some general rules. For example, taking glucocorticoids in the morning is an effective measure to reduce the side effects of adrenal suppression. Again, in asthmatic patients, theophylline is recommended in the evening to increase bronchodilation and reduce side effects. In another study, it was stated that the administration of theophylline in the morning was more effective. It is known that the administration of anti-h1 and anti-h2 antihistamines in the evening is better tolerated. In a controlled randomized trial, the use of antihistamine therapy in the evening in patients with severe allergic rhinitis showed better results than the use of it in the morning (Smolensky & Peppas, 2007). Again, it is a known situation that statin group drugs should be taken in the evening. In this sense, chronotherapy is an application that makes significant changes in the pharmacodynamics and pharmacokinetics of drugs and affects their efficacy and tolerability.

Cancer and Chronotherapy

The correct timing of the chemotherapeutic dose is particularly important as they are usually administered at the maximum tolerable dose. The administration of chemotherapy drugs with a chronotherapeutic approach in a time frame in which side effects are less visible is important in terms of dosing and adverse events. Likewise, scheduling and planning of radiotherapy is also important. Already in tumor tissues, the circadian rhythm is disturbed (Kettner et al., 2014). Ensuring that the circadian synchronization between healthy and cancer cells is different can be used as a timing for treatment, especially to maintain healthy cells, when targeting cancer cells.

The circadian timing system rhythmically controls both drug metabolism and cellular detoxification, thereby altering drug interactions with its molecular targets, and DNA repair and apoptosis in healthy tissues around the clock. CTS also regulates the healthy cell cycle (Antoch & Kondratov, 2013). Since many anticancer drugs target a specific stage of the cell division cycle, clock-controlled cell proliferation events also represent a critical determinant of anticancer drug cytotoxicity (Granda et al., 2005; Tampellini et al., 1998; Smaaland et al., 2002). Both orders of mechanisms are responsible for large and predictable changes in the tolerability of anticancer drugs. In contrast, cell divisions often occur asynchronously in cancer tissues (Fu and Lee, 2003; Le´vi et al., 2007a). The temporal separation between healthy and cancer tissues provides the main rationale for cancer chronotherapy, which aims to minimize treatment toxicities while maximizing effectiveness by appropriately timing treatment delivery (Le´vi & Okyar, 2011). However, there may be circadian regulation of malignant tumors that may involve CTS control of vascular endothelial growth factor-mediated neo-angiogenesis (Koyanagi et al., 2003; Le´vi et al., 2010).

The tolerance rhythms of more than 40 anticancer drugs, including cytokines, cytostatics, antiangiogenic agents, and cell cycle inhibitors, in mice or rats have been synchronized with a 12-h light and 12-h dark alternation (Le´vi et al., 2010). Fatal toxicity and/or body weight loss following anticancer drug administration often varies two- to tenfold as a function of circadian timing (Le´vi & Schibler, 2007). Experimental evidence suggests that both dose and circadian timing together play a critical role in the antitumor efficacy of 28 anticancer agents in mice, using tumor growth inhibition or increase in survival as established measures of treatment efficacy in experimental systems (Le´vi et al., 2010).

Inside each cell there is a molecular clock consisting of a series of feedback loops that create oscillations in gene expression at mRNA and protein levels over a period of approximately 24 h (Ko & Takahashi, 2006).

These clock genes control the rhythmic expression of up to 10% of the transcriptome (Panda et al., 2002; Storch et al., 2002). Additionally, some posttranslational rhythms appear to be independent of transcriptional rhythms (O'Neill et al., 2011). Additionally, non-genetic circadian clocks have recently been identified in red blood cells (O'Neill & Reddy, 2011). Neither the mechanistic connections between these different circadian oscillators nor their relevance to cancer chronotherapy are currently known.

Cancer chronotherapeutics have revealed the important role of circadian timing for both chronotolerance and chronoefficiency. A striking principle is the ordinary coincidence of chronotolerance and chronoefficiency, which runs counter to the principles governing conventional cancer treatments. Chronotherapeutics, therefore, allow the design of a new strategy aimed at jointly enhancing host tolerability and antitumor efficacy through appropriate dosing and timing of anticancer drugs. This aim requires comprehensive attention to gender, because male and female mice, as well as cancer patients, may respond differently to the same chronotherapy program (Giacchetti et al., 2006, 2012; Le´vi et al., 2007b; Ahowesso et al., 2011; Okyar et al., 2011).

Both experimental and clinical data support the suitability of a robust circadian timing system to enhance both host control of cancer progression and treatment tolerability. Thus, circadian disruption has been shown to accelerate cancer progression in experimental models and is an independent survival prognostic factor in patients with different cancer types and stages (Mormont et al., 2000; Sephton et al., 2000; Innominato et al., 2009). However, the treatment itself may alter the circadian timing system, and this may also provide independent prognostic information regarding patient survival (Ortiz-Tudela et al., 2011; Savard et al., 2009; Innominato et al., 2012). These data demonstrate the necessity of minimizing circadian disruption to increase the effectiveness of chronotherapy.

Therefore, reliable and noninvasive circadian biomarkers, such as those provided by rest-activity and temperature monitoring, are necessary in the perspective of fully exploiting the circadian timing system to optimize cancer treatments.

Cancer and chronotherapy have been seriously recently researched. In a retrospective study of 617 patients between 2012 and 2015, it was shown that acute complications were fewer in patients who received radiotherapy during the day than in patients who received it at night (Brolese et al., 2021). In another study, cisplatin was administered to mice with breast cancer, divided into two groups: normal time and jet-lag protocol, and the results were evaluated. Treatment has been shown to be less successful in mice receiving the jet-lag protocol (Koritala et al., 2022). When resistance was encountered in tanstuzumab treatment used in Her-2 positive gastric cancer patients, a problem was detected in the hexokinase pathway, which has a high glycolytic effect. By inhibiting circadian release and inhibiting the activity of PER-1, its resistance to transtuzumab was reduced. Additionally, it was observed that the synergistic effect of trantuzumab was increased by inhibiting metformin treatment via hexokinase and PER-1 (Wang et al., 2022). In the phase 1 study where the effective dose of capecitabine was investigated, the same effect was observed when the drug dose was reduced by 20% when the dose was divided in the morning and evening, compared to taking a single dose per day (Roosendaal et al., 2020). As a result, it seems reasonable to work on chronotherapeutic methods to benefit from cancer treatments more effectively and in sufficient doses.

Rheumatology and Chronotherapy

Susceptibility to infection is closely related to chronotherapy because immunological processes, and systemic proinflammatory cytokine levels are under circadian control (Labrecque & Cermakian, 2015). In diseases of the immune system, such as osteoarthritis and rheumatoid arthritis, the intensity of symptoms varies throughout the day (Curtis et al., 2015). Anti-inflammatory drugs play an important role in the fight against rheumatologic diseases. In this sense, circadian drug timing is important in terms of drug effectiveness, pharmacokinetics, pharmacodynamics, and tolerability. For example, in osteoarthritis patients, ketoprofen and indomethacin, which are anti-inflammatory drugs administered in the evening, were found to have better tolerability (Clench et al., 1981; Guissou et al., 1983; Ollagnier et al., 1987). The incidence of gastrointestinal and central nervous system side effects was lower in the evening dose compared to the dose taken in the morning (35% vs. 7%). While morning exacerbation was more common in anti-inflammatory drugs taken during the day due to mechanical pain, it was understood that morning exacerbations were better in evening use (Levi et al., 1985).

Chronotherapy and Cardiovascular Diseases

In the cardiovascular system, there are biochemical, physiological, and molecular parameters synchronized with the circadian rhythm. These include; blood pressure, heart rate, peripheral vascular resistance, blood volume, sodium within the cell, potassium ion concentrations, plasma levels of circulating albumin and proteins, clock genes and proteins in the heart and arteries (Hermida et al., 2007; Smolensky et al., 2016). We can better understand myocardial infarction and sudden deaths, which we usually see many times in the morning, with the circadian timing system. Statistical and mathematical modeling approaches have begun to address this problem in chronotherapy (Fijorek et al., 2013).

The effectiveness of various drugs in cardiovascular diseases is greatly different according to the timing of administration (Smolensky et al., 2007). Compared to the morning medication against hypertension, bedtime medication resulted in lower cardiovascular risk and better control of blood pressure (Smolensky et al., 2016). For this purpose, some companies have produced the form of valsartan, which is released towards the morning in the evening intake (Biswas & Kuotsu, 2017). For cardiovascular drugs, they developed the form that affects plasma drug levels through pharmacodynamics and pharmacokinetics using the QT interval with the logic of circadian control modeling. In another study, a model was developed that integrates variations in intraday variability to predict drug-induced QT prolongation (Huh & Hutmacher, 2015). The development of such models will facilitate the personalized evaluation of cardiovascular diseases.

Chronotherapy and Metabolic Diseases

Since both the suprachiasmatic nucleus and cellular rhythm transmitters regulate metabolic processes, chronotherapy has a high effect on energy metabolism (Dumbell et al., 2016). Many metabolic diseases, such as diabetes and obesity, are under circadian control (Qian & Scheer, 2016). Recently, the dynamics of circadian processes that study energy metabolism with a systemic approach have been investigated. Since white adipose tissue plays a role in many metabolic disorders, he developed a mechanical model of the regulation of adipokine expression in these tissues by the circadian timing system. Additionally, this model includes the free fatty acid and insulin system. This study gave information about the chronopharmacology of methylprednisolone, which directs the modification of glucose, free fatty acid, insulin, and plasma circadian profiles after drug administration with a systemic chronopharmacological approach (Sukumaran et al., 2011). Diabetes-related insulin pumps and implanted artificial pancreas are now available (Denecke, 2015; Visentin et al., 2015). In order for the treatment to be optimal, it is necessary to both model and statistically verify the age, sex, and biological rhythm of the patient (Holterhus et al., 2013; Klonoff & Perz, 2010).

Systemic Chronotherapeutic Approach

The effects of diseases and drugs on the circadian timing system need to be functionally explained. Disruption of the circadian rhythm causes non-physiological changes. If we want to correct the pathological changes, it is wise to plan according to the disturbed circadian rhythm. Drugs, diseases, and molecular mechanisms affecting circadian timing should be evaluated separately, and treatment planning should be planned according to these variables. Recently, a mathematical model of intermittent fasting and nutrition has been developed in relation to the circadian clock at the molecular level (Woller et al., 2016). It is particularly noteworthy in cancer chronotherapeutic because of the interesting effect of diet on anti-cancer treatment (Bass, 2012; Longo & Panda, 2016; Vernieri et al., 2016). In another study, the relationship between DNA damage caused by ionizing radiation, and circadian rhythm dexamethasone exposure was examined at the molecular level. To understand the logic of this result, he investigated the mathematical model that represents intracellular pathways activated by DNA damage in cells cultured with dexamethasone. They concluded that DNA damage due to radiation phosphorylated PER proteins on the occasion of CHK2 kinase but did not interact with PER in the complex with BMAL1/CLOCK dimers (Hong et al., 2009). PER, which forms the basis for an autocatalytic process, stabilizes itself by forming complexes. Incorporating this important feedback mechanism into the model was valuable and necessary for mathematical modeling.

Do Chronotherapeutic Applications According to Circadian Timing Provide Effective Benefits?

This question is very meaningful and excites clinicians. In fact, the importance of circadian timing has increased a lot in recent years. Many publications on chronotherapy and circadian rhythm are gradually taking their place in the literature. The chronotherapeutic approach can help by effectively using the biological clock to deliver the right stimuli to the patient in need in a timely manner. Behavioral and pharmacological intervention can be significantly benefited from a chronotherapeutic approach to diseases, and more clinical studies are needed to support this. The light-dark cycle, the timing of meals, sociological interactions, physical activities, and many more stimuli create a synchronized effect on the biological clock. The pacemaker effect of circadian timing shows us that human beings and the environment are related to each other, a fact that affects brain transmitter function and the transcription of clock genes (Benedetti et al., 2007). It is clear that most diseases and treatments are influenced by these stimuli.

Behavioral Chronotherapeutic Examples

The regulation of sleep-wake and light-dark cycles is actively used as a chronotherapeutic approach to the circadian system. It is actively used as light therapy, dawn simulation, especially in sleep disorders and mood disorders (Wirz-Justice, 2009). The fact that these treatments are also useful in cancer surprises clinicians (Jeste et al., 2013; Neikrug et al., 2012; Valdimarsdottir et al., 2014). These techniques are very easy to apply and have no side effects.

In fact, the logic is this: to regulate body functions according to the circadian rhythm according to the correct timing of sleep and light. Bagheri et al. first studied circadian rhythm and light exposure (Bagheri et al., 2008). As a result of this study, they saw that light acts on clock gene transcription and mRNA. Significant improvements in sleep disorders and mood disorders have been identified with light therapy (Cardinali et al., 2021).

Dean et al. studied a mathematical modeling against the jet-lag problem (Dean et al., 2009). Thanks to the algorithm developed, rapid circadian re-drift and improvement of neurobehavioral performance resulted in (Dean et al., 2009). In a similar study, Serkh et al. made the most effective use of the human circadian system and performed chronotherapy with light (Serkh & Forger, 2014).

Nutrition is also very important at the circadian clock. Fasting in rodents has been observed to alter the molecular clock mechanism in peripheral tissues (Damiola et al., 2000; Longo & Panda, 2016; Sherman et al., 2012). Restriction of feeding time in mice exposed to jet-lag resulted in positive development along with increasing body temperature circadian (Chen et al., 2004). Anorexia is an eating disorder characterized by circadian disorder that can also be seen in cancer patients and some other chronic patients (Innominato et al., 2009). Appetite can be increased by using anomerilin, which is ghrelin-mimetic with appetizing effects in cancer (Fearon et al., 2016). There are also preclinical studies for the use of a melanocortin-4 receptor agonist in cancer cachexia (Peter et al., 2013). These pathways can be used for chronotherapeutic purposes to increase appetite and adjust the timing of food intake (Mattson et al., 2014; Zarrinpar et al., 2016).

To summarize, light therapy in behavioral chronotherapy; While physical exercise affects sleep patterns, mood, social life, and family life, chronotherapy approaches to nutrition such as intermittent fasting affect the circadian rhythm due to metabolism.

Pharmacological Chronotherapeutic Samples

Behavioral chronotherapeutic applications can be supported by pharmacological therapies. Melatonin and melatonin receptor agonist pharmacological agents can be used in appropriate patient profiles in sleep regulation (Kuriyama et al., 2014; Lemoine & Zisapel, 2012; Rajaratnam et al., 2009; Wilt et al., 2016). Cancer patients and many patients with chronic conditions who have sleep problems benefit from cognitive behavioral therapy and pharmacological therapy (Baglioni et al., 2011; Bootzin & Epstein, 2011; Langford et al., 2012). Cognitive behavioral therapy is preferred for treatment in patients with sleep disorders (Johnson et al., 2016). In some cases, alternative therapies such as behavioral therapy, yoga, and tai chi may give better results than pharmacological treatments (Mustian et al., 2007; Saligan et al., 2015). The efficacy of pharmacological agents in insomnia seems to be more limited compared to integrative approaches (Irwin et al., 2014). However, pharmacotherapy and integrative approaches have been shown to be much more beneficial when applied together.

Psychotherapy and pharmacotherapy are more effective when used together in patients with depression. Therefore, it is very useful to apply cognitive behavioral therapy, mindfulness, and psychodynamic therapy in addition to antidepressant drugs in patients who are depressed due to cancer or other reasons (Hirschfeld et al., 1997; Mann, 2005; Walker et al., 2014). When we look at it from circadian logic, social rhythm therapy has valuable and interesting results in bipolar disorder (Frank, 2007). This intervention is satisfactory in its application in psychiatric disorders associated with the deterioration of the circadian rhythm and has no side effects.

Melatonin and melatonin receptor agonists are used for sleep problems. A mathematical model of circadian endogenous production and clearance of melatonin was established (St Hilaire et al., 2007). The study looks at saliva levels to determine the circadian phases of melatonin. Additionally, in a mathematical modeling, pharmacokinetics were supported to include phase shift effects through the receptors of exogenously given melatonin in the suprachiasmatic nucleus (Breslow et al., 2013). There is also a more complex physiologically based model of the pharmacokinetics of exogenous melatonin given throughout the body (Peng et al., 2013). These models are intended to benefit by personalizing it, planning the delivery of melatonin, and the balance of exposure to light.

Another exciting issue is the study of molecular circadian genes. Chronotherapy is the planning of circadian core clock genes by targeting agonists or antagonists (Schroeder & Colwell, 2013). Simultaneous administration of CK1δ/ε inhibitor attempted to demonstrate a pharmacological systems approach using circadian timing (Kim et al., 2013). PF-670462 A molecular clock model of the suprachiasmatic nucleus containing brain and plasma pharmacokinetics and drug inhibition of CK1δ/ε was designed. Modeled in mice, a constant delay in activity was observed with chronic CK1δ/ε inhibition in the first hours of the LD12:12 cycle. It was determined that the timing was not the same result as the drug given in a different time frame.

All of the approaches we have mentioned here have the aim of regaining a healthy circadian function. Since there may be many reasons to disrupt the circadian rhythm, it is necessary to evaluate it in many ways and to handle it with a systemic and holistic approach without skipping personal differences in order to achieve the same function again. For this, we have pharmacological agents, behavioral therapies, and integrative approaches. Approaching patients with a holistic approach by evaluating the personal ground well will constitute the best clinical response.

Conclusion

With a better understanding of the concept of circadian rhythm, the importance of chronotherapy approaches is increasing day by day. With a better understanding of these concepts, it is emerging as a necessity that individual-specific approaches increase. By blending mathematical modeling with clinical experience using technological developments, creating an individual-specific chronotherapy plan will provide much more efficient results. While exhibiting these approaches, behavioral therapies, pharmacological agents, and integrative approaches will strengthen our hands. In order for this field to develop much more, there should be a circadian rhythm from the perspective of clinicians, planning should be looked at from this point of view, and studies in this field should be increased.

References

Ahowesso, C., Li, X. M., Zampera, S., Peteri-Brunbäck, B., Dulong, S., Beau, J., Hossard V, Filipski E, Delaunay F, Claustrat B, & Lévi, F. (2011). Sex and dosing-time dependencies in irinotecan-induced circadian disruption. *Chronobiology international*, *28*(5), 458-470. https://doi.org/10.3109/07420528.2011.569043.

Antoch, M. P., & Kondratov, R. V. (2013). Pharmacological modulators of the circadian clock as potential therapeutic drugs: focus on genotoxic/anticancer therapy. *Circadian clocks*, 289-309. https://doi.org/10.1007/978-3-642-25950-0_12.

Bagheri, N., Stelling, J., & Doyle III, F. J. (2008). Circadian phase resetting via single and multiple control targets. *PLoS computational biology*, *4*(7), e1000104. https://doi.org/10.1371/journal.pcbi.1000104.

Baglioni, C., Battagliese, G., Feige, B., Spiegelhalder, K., Nissen, C., Voderholzer, U., Lombardo, C., & Riemann, D. (2011). Insomnia as a predictor of depression: a meta-analytic evaluation of longitudinal epidemiological studies. *Journal of affective disorders*, *135*(1-3), 10-19. https://hdl.handle.net/11573/470069.

Bass, J. (2012). Circadian topology of metabolism. *Nature*, *491*(7424), 348-356. https://doi.org/10.1038/nature11704.

Benedetti, F., Barbini, B., Colombo, C., & Smeraldi, E. (2007). Chronotherapeutics in a psychiatric ward. *Sleep medicine reviews*, *11*(6), 509-522. https://doi.org/10.1016/j.smrv.2007.06.004.

Biswas, N., & Kuotsu, K. (2017). Chronotherapeutically modulated pulsatile system of valsartan nanocrystals—an in vitro and in vivo evaluation. *AAPS PharmSciTech*, *18*, 349-357. https://doi.org/10.1208/s12249-016-0511-5.

Bootzin, R. R., & Epstein, D. R. (2011). Understanding and treating insomnia. *Annual Review of Clinical Psychology*, *7*, 435-458. https://doi.org/10.1146/annurev.clinpsy.3.022806.091516.

Breslow, E. R., Phillips, A. J., Huang, J. M., St. Hilaire, M. A., & Klerman, E. B. (2013). A mathematical model of the circadian phase-shifting effects of exogenous melatonin. *Journal of biological rhythms*, *28*(1), 79-89. https://doi.org/10.1177/0748730412468081.

Brolese, E. K., Cihoric, N., Bojaxhiu, B., Sermaxhaj, B., Schanne, D. H., Mathier, E., Lippmann J, Shelan M, Eller Y, Aebersold DM, Giger R, & Elicin O. (2021). The impact of delivery daytime and seasonality of radiotherapy for head and neck cancer on toxicity burden. *Radiother Oncol., 158*, 162-166.

Buhr, E. D., & Takahashi, J. S. (2013). Molecular components of the Mammalian circadian clock. *Circadian clocks*, 3-27. https://doi.org/10.1007/978-3-642-25950-0_1.

Buttgereit, F., Doering, G., Schaeffler, A., Witte, S., Sierakowski, S., Gromnica-Ihle, E., Jeka, S., Krueger, K., Szechinski, J., & Alten, R. (2008). Efficacy of modified-release versus standard prednisone to reduce duration of morning stiffness of the joints in rheumatoid arthritis (CAPRA-1): a double-blind, randomised controlled trial. *The Lancet*, *371*(9608), 205-214. https://doi.org/10.1016/S0140-6736(08)60132-4.

Buttgereit, F., Smolen, J. S., Coogan, A. N., & Cajochen, C. (2015). Clocking in: chronobiology in rheumatoid arthritis. *Nature Reviews Rheumatology*, *11*(6), 349-356. https://doi.org/10.1038/nrrheum.2015.31.

Cardinali, D. P., Brown, G. M., & Pandi-Perumal, S. R. (2021). Chronotherapy. *Handbook of Clinical Neurology*, *179*, 357-370. https://doi.org/10.1016/B978-0-12-819975-6.00023-6.

Chen, L., Wu, W., Dentchev, T., Zeng, Y., Wang, J., Tsui, I., Tobias, J. W., Bennett, J., Baldwin, D., & Dunaief, J. L. (2004). Light damage induced changes in mouse retinal gene expression. *Experimental eye research*, *79*(2), 239-247. https://doi.org/10.1016/j.exer.2004.05.002.

Chu, I. M., Hengst, L., & Slingerland, J. M. (2008). The Cdk inhibitor p27 in human cancer: prognostic potential and relevance to anticancer therapy. *Nature Reviews Cancer*, *8*(4), 253-267. https://doi.org/10.1038/nrc2347.

Clench, J., Reinberg, A., Dziewanowska, Z., Ghata, J., & Smolensky, M. (1981). Circadian changes in the bioavailability and effects of indomethacin in healthy subjects. *European journal of clinical pharmacology*, *20*, 359-369. https://doi.org/10.1007/BF00615406.

Curtis, A. M., Fagundes, C. T., Yang, G., Palsson-McDermott, E. M., Wochal, P., McGettrick, A. F., Foley, N. H., Early, J. O., Chen, L., & Zhang, H. (2015). Circadian control of innate immunity in macrophages by miR-155 targeting Bmal1. *Proceedings of the National Academy of Sciences*, *112*(23), 7231-7236. https://doi.org/10.1073/pnas.1501327112.

Dallmann, R., Okyar, A., & Lévi, F. (2016). Dosing-time makes the poison: circadian regulation and pharmacotherapy. *Trends in molecular medicine*, *22*(5), 430-445. https://doi.org/10.1016/j.molmed.2016.03.004.

Damiola, F., Le Minh, N., Preitner, N., Kornmann, B., Fleury-Olela, F., & Schibler, U. (2000). Restricted feeding uncouples circadian oscillators in peripheral tissues from the central pacemaker in the suprachiasmatic nucleus. *Genes & development*, *14*(23), 2950-2961. https://doi.org/10.1101/gad.183500. Genes & Dev. 2000. 14: 2950-2961.

Dean, D. A., Forger, D. B., & Klerman, E. B. (2009). Taking the lag out of jet lag through model-based schedule design. *PLoS computational biology*, *5*(6), e1000418. https://doi.org/10.1371/journal.pcbi.1000418.

Denecke, C. (2015). The bionic pancreas: novel perspectives on insulin replacement therapies. *Transplantation*, *99*(2), 268-269. *https://doi.org/*10.1097/TP.0000000000000544.

Dumbell, R., Matveeva, O., & Oster, H. (2016). Circadian clocks, stress, and immunity. *Frontiers in endocrinology*, *7*, 37. https://doi.org/10.3389/fendo.2016.00037.

Ertel, R. J., & Ungar, F. (1964). In vitro effect of 2-methyl-l, 2-bis (3-pyridyl)-l-propanone (Su-4885) and NADPH in the mouse adrenal. *Endocrinology*, *75*(6), 949-956. https://doi.org/10.1210/endo-75-6-949.

Fearon, K., Currow, D., Temel, J., Giorgino, R., Friend, J., & Abernethy, A. (2016). OR45: Body composition in non-small cell lung cancer (Nsclc) patients with cachexia and improved anorexia-cachexia symptoms: anamorelin phase 3 trials pooled analysis. *Clinical Nutrition*. http://hdl.handle.net/10453/154248.

Fijorek, K., Puskulluoglu, M., & Polak, S. (2013). Circadian models of serum potassium, sodium, and calcium concentrations in healthy individuals and their application to cardiac electrophysiology simulations at individual level. *Computational and mathematical methods in medicine*, *2013*. https://doi.org/10.1155/2013/429037.

Frank, E. (2007). *Treating bipolar disorder: A clinician's guide to interpersonal and social rhythm therapy*. Guilford Press.

Fu, L., & Lee, C. C. (2003). The circadian clock: pacemaker and tumour suppressor. *Nature Reviews Cancer*, *3*(5), 350-361. https://doi.org/10.1038/nrc1072.

Gery, S., Gombart, A. F., Yi, W. S., Koeffler, C., Hofmann, W. K., & Koeffler, H. P. (2005). Transcription profiling of C/EBP targets identifies Per2 as a gene implicated in myeloid leukemia. *Blood*, *106*(8), 2827-2836. https://doi.org/10.1182/blood-2005-01-0358.

Giacchetti, S., Dugué, P., Innominato, P., Bjarnason, G., Focan, C., Garufi, C., Tumolo, S., Coudert, B., Iacobelli, S., & Smaaland, R. (2012). Sex moderates circadian chemotherapy effects on survival of patients with metastatic colorectal cancer: a meta-analysis. *Annals of oncology*, *23*(12), 3110-3116. https://doi.org/10.1093/annonc/mds148.

Giacchetti, S., Bjarnason, G., Garufi, C., Genet, D., Iacobelli, S., Tampellini, M., Smaaland R, Focan C, Coudert B, Humblet Y, Canon JL, Adenis A, Lo Re G, Carvalho C, Schueller J, Anciaux N, Lentz MA, Baron B, Gorlia T,& Lévi, F. (2006). Phase III trial comparing 4-day chronomodulated therapy versus 2-day conventional delivery of fluorouracil, leucovorin, and oxaliplatin as first-line chemotherapy of metastatic colorectal cancer: the European Organisation for Research and Treatment of Cancer Chronotherapy Group. *Journal of clinical oncology*, *24*(22), 3562-3569. https://doi.org/10.1200/JCO.2006.06.1440.

Guissou, P., Cuisinaud, G., Llorca, G., Lejeune, E., & Sassard, J. (1983). Chronopharmacokinetic study of a prolonged release form of indomethacin. *European journal of clinical pharmacology*, *24*, 667-670. https://doi.org/10.1007/BF00542219.

Halberg, F., Haus, E., Cardoso, S., Scheving, L., Kühl, J., Shiotsuka, R., Rosene, G., Pauly, J., Runge, W., & Spalding, J. (1973). Toward a chronotherapy of neoplasia: tolerance of treatment depends upon host rhythms. *Experientia*, *29*, 909-934. https://doi.org/10.1007/BF01930381.

Haus, E., Halberg, F., Scheving, L. E., Pauly, J. E., Cardoso, S., Kühl, J. F., Sothern, R. B., Shiotsuka, R. N., & Hwang, D. S. (1972). Increased tolerance of leukemic mice to arabinosyl cytosine with schedule adjusted to circadian system. *Science*, *177*(4043), 80-82. https://doi.org/10.1126/science.177.4043.80.

Hawkins, R., Kripke, D. F., & Janowsky, D. S. (1978). Circadian rhythm of lithium toxicity in mice. *Psychopharmacology*, *56*, 113-114. https://doi.org/10.1007/BF00571418.

Hermida, R. C., Ayala, D. E., & Portaluppi, F. (2007). Circadian variation of blood pressure: the basis for the chronotherapy of hypertension. *Advanced drug delivery reviews*, *59*(9-10), 904-922. https://doi.org/10.1016/j.addr.2006.08.003.

Hirschfeld, R. M., Keller, M. B., Panico, S., Arons, B. S., Barlow, D., Davidoff, F., Endicott, J., Froom, J., Goldstein, M., & Gorman, J. M. (1997). The National Depressive and Manic-Depressive Association consensus statement on the undertreatment of depression. *Jama*, *277*(4), 333-340. https://doi.org/10.1001/jama.1997.03540280071036.

Holterhus, P.-M., Bokelmann, J., Riepe, F., Heidtmann, B., Wagner, V., Rami-Merhar, B., Kapellen, T., Raile, K., Quester, W., & Holl, R. W. (2013). Predicting the optimal basal insulin infusion pattern in children and adolescents on insulin pumps. *Diabetes Care*, *36*(6), 1507-1511. https://doi.org/10.2337/dc12-1705.

Hong, C. I., Zámborszky, J., & Csikász-Nagy, A. (2009). Minimum criteria for DNA damage-induced phase advances in circadian rhythms. *PLoS computational biology*, *5*(5), e1000384. https://doi.org/10.1371/journal.pcbi.1000384.

Hua, H., Wang, Y., Wan, C., Liu, Y., Zhu, B., Wang, X., Wang, Z., & Ding, J. M. (2007). Inhibition of tumorigenesis by intratumoral delivery of the circadian gene mPer2 in C57BL/6 mice. *Cancer gene therapy*, *14*(9), 815-818.

Huh, Y., & Hutmacher, M. (2015). Evaluating the use of linear mixed-effect models for inference of the concentration-QTc slope estimate as a surrogate for a biological QTc model. *CPT: Pharmacometrics & Systems Pharmacology*, *4*(1), 1-9. https://doi.org/10.1002/psp4.14. https://doi.org/10.1038/sj.cgt.7701061.

Innominato, P. F., Mormont, M. C., Rich, T. A., Waterhouse, J., Lévi, F. A., & Bjarnason, G. A. (2009). Circadian disruption, fatigue, and anorexia clustering in advanced cancer patients: implications for innovative therapeutic approaches. *Integrative cancer therapies*, *8*(4), 361-370. https://doi.org/10.1177/1534735409355293.

Innominato, P. F., Lévi, F. A., & Bjarnason, G. A. (2010). Chronotherapy and the molecular clock: Clinical implications in oncology. *Advanced drug delivery reviews*, *62*(9-10), 979-1001. https://doi.org/10.1016/j.addr.2010.06.002.

Irwin, M. R., Olmstead, R., Carrillo, C., Sadeghi, N., Breen, E. C., Witarama, T., Yokomizo, M., Lavretsky, H., Carroll, J. E., & Motivala, S. J. (2014). Cognitive behavioral therapy vs. Tai Chi for late life insomnia and inflammatory risk: a randomized controlled comparative efficacy trial. *Sleep*, *37*(9), 1543-1552. https://doi.org/10.5665/sleep.4008.

Jeste, N., Liu, L., Rissling, M., Trofimenko, V., Natarajan, L., Parker, B. A., & Ancoli-Israel, S. (2013). Prevention of quality-of-life deterioration with light therapy is associated with changes in fatigue in women with breast cancer undergoing chemotherapy. *Quality of Life Research*, *22*, 1239-1244. https://doi.org/10.1007/s11136-012-0243-2.

Johnson, J. A., Rash, J. A., Campbell, T. S., Savard, J., Gehrman, P. R., Perlis, M., Carlson, L. E., & Garland, S. N. (2016). A systematic review and meta-analysis of randomized controlled trials of cognitive behavior therapy for insomnia (CBT-I) in cancer survivors. *Sleep medicine reviews*, *27*, 20-28. https://doi.org/10.1016/j.smrv.2015.07.001.

Kettner, N. M., Katchy, C. A., & Fu, L. (2014). Circadian gene variants in cancer. *Annals of medicine*, *46*(4), 208-220. https://doi.org/10.3109/07853890.2014.914808.

Koyanagi, S., Tanigawa, N., Nakagawa, H., Soeda, S., & Shimeno, H. (2003). Oversulfation of fucoidan enhances its anti-angiogenic and antitumor activities. *Biochemical pharmacology*, *65*(2), 173-179. https://doi.org/10.1016/s0006-2952(02)01478-8.

Ko, C. H., & Takahashi, J. S. (2006). Molecular components of the mammalian circadian clock. *Human molecular genetics*, *15*(suppl_2), R271-R277. https://doi.org/10.1093/hmg/ddl207.

Koritala, B. S., Porter, K. I., Sarkar, S., Gaddameedhi, S. J. T., & Pharmacology, A. (2022). Circadian disruption and cisplatin chronotherapy for mammary carcinoma. *436*, 115863.

Kim, J. K., Forger, D., Marconi, M., Wood, D., Doran, A., Wager, T., Chang, C., & Walton, K. (2013). Modeling and validating chronic pharmacological manipulation of circadian rhythms. *CPT: Pharmacometrics & Systems Pharmacology*, 2(7), 1-11. https://doi.org/10.1038/psp.2013.34.

Klonoff, D. C., & Perz, J. F. (2010). Assisted monitoring of blood glucose: special safety needs for a new paradigm in testing glucose. In (Vol. 4, pp. 1027-1031): SAGE Publications Sage CA: Los Angeles, CA. https://doi.org/10.1177/193229681000400501.

Kuriyama, A., Honda, M., & Hayashino, Y. (2014). Ramelteon for the treatment of insomnia in adults: a systematic review and meta-analysis. *Sleep medicine*, *15*(4), 385-392. https://doi.org/10.1016/j.sleep.2013.11.788.

Labrecque, N., & Cermakian, N. (2015). Circadian clocks in the immune system. *Journal of biological rhythms*, *30*(4), 277-290. https://doi.org/10.1177/0748730415577723.

Langford, D. J., Lee, K., & Miaskowski, C. (2012). Sleep disturbance interventions in oncology patients and family caregivers: a comprehensive review and meta-analysis. *Sleep medicine reviews*, *16*(5), 397-414. https://doi.org/10.1016/j.smrv.2011.07.002.

Lemoine, P., & Zisapel, N. (2012). Prolonged-release formulation of melatonin (Circadin) for the treatment of insomnia. *Expert opinion on pharmacotherapy*, *13*(6), 895-905. https://doi.org/10.1517/14656566.2012.667076.

Lenox, R. H., & FRAZIER, T. W. (1972). Methadone induced mortality as a function of the circadian cycle. *Nature*, *239*(5372), 397-398. https://doi.org/10.1038/239397a0.

Levi, F., Louarn, C. L., & Reinberg, A. (1985). Timing optimizes sustained-release indomethacin treatment of osteoarthritis. *Clinical Pharmacology & Therapeutics*, *37*(1), 77-84. https://doi.org/10.1038/clpt.1985.15.

Lévi, F., Okyar, A., Dulong, S., Innominato, P. F., & Clairambault, J. (2010). Circadian timing in cancer treatments. *Annual review of pharmacology and toxicology*, *50*, 377-421. https://doi.org/10.1146/annurev.pharmtox.48.113006.094626.

Levi, F., & Schibler, U. (2007). Circadian rhythms: mechanisms and therapeutic implications. *Annu. Rev. Pharmacol. Toxicol.*, *47*, 593-628. https://doi.org/10.1146/annurev.pharmtox.47.120505.105208.

Longo, V. D., & Panda, S. (2016). Fasting, circadian rhythms, and time-restricted feeding in healthy lifespan. *Cell metabolism*, *23*(6), 1048-1059. https://doi.org/10.1016/j.cmet.2016.06.001.

Lutsch, E. F., & Morris, R. W. (1967). Circadian periodicity in susceptibility to lidocaine hydrochloride. *Science*, *156*(3771), 100-102. https://doi.org/10.1126/science.156.3771.100.

Mann, J. J. (2005). The medical management of depression. *New England Journal of Medicine*, *353*(17), 1819-1834. https://doi.org/10.1056/NEJMra050730.

Mattson, M. P., Allison, D. B., Fontana, L., Harvie, M., Longo, V. D., Malaisse, W. J., Mosley, M., Notterpek, L., Ravussin, E., & Scheer, F. A. (2014). Meal frequency and timing in health and disease. *Proceedings of the National Academy of Sciences*, *111*(47), 16647-16653. https://doi.org/10.1073/pnas.1413965111.

Morris, R. W., & Lutsch, E. F. (1967). Susceptibility to morphine-induced analgesia in mice. *Nature*, *216*(5114), 494-495. https://doi.org/10.1038/216494a0.

Mormont, M. C., Waterhouse, J., Bleuzen, P., Giacchetti, S., Jami, A., Bogdan, A., Lellouch J, Misset JL, Touitou Y, & Lévi, F. (2000). Marked 24-h rest/activity rhythms are associated with better quality of life, better response, and longer survival in patients with metastatic colorectal cancer and good performance status. *Clinical cancer research*, *6*(8), 3038-3045. PMID: 10955782.

Mustian, K. M., Morrow, G. R., Carroll, J. K., Figueroa-Moseley, C. D., Jean-Pierre, P., & Williams, G. C. (2007). Integrative nonpharmacologic behavioral interventions for the management of cancer-related fatigue. *The oncologist*, *12*(S1), 52-67. https://doi.org/10.1634/theoncologist.12-S1-52.

Neikrug, A. B., Rissling, M., Trofimenko, V., Liu, L., Natarajan, L., Lawton, S., Parker, B. A., & Ancoli-Israel, S. (2012). Bright light therapy protects women from circadian rhythm desynchronization during chemotherapy for breast cancer. *Behavioral sleep medicine*, *10*(3), 202-216. https://doi.org/10.1080/15402002.2011.634940.

Okyar, A., Piccolo, E., Ahowesso, C., Filipski, E., Hossard, V., Guettier, C., La Sorda R, Tinari N, Iacobelli S, & Levi, F. (2011). Strain-and sex-dependent circadian changes in abcc2 transporter expression: implications for irinotecan chronotolerance in mouse ileum. *PloS one*, *6*(6), e20393. https://doi.org/10.1371/journal.pone.0020393.

Ollagnier, M., Decousus, H., Cherrah, Y., Levi, F., Mechkouri, M., Queneau, P., & Reinberg, A. (1987). Circadian changes in the pharmacokinetics of oral ketoprofen. *Clinical pharmacokinetics*, *12*(5), 367-377. https://doi.org/10.2165/00003088-198712050-00003.

Ortiz-Tudela, E., De la Fuente, M., & Mendiola, P. (2011). Chronodisruption and ageing. *Revista Espanola de Geriatria Y Gerontologia*, *47*(4), 168-173. https://doi.org/10.1016/j.regg.2011.09.013.

Panda, S., Sato, T. K., Castrucci, A. M., Rollag, M. D., DeGrip, W. J., Hogenesch, J. B., Provencio, I., & Kay, S. A. (2002). Melanopsin (Opn4) requirement for normal light-induced circadian phase shifting. *Science*, *298*(5601), 2213-2216. https://doi.org/10.1126/science.1076848.

Peng, H. T., Bouak, F., Vartanian, O., & Cheung, B. (2013). A physiologically based pharmacokinetics model for melatonin—effects of light and routes of administration. *International journal of pharmaceutics*, *458*(1), 156-168. https://doi.org/10.1016/j.ijpharm.2013.09.033.

Peter, J.-C., Rossez, H., Weckering, M., Zipfel, G., Lecourt, A. C., Owen, J. B., Banks, W. A., & Hofbauer, K. G. (2013). Protective effects of an anti-melanocortin-4 receptor scFv derivative in lipopolysaccharide-induced cachexia in rats. *Journal of cachexia, sarcopenia and muscle*, *4*, 79-88. https://doi.org/10.1007/s13539-012-0084-4.

Qian, J., & Scheer, F. A. (2016). Circadian system and glucose metabolism: implications for physiology and disease. *Trends in Endocrinology & Metabolism*, *27*(5), 282-293. https://doi.org/10.1016/j.tem.2016.03.005.

Rajaratnam, S. M., Polymeropoulos, M. H., Fisher, D. M., Roth, T., Scott, C., Birznieks, G., & Klerman, E. B. (2009). Melatonin agonist tasimelteon (VEC-162) for transient insomnia after sleep-time shift: two randomised controlled multicentre trials. *The Lancet*, *373*(9662), 482-491. https://doi.org/10.1016/S0140-6736(08)61812-7.

Roosendaal, J., Jacobs, B. A., Pluim, D., Rosing, H., de Vries, N., van Werkhoven, E., Nuijen B, Beijnen JH, Huitema ADR, Schellens JHM, & Marchetti S. (2020). Phase I pharmacological study of continuous chronomodulated capecitabine treatment. *Pharm Res., 37*, 1-10.

Saligan, L. N., Olson, K., Filler, K., Larkin, D., Cramp, F., Sriram, Y., Escalante, C. P., Del Giglio, A., Kober, K. M., & Kamath, J. (2015). The biology of cancer-related fatigue: a review of the literature. *Supportive Care in Cancer, 23*, 2461-2478. https://doi.org/10.1007/s00520-015-2763-0.

Savard, J., Liu, L., Natarajan, L., Rissling, M. B., Neikrug, A. B., He, F., Dimsdale JE, Mills PJ, Parker BA, Sadler GR, & Ancoli-Israel, S. (2009). Breast cancer patients have progressively impaired sleep-wake activity rhythms during chemotherapy. *Sleep, 32*(9), 1155-1160. https://doi.org/10.1093/sleep/32.9.1155.

Schroeder, A. M., & Colwell, C. S. (2013). How to fix a broken clock. *Trends in pharmacological sciences, 34*(11), 605-619. https://doi.org/10.1016/j.tips.2013.09.002.

Sephton, S. E., Sapolsky, R. M., Kraemer, H. C., & Spiegel, D. (2000). Diurnal cortisol rhythm as a predictor of breast cancer survival. *Journal of the National Cancer Institute, 92*(12), 994-1000. https://doi.org/10.1093/jnci/92.12.994.

Selfridge, J. M., Gotoh, T., Schiffhauer, S., Liu, J., Stauffer, P. E., Li, A., Capelluto, D. G., & Finkielstein, C. V. (2016). Chronotherapy: intuitive, sound, founded… but not broadly applied. *Drugs, 76*, 1507-1521. https://doi.org/10.1007/s40265-016-0646-4.

Serkh, K., & Forger, D. B. (2014). Optimal schedules of light exposure for rapidly correcting circadian misalignment. *PLoS computational biology, 10*(4), e1003523. https://doi.org/10.1371/journal.pcbi.1003523.

Sherman, H., Genzer, Y., Cohen, R., Chapnik, N., Madar, Z., & Froy, O. (2012). Timed high-fat diet resets circadian metabolism and prevents obesity. *The FASEB Journal, 26*(8), 3493-3502. https://doi.org/10.1096/fj.12-208868.

Smaaland, R., Sothern, R. B., Laerum, O. D., & Abrahamsen, J. F. (2002). Rhythms in human bone marrow and blood cells. *Chronobiology international, 19*(1), 101-127. https://doi.org/10.1081/cbi-120002594.

Smolensky, M. H., Hermida, R. C., Castriotta, R. J., & Portaluppi, F. (2007). Role of sleep-wake cycle on blood pressure circadian rhythms and hypertension. *Sleep medicine, 8*(6), 668-680. https://doi.org/10.1016/j.sleep.2006.11.011.

Smolensky, M. H., Hermida, R. C., Reinberg, A., Sackett-Lundeen, L., & Portaluppi, F. (2016). Circadian disruption: new clinical perspective of disease pathology and basis for chronotherapeutic intervention. *Chronobiology international, 33*(8), 1101-1119. https://doi.org/10.100/07420528.2016.1184678.

Smolensky, M. H., & Peppas, N. A. (2007). Chronobiology, drug delivery, and chronotherapeutics. *Advanced drug delivery reviews, 59*(9-10), 828-851. https://doi.org/10.1016/j.addr.2007.07.001.

St Hilaire, M. A., Gronfier, C., Zeitzer, J. M., & Klerman, E. B. (2007). A physiologically based mathematical model of melatonin including ocular light suppression and interactions with the circadian pacemaker. *Journal of pineal research, 43*(3), 294-304. https://doi.org/10.1111/j.1600-079X.2007.00477.x.

Sukumaran, S., Jusko, W. J., DuBois, D. C., & Almon, R. R. (2011). Mechanistic modeling of the effects of glucocorticoids and circadian rhythms on adipokine expression. *Journal of Pharmacology and Experimental Therapeutics*, *337*(3), 734-746. https://doi.org/10.1124/jpet.111.179960.

Tampellini, M., Filipski, E., Liu, X. H., Lemaigre, G., Li, X. M., Vrignaud, P., François, E., Bissery, M. C., & Lévi, F. (1998). Docetaxel chronopharmacology in mice. *Cancer research*, *58*(17), 3896-3904. PMID: 9731500.

Valdimarsdottir, H., Davidson, W., Redd, W., Wu, L., & Ancoli-Israel, S. (2014). Bright Light Therapy, Cancer Related Fatigue And Circadian Activity Rhythm. *International Journal Of Behavioral Medicine, 21,* 70.

Vernieri, C., Casola, S., Foiani, M., Pietrantonio, F., de Braud, F., & Longo, V. (2016). Targeting Cancer Metabolism: Dietary and Pharmacologic InterventionsAnticancer Metabolic Therapies. *Cancer discovery*, *6*(12), 1315-13 https://doi.org/10.1158/2159-8290.CD-16-0615.

Visentin, R., Dalla Man, C., Kudva, Y. C., Basu, A., & Cobelli, C. (2015). Circadian variability of insulin sensitivity: physiological input for in silico artificial pancreas. *Diabetes technology & therapeutics*, *17*(1), 1-7. https://doi.org/10.1089/dia.2014.0192.

Walker, J., Hansen, C. H., Martin, P., Symeonides, S., Ramessur, R., Murray, G., & Sharpe, M. (2014). Prevalence, associations, and adequacy of treatment of major depression in patients with cancer: a cross-sectional analysis of routinely collected clinical data. *The Lancet Psychiatry*, *1*(5), 343-350. https://doi.org/10.1016/S2215-0366(14)70313-X.

Wang, J., Huang, Q., Hu, X., Zhang, S., Jiang, Y., Yao, G., Hu K, Xu X, Liang B, Wu Q, Ma Z, Wang Y, Wang C, Wu Z, Rong X, Liao W, & Shi M. (2022). Disrupting circadian rhythm via the PER1–HK2 axis reverses trastuzumab resistance in gastric cancer. *82*(8), 1503-1517.

Wilt, T. J., MacDonald, R., Brasure, M., Olson, C. M., Carlyle, M., Fuchs, E., Khawaja, I. S., Diem, S., Koffel, E., & Ouellette, J. (2016). Pharmacologic treatment of insomnia disorder: an evidence report for a clinical practice guideline by the American College of Physicians. *Annals of internal medicine*, *165*(2), 103-112. https://doi.org/10.7326/M15-1781.

Wirz-Justice, A. (2009). From the basic neuroscience of circadian clock function to light therapy for depression: on the emergence of chronotherapeutics. *Journal of affective disorders*, *116*(3), 159. https://doi.org/10.1016/j.biopsych.2009.02.018.

Woller, A., Duez, H., Staels, B., & Lefranc, M. (2016). A mathematical model of the liver circadian clock linking feeding and fasting cycles to clock function. *Cell reports*, *17*(4), 1087-1097. https://doi.org/10.1016/j.celrep.2016.09.060.

Zarrinpar, A., Chaix, A., & Panda, S. (2016). Daily eating patterns and their impact on health and disease. *Trends in Endocrinology & Metabolism*, *27*(2), 69-83. https://doi.org/10.1016/j.tem.2015.11.007.

Zhu, Y., Stevens, R. G., Leaderer, D., Hoffman, A., Holford, T., Zhang, Y., Brown, H. N., & Zheng, T. (2008). Non-synonymous polymorphisms in the circadian gene NPAS2 and breast cancer risk. *Breast cancer research and treatment*, *107*, 421-425. https://doi.org/10.1007/s10549-007-9565-0.

Index

M

N

O

P

R